Advances in Diagnosis and Management of Cutaneous Adverse Drug Reactions

Neil H. Shear • Roni P. Dodiuk-Gad
Editors

Advances in Diagnosis and Management of Cutaneous Adverse Drug Reactions

Current and Future Trends

Adis

Editors
Neil H. Shear, MD, FRCPC
University of Toronto Medical School
Sunnybrook Health Sciences Centre
Toronto, ON
Canada

Roni P. Dodiuk-Gad, MD
Department of Dermatology
Emek Medical Center
Afula
Israel

Bruce Rappaport Faculty of Medicine
Technion-Institute of Technology
Haifa
Israel

Sunnybrook Health Sciences Centre
University of Toronto Medical School
Toronto, ON
Canada

Editorial Assistants
Cristina Olteanu, MD
Dermatology Resident
University of Alberta
Canada

Rena Hashimoto, MD
Clinical instructor
Department of Dermatology
Keio University Hospital
Tokyo
Japan

ISBN 978-981-13-1488-9 ISBN 978-981-13-1489-6 (eBook)
https://doi.org/10.1007/978-981-13-1489-6

Library of Congress Control Number: 2018960934

This Adis imprint is published by the registered company Springer Nature Singapore Pte Ltd.
The registered company address is: 152 Beach Road, #21-01/04 Gateway East, Singapore 189721, Singapore

Preface

The purpose of this text is to update clinicians who are faced with a patient who suffers a suspected drug-induced rash. This problem is common in clinical practice and yet almost always a challenge and filled with complex considerations.

The number of chapters reflects the variable clinical situations where cutaneous adverse drug-reactions (cADRs) can occur. The authors are global leaders in their field and the information presented is done with a clinical perspective and up-to-date.

The editorial team cares deeply that patients who have drug-induced diseases of the skin are treated by the most knowledgeable and committed physicians. These doctors want to optimize their care so that patients are diagnosed properly, treated effectively, and have a knowledge base that allows them to safely navigate their future care.

The maturation of the cADR field has taken decades. We now have clearer classifications, better understanding of the mechanisms at play, and thoughtful insights into the research that needs to be done. It might be said that the skin is body's playground for drugs. And, as with a playground, problems can and do arise.

Our text cannot be considered a comprehensive compendium; there are other resources for that. But it is hoped that the reader will learn about the epidemiology, causes, and treatments around cADRs.

We will say that the nomenclature around drug-induced disease in general is a mess. Therefore, we have tried to stick to currently used terms for uniformity and continuity. What is called SJS/TEN in the chapters is more often called TENS (toxic epidermal necrolysis spectrum) by the editors. DRESS or DIHS is referred to as DReSS by the editors (the lower case e is a reminder that eosinophilia is not a necessary criterion and that other hematologic abnormalities are seen). We did not remove suggested improvements by the authors (such as EN for TEN).

If there are omissions and errors, we hope they are minor and are very open to feedback.

Finally, we must personally acknowledge the authors, our families, and our patients.

We hope that readers will become as enthralled with the complexity and importance of cADR care as much as we have.

Toronto, ON, Canada — Neil H. Shear
Haifa, Israel — Roni P. Dodiuk-Gad

Contents

Acknowledgments

We have the greatest appreciation for our leading editorial assistant, Dr. Cristina Olteanu. She was a dominant player in editing of this book. She participated in all of the editing process including planning of the book outline to the last stages of editing and formatting. Dr. Olteanu invested hundreds of hours in reading the chapters submitted, conducting editing, and correspondence with the authors. Her voice and contribution can be seen in each chapter of the book. Her job description was editorial assistant, but we felt she was actually working as an editor. There are not enough words to express our gratitude to her dedication, professionalism, and hard work in creating this important project. Above all, she was a great companion to work with in the challenging road in creating this book.

We would also like to thank our editorial assistant, Dr. Rena Hashimoto, for her detailed review of the chapters and editing of the book. Her dedication to the team and time invested in this project is truly invaluable.

This book is a result of fruitful international contributions of global opinion leaders in the field of adverse drug reactions. We are deeply grateful and honoured to have the privilege of gathering their knowledge into the first edition of this book with the united mission of advancing the field. We hope that this book will serve as a teaching resource to various fields in medicine including dermatology, immunology, paediatrics, and family medicine.

We would like to thank our publisher Springer Nature; the Responsible Editors, Cameron Wright and Jo Grant. Commissioning Editor, Nitin Joshi; and the Project Coordinator, Prasad Gurunadham.

We would like to express our gratitude to our patients for sharing with us their medical experience of having cutaneous adverse drug reactions, which both inspired us and contributed tremendously to our sense of responsibility in pursuing the advancement of this field.

Last but not least, we thank our dear families for their unconditional support, love, and encouragement to dedicate ourselves to this important project.

Editorial Team

Lead Editors

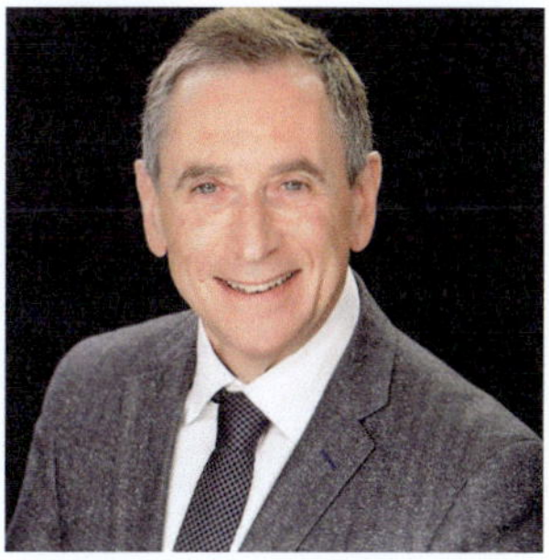

Neil H. Shear, MD, FRCPC
Sunnybrook Health Sciences Centre, University of Toronto Medical School, Toronto, ON, Canada

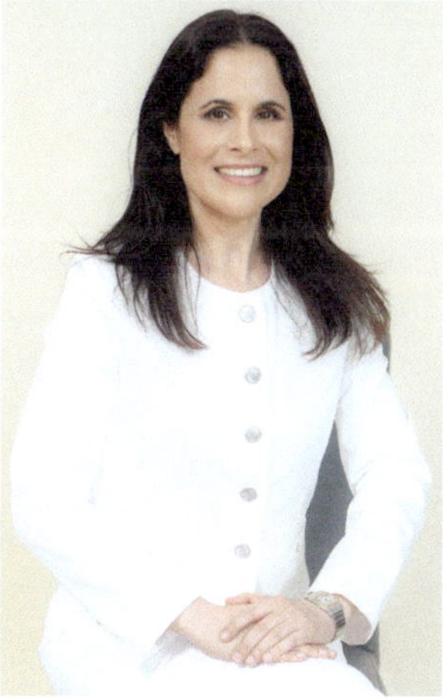

Roni P. Dodiuk-Gad, MD
Department of Dermatology, Emek Medical Center, Afula, Israel
Bruce Rappaport Faculty of Medicine, Technion-Institute of Technology, Haifa, Israel
Sunnybrook Health Sciences Centre, University of Toronto Medical School, Toronto, ON, Canada

Editorial Assistants

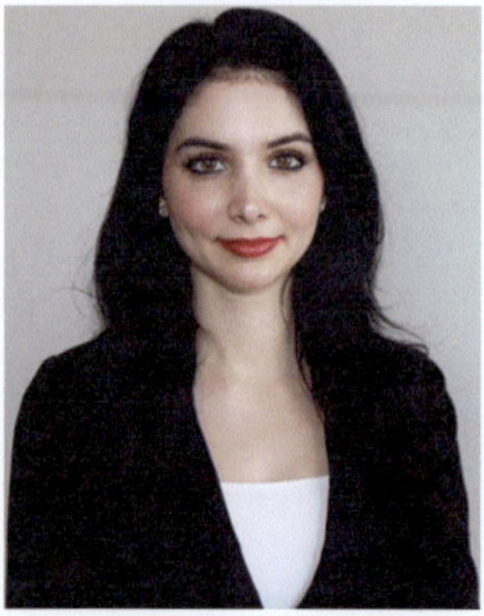

Cristina Olteanu, MD
University of Alberta, Edmonton, AB, Canada

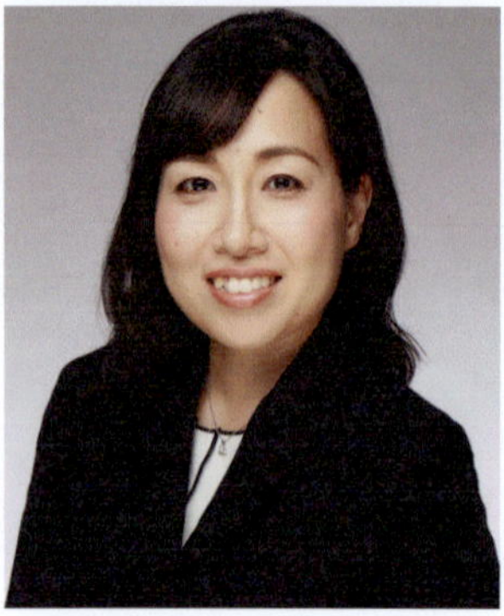

Rena Hashimoto, MD
Department of Dermatology, Keio University Hospital, Tokyo, Japan

Part I

Introduction

Introduction: Classification, Terminology, Epidemiology, and Etiology of Cutaneous Adverse Drug Reactions

1

Maja Mockenhaupt

Abbreviations

ADR	Adverse drug reactions
AGEP	Acute generalized exanthematous pustulosis
BSA	Body surface area
cADR	Cutaneous adverse drug reactions
DIHS	Drug-induced hypersensitivity syndrome
DRESS	Drug reaction with eosinophilia and systemic symptoms
E(E)M	Erythema (exsudativum) multiforme
EMM	EM majus
EN	Epithelial necrolysis
FDE	Fixed drug eruption
GBFDE	Generalized bullous fixed drug eruption
HSS	Hypersensitivity syndrome
MPE	Maculopapular exanthema
NSAIDs	Nonsteroidal anti-inflammatory drugs
SCAR	Severe cutaneous adverse reactions
SJS	Stevens–Johnson syndrome
TEN	Toxic epidermal necrolysis
WHO	World Health Organization

M. Mockenhaupt (✉)
Dokumentationszentrum schwerer Hautreaktionen (dZh), Department of Dermatology, Medical Center and Medical Faculty—University of Freiburg, Freiburg, Germany
e-mail: dzh@uniklinik-freiburg.de

N. H. Shear, R. P. Dodiuk-Gad (eds.), *Advances in Diagnosis and Management of Cutaneous Adverse Drug Reactions*, https://doi.org/10.1007/978-981-13-1489-6_1

Key Points

- Epidemiologic studies on cADR are important to evaluate their impact in dermatology and health care in general as well as their burden for affected patients.
- For milder, non-life-threatening ADR, only rough incidence estimates exist, whereas for severe cADR incidence rates have been calculated.
- A clear clinical diagnosis and classification are of major importance in the field of cADR before causality can be assessed in the individual case and before epidemiologic investigations can be done.
- The time latency between the beginning of drug use and reaction onset differs considerably among the reaction types. In SCAR the inducing agent has not been used before and resembles the first continuous use of the medication.
- Antibiotics are the most frequent inducers of MPE or AGEP, but they have a lower risk to cause SJS/TEN or DRESS.
- "High-risk" drugs for SJS/TEN are allopurinol, anti-infective sulfonamides, certain antiepileptic drugs, nevirapine, and oxicam-NSAIDs, some of which may also cause DRESS.

1.1 Introduction

Based on the definition of the World Health Organization (WHO), an adverse drug reaction (ADR) is "a response to a medicine which is noxious and unintended, and which occurs at doses normally used in man" (World Health Organization 1972). Most ADR (up to 80%) are dose-dependent and predictable, whereas the remaining 20% occur independently of the doses taken and are not predictable. These may be immunologically mediated reactions, which are often referred to as "drug allergy" and which either involve IgE or T-cells. In contrast, non-immunologically mediated reactions are also called "idiosyncratic" (Johansson et al. 2004). A review of all published epidemiological studies quantifying ADR in Europe showed that the median percentage of hospital admissions due to ADR was 3.5%, whereas the median percentage of patients that experienced ADR while hospitalized was 10.1% (Bouvy et al. 2015). Only very limited data is available for ADR that occur and are treated outside the hospital.

Since a large proportion of ADR affects the skin, epidemiological studies have been performed in relation to cutaneous manifestations. However, these studies often comprise various cutaneous ADR of different mechanisms and clinical appearance. Except for anaphylaxis of different etiologies, systematic large-scale epidemiological studies have only been performed for severe cutaneous adverse reactions (SCAR) allowing to obtain reliable data on incidence and demography. In contrast, few studies on the epidemiology of milder cutaneous ADR have been undertaken and published.

1.2 Classification and Terminology

The majority of adverse drug reactions affecting the skin are nonserious and not life-threatening eruptions. However, many patients with such a reaction are admitted to the hospital, because in the beginning a serious and life-threatening condition is suspected or cannot be excluded.

1.2.1 Nonserious Cutaneous ADR

Milder, non-life-threatening cutaneous ADR include maculopapular exanthema (MPE), fixed drug eruption (FDE), morbilliform eruption, urticaria, purpura, vasculitis, and many other clinical manifestations. These reactions, except perhaps FDE, are not exclusively caused by medications but can also be induced by various kinds of infections. In some of them, infections even seem to be the more likely etiology, e.g., in urticaria or vasculitis, whereas others almost obligatory occur when both certain infections and specific medications are present, e.g., EBV infection and aminopenicillins leading to MPE (Bork 2009). The clinical pattern of these frequently occurring, less severe conditions is known by many physicians, but it may be difficult to differentiate in the early phase whether the eruption is benign or whether it may be the beginning of a severe condition. Therefore, the entire skin of the patient has to be inspected, and signs for severity have to be looked for. Such danger signs are, e.g., little crusts in SJS/TEN, even before skin detachment is obvious, and mucosal symptoms like burning or soreness reported by the patient before lesions are seen. Fever and constitutional symptoms are often a marker for a more severe type of ADR (Paulmann and Mockenhaupt 2016). The patient should be examined again the next day, since the clinical pattern may progress or change rapidly. To confirm the clinical diagnosis, the evaluation by a dermatologist and the result of a skin biopsy are needed. Whether a drug caused a specific reaction or not is sometimes difficult to determine, and a detailed medication history has to be obtained. Further allergy work-up, such as skin tests, may follow 2–4 months after the skin eruption has resolved (see Chap. 18).

1.2.2 Serious Cutaneous ADR

These life-threatening conditions are also called severe cutaneous adverse reactions (SCAR). They include Stevens–Johnson syndrome (SJS) and toxic epidermal necrolysis (TEN), but also acute generalized exanthematous pustulosis (AGEP) and drug reaction with eosinophilia and systemic symptoms (DRESS) (Paulmann and Mockenhaupt 2016). The precondition for these studies and the analysis of data were a clinical consensus definition of skin reactions in the spectrum of SJS/TEN (Bastuji-Garin et al. 1993). In addition, well-defined diagnostic scores were elaborated for DRESS and AGEP (Kardaun et al. 2013; Sidoroff et al. 2007).

1.2.2.1 SJS/TEN

These reactions are characterized by erythematous skin and extensive detachment of epidermis as well as hemorrhagic erosions of mucous membranes (Fig. 1.1) (Mockenhaupt 2009). SJS and TEN are considered as a single disease entity of different severity but with common causes and mechanisms. The differentiation is made based on the extent of skin detachment, that is, limited to less than 10% of the body surface area (BSA) in SJS, widespread with more than 30% of the BSA in TEN, and in-between defined as SJS/TEN overlap (Fig. 1.1) (Bastuji-Garin et al. 1993; Auquier-Dunant et al. 2002). Nikolsky sign is positive revealing a "wet" ground when the necrotic epidermis is slightly pushed away (Salopek 1997). The

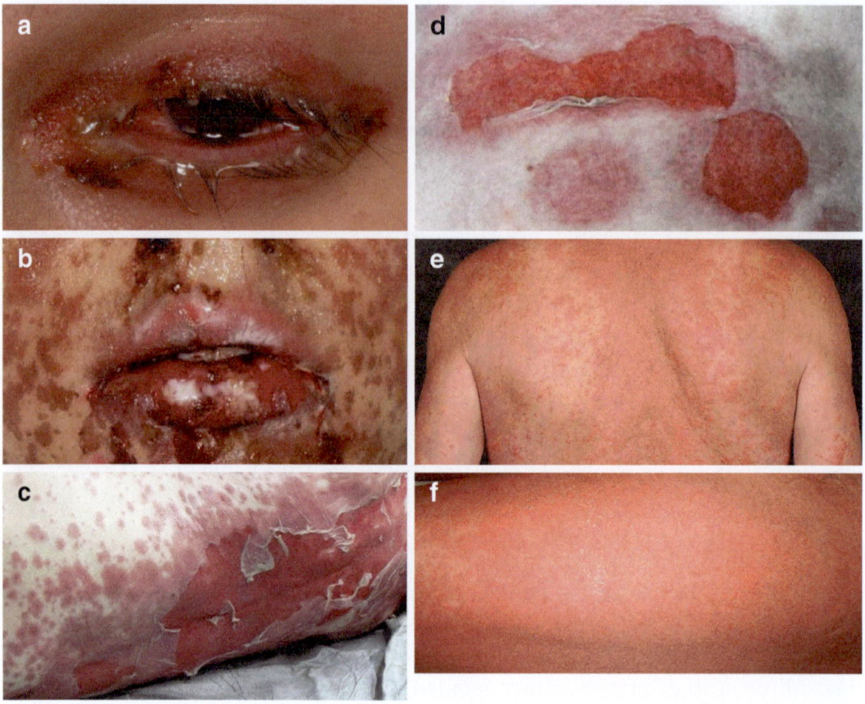

Fig. 1.1 Clinical pictures of patients with SJS/TEN (**a**–**c**), GBFDE (**d**), DRESS (**e**), and AGEP (**f**)

histopathology shows subepidermal blistering and necrotic keratinocytes either in wide dissemination or full-thickness necrosis of the epidermis, which is due to extensive apoptosis (Ziemer and Mockenhaupt 2011). Recently, the denomination of "epidermal" or "epithelial necrolysis" (EN) has been suggested for SJS/TEN (see Chap. 6).

Based on the almost identical histopathology of SJS/TEN and erythema (exsudativum) multiforme (E(E)M), SJS/TEN is often thought to be part of a broader EM spectrum (Mockenhaupt 2009). For decades EM with mucosal involvement (EM majus, EMM) was considered as Stevens-Johnson syndrome leading to false assessment of the etiology, which in EMM are predominantly infections and not medications (Auquier-Dunant et al. 2002; Schröder et al. 1999). However, a consensus definition allows differentiating SJS from EMM based on the clinical presentation (Bouvy et al. 2015; Fagot et al. 2001).

Besides EMM, multiforme-like drug eruption is often confused with SJS/TEN in the initial state or EMM. Histologically, it reflects what used to be called the dermal type of EM. Clinically, it is less severe, and blisters may be due to edema with mucous membranes spared (Ziemer and Mockenhaupt 2011; Ziemer et al. 2007). Another important differential diagnosis is generalized bullous fixed drug eruption (GBFDE), which is usually characterized by well-defined round or oval patches of dusky violaceous or brownish color. Blisters develop on these patches, but typically skin detachment does not affect more than 10% of the BSA (Kauppinen 1972; Lipowicz et al. 2013). However, the reaction may also present with diffuse erythema and blisters, which will show demarcation during the course. Nikolsky sign is positive on the areas with marked erythema but not beyond. Patients with GBFDE rarely have fever and mucosal involvement, but may present with periorificial erosions. Previous eruptions are frequent in patients' history and support the clinical diagnosis, which histologically shows the same features as SJS/TEN (Table 1.1, Fig. 1.1). Only in repeated events the skin biopsy may reveal pigment changes, which are rarely present in the histopathology of an acute reaction (Ziemer and Mockenhaupt 2011).

1.2.2.2 DRESS

For many years the term drug hypersensitivity syndrome summarized numerous severe drug reactions (Shear and Spielberg 1988). However, about 20 years ago, efforts were made to separate a specific entity of "drug hypersensitivity syndrome" from other ADR (Bocquet et al. 1996), which was later renamed in Europe as drug

Table 1.1 Comparison of main features in SJS/TEN, GBFDE, DRESS, and AGEP

Features/diagnosis	SJS/TEN	GBFDE	DRESS	AGEP
Fever	+++	(+)	+++	+++
Facial edema	–	–	+++	++
Pustules	–	–	+	+++
Blisters	+++	++	+[a]	+[a]
Target lesions/macules	+++	–	±	±
Mucosal involvement	+++	±	±	±
Histological findings	Epidermal necrosis	Epidermal necrosis	Lymphocytic infiltrate	Subcorneal pustules
Lymph node enlargement	–	–	+++	+
Lymph node histology	–	–	Lymphoid hyperplasia	–
Hepatitis	+	–	+++	++
Other organ involvements	+[b]	–	+++[c]	+
Neutrophils (in the peripheral blood)	↓	↓	(↑)	↑↑↑
Eosinophils (in the peripheral blood)	–	–	↑↑↑	↑
Atypical lymphocytes	–	–	++	+
Time between beginning of drug use and reaction onset	1–4 weeks	1–2 days	2–8 weeks	1–2 days 9–11 days
Typical duration of the reaction (skin, mucosa)	2–3 weeks	1–2 weeks	Several weeks	1 week
Previous event (of the same type)	–	++	–	–

[a]Tension blisters due to edema
[b]Tracheobronchial necrosis, tubular nephritis
[c]Interstitial nephritis, interstitial pneumonia

reaction with eosinophilia and systemic symptoms (DRESS) and in Japan as drug-induced hypersensitivity syndrome (DIHS) (Kardaun et al. 2013; Shiohara et al. 2012). DRESS/DIHS is characterized by a highly variable skin eruption, multi-organ involvement, lymphocyte activation (lymph node enlargement, lymphocytosis, atypical lymphocytes), eosinophilia, and frequent virus reactivation (Table 1.1, Fig. 1.1) (Kardaun et al. 2013; Shiohara et al. 2012). The histopathology of a skin biopsy reflects the skin pattern and is thus as variable as the clinical lesions (Ziemer and Mockenhaupt 2011). However, it should be performed to exclude potential differential diagnoses. From a skin perspective, a wide range of differential diagnoses have to be considered, especially due to the fact that the cutaneous lesions may vary from macular, papular, pustular, purpuric, urticarial to infiltrated plaques and even erythroderma. Cutaneous edema frequently leads to tension blisters, which may raise the suspicion of SJS/TEN (Paulmann and Mockenhaupt 2016).

The main features such as skin eruption, fever, and organ involvement can also be attributed to a wide range of infections and to concomitant and underlying diseases. Therefore, each symptom has to be thoroughly investigated for its relation to the reaction. Since the various signs and symptoms may develop consecutively over time, they may be easily overlooked, especially when they are asymptomatic like eosinophilia and atypical lymphocytes or sometimes increased liver enzymes. Obvious symptoms and visible skin lesions may occur at different time points in the course of the disease than elevated specific laboratory values (Paulmann and Mockenhaupt 2016; Kardaun et al. 2013). In order to make a correct diagnosis, a score was developed that has to be applied very strictly. In order to give a score point for liver involvement, liver enzymes need to be elevated at least twofold on at least two different dates. Similar rules define kidney involvement and lymphadenopathy can only be considered a relevant criterion of DRESS when present in different body sites. Unfortunately, the score is frequently applied inappropriately leading to a milder eruption with, e.g., slightly elevated liver enzymes or eosinophilia being called DRESS (Paulmann and Mockenhaupt 2016; Kardaun et al. 2007) (see Chap. 7).

1.2.2.3 AGEP

Acute generalized exanthematous pustulosis is characterized by the sudden occurrence of dozens of sterile, non-follicular pinhead-sized pustules on edematous erythema predominantly in the main body folds. The reaction is frequently accompanied by fever and leukocytosis, especially neutrophilia. The pustules appear within only a few hours and resolve within a few days leaving a typical post-pustular desquamation. Complications are rare but may occur in patients with underlying diseases and overall poor medical condition (Table 1.1, Fig. 1.1) (Sidoroff et al. 2007).

The histopathology reveals subcorneal and/or intraepidermal pustules, a sometimes pronounced edema in the papillary dermis and perivascular infiltrates consisting of neutrophils and some eosinophils. In the pustular stage, the most difficult differential diagnosis is generalized pustular psoriasis, which in the acute stage rarely displays psoriatic changes such as acanthosis in the histopathology (Ziemer and Mockenhaupt 2011). Several reports have been published suggesting that AGEP may turn into TEN, because Nikolsky phenomenon appeared positive. When pustules are confluent, this may indeed imitate a Nikolsky-like pattern, but the intraepidermal subcorneal separation does not change to the subepidermal blistering with necrotic keratinocytes in SJS/TEN.

The presence of pustules frequently leads to a misdiagnosis of an infectious condition and explains how an ADR may be overlooked. A diagnostic score has been elaborated to standardize the diagnosis of AGEP (Sidoroff et al. 2007) (see Chap. 8).

1.3 Epidemiology and Etiology

1.3.1 Epidemiological Studies on Cutaneous ADR

Most published reports of adverse drug reactions are summaries related to observations in a specific setting in a certain time period, e.g., a teaching hospital over a period of 10 years (Bouvy et al. 2015). Most often various types of ADR are comprised, sometimes differentiated in cutaneous and non-cutaneous. However, rarely a differentiation is made between serious and nonserious cutaneous ADR. Since serious cutaneous ADR are rare, the vast majority of reactions reported in the literature represent milder, non-life-threatening reactions (Bork 2009).

Studies monitoring cutaneous ADR, e.g., the Boston Collaborative Drug Surveillance Program, provided important information on the type of reaction and the potentially culprit medications, but they were not designed to estimate incidence or prevalence of the reactions. In later years, two prospective studies have been undertaken to investigate the epidemiology of cutaneous ADR in a hospital setting. The first study from France analyzed cutaneous ADR due to systemic drugs in a specific hospital over a period of 6 months. All patients were examined and clinically diagnosed by a dermatologist, whereas medication intake was reviewed by a pharmacologist. Based on 48 inpatients with a diagnosis of cADR, the prevalence was calculated as 3.6 per 1000 hospitalized patients (Fiszenson-Albala et al. 2003). The second study from Mexico was a prospective cohort study over 10 months and revealed a prevalence of 7 per 1000 hospitalized patients with cADR (35/4765 inpatients) (Hernández-Salazar et al. 2006). Among 55,432 admissions in a period of 7 months, 2682 cases of ADR, both cutaneous and non-cutaneous, were identified by a mandatory electronic reporting system for immunologically mediated drug reactions in South Korea. After review by allergists, 532 were classified as "significant drug hypersensitivity reactions," 100 of these were new events, of which 70% had cutaneous manifestations. The overall incidence of ADR was estimated as 1.8 per 1000 hospital admissions (Park et al. 2008).

1.3.2 Epidemiological Studies on Serious Cutaneous ADR

Several epidemiologic studies on severe cutaneous adverse reactions (SCAR) were undertaken in Europe in the past 25–30 years. First, two hospital-based retrospective studies were performed in France and Germany over a period of 5 years in the

1980s (Roujeau et al. 1995; Schöpf et al. 1991). Second, a prospective population-based registry on severe skin reactions was initiated in Germany in 1990 with the aim to ascertain all hospitalized cases of SJS/TEN (Rzany et al. 1996). In parallel, an international case-control study on severe cutaneous adverse reactions—also called SCAR study—was conducted in France, Germany, Italy, and Portugal between 1989 and 1995 (Roujeau et al. 1995). This study was followed by the European ongoing case-control surveillance of SCAR—also referred to as EuroSCAR—which was undertaken in Austria, France, Germany, Israel, Italy, and the Netherlands from 1997 to 2001 (Mockenhaupt et al. 2008). Besides SJS/TEN, acute generalized exanthematous pustulosis (AGEP) was investigated (Sidoroff et al. 2001). The European registry on SCAR to drugs and collection of biological samples—also called RegiSCAR—was established in 2003 and initially collected cases of SJS/TEN, AGEP, and DRESS in the same six countries as the EuroSCAR study, but later expanded to further countries such as Taiwan, the United Kingdom, South Africa, and Spain (Sekula et al. 2013). These epidemiologic studies first established clinical networks for active and prospective case ascertainment.

For the *German Registry*, a population-based approach was chosen with a network of approximately 1700 hospitals including all hospitals and departments that are likely to treat patients with SJS/TEN, such as departments of dermatology and pediatrics, burn units, and departments of internal medicine with intensive care facilities. Potential cases are reported by phone, fax, or e-mail to the registry center. When the inclusion criteria are met, a visit of the patient by a trained investigator in the reporting/treating hospital is scheduled.

In order to achieve a high coverage rate, all departments receive quarterly letters addressed to a nominated contact person. Prepaid postcards asking whether cases of SCAR occurred in the past 3–4 months that have not yet been reported are added to these letters and should be returned. A high percentage of postcards is returned to the registry center, but departments that do not respond over a certain period of time receive a reminder phone call. Due to such active and systematic ascertainment, the registry is considered to be exhaustive for detection of SJS/TEN cases in Germany (Paulmann and Mockenhaupt 2016; Roujeau et al. 1995).

For the *SCAR- and EuroSCAR-studies*, cases from the German Registry were included, whereas specific networks were established in the other participating countries. These were not operating nationwide but followed the same rules for case ascertainment. However, only prospectively ascertained and directly interviewed community cases of SJS/TEN (i.e., patients who developed the reaction in the community and were admitted due to SCAR) were included. For the case-control analysis, three control patients were matched on age, gender, region, and date of interview to each case patient. Controls were patients hospitalized for acute conditions including acute infections, trauma, and abdominal emergencies, which were not related to an underlying chronic disease. Both cases and controls were validated and checked for appropriateness of diagnosis and eligibility, and inappropriate controls were excluded (Roujeau et al. 1995; Mockenhaupt et al. 2008; Sidoroff et al. 2001).

In the current *RegiSCAR project*, reactions developing in patients already hospitalized for another disease are also included (so-called in hospital cases). In addition to SJS/TEN, further reactions such as DRESS and AGEP and most recently GBFDE are included in the study. Initially, the networks of the German Registry and the EuroSCAR study were used for the RegiSCAR project, but the network expanded to new research teams in further countries, as described above. Within RegiSCAR a cohort of SJS/TEN patients was followed for long-term sequelae and quality of life after the reaction; a cohort of DRESS patients is still investigated. Furthermore, blood samples are taken and stored centrally for pathophysiologic and genetic investigations (Sekula et al. 2013).

All patients with SCAR included in these studies were/are seen and interviewed by a trained health-care professional (physician, pharmacist, study nurse, biologist) using a standardized questionnaire. The interview includes questions regarding the current illness, demographic data, recent and past medical history, recent infections, as well as detailed information on medication use. All collected cases are reviewed by a dermatologic expert committee with no information on exposures using clinical data, photographs, and histopathology for clinical case validation. Cases are classified as "definite," "probable," or "possible" severe skin reactions or are excluded based on the consensus definition for SJS/TEN and the specific score systems for AGEP and DRESS (Bastuji-Garin et al. 1993; Kardaun et al. 2013; Sidoroff et al. 2007).

1.3.3 Incidence and Demographic Data

1.3.3.1 SJS/TEN

The retrospective studies performed in the 1980s provided incidence estimates of 1.2 per 1 million inhabitants per year for TEN in France and of 0.93 per 1 million per year in Germany, although data were not primarily collected for that purpose (Schöpf et al. 1991; Roujeau et al. 1990). Incidences between 1.4 and 6 per million person years were reported for SJS and TEN in other countries (Strom et al. 1991). The huge variation among incidence rates may be caused by various factors, such as smaller reference populations, different diagnostic criteria, methodological issues, e.g., the use of automated data bases with variable coding to identify cases.

Over the past 25 years, the prospective population-based registry in Germany has calculated an incidence of one to two cases of SJS/TEN per 1 million population per year (varying between 1.53 and 1.89) (Mockenhaupt 2009; Rzany et al. 1996). Approximately one third of cases developed in the hospital, while the other two thirds in the community, i.e., the reaction itself, led to hospital admission. SJS/TEN occurring in the hospital reveals more underlying diseases in the affected patient, a higher number of drugs before reaction onset, and an overall poorer prognosis (data of the German Registry).

SJS/TEN occurs in all age groups. In the German Registry, the average age of patients with validated SJS/TEN was 53.4 years (1–94 years) for over 2200 patients. Thirty-six percent of SJS patients were ≤40 years of age, whereas 75% of the patients with SJS/TEN overlap and 72% of the patients with TEN were >40 years of age. In contrast, 83% of the patients with EM majus were ≤40 years of age (Paulmann and Mockenhaupt 2016).

Among patients with SJS/TEN in Europe, about 5% have been shown to be HIV infected, with a lower percentage in recent years. Although the distribution of age and gender differs from that of non-HIV-infected patients, mortality rate and outcome are comparable (Bork 2009; Mockenhaupt et al. 2008).

The reason for death in patients with SJS/TEN is often difficult to determine, but death within 6 weeks after the onset of the reaction is considered to be related to the reaction. Thus, 9% of the patients with SJS, 29% of patients with SJS/TEN overlap, and 48% of those with TEN, altogether almost 25%, died in that large cohort (Mockenhaupt 2009).

In recent years the average age of patients with SJS/TEN observed by the German Registry has increased as well as the mortality rate, probably reflecting the increasing age of patients in an older general population, accompanied by a higher rate of underlying diseases. Based on the RegiSCAR cohort study, risk factors for death in the acute stage of the disease are large amount of skin detachment, old age, and renal failure, whereas death in the first year after SJS/TEN is related to preexisting conditions such as hepatic insufficiency and active malignant disease (Sekula et al. 2013).

1.3.3.2 GBFDE

Few studies beyond case reports have so far been undertaken for generalized bullous fixed drug eruption (GBFDE), and incidence data are not available. In fact, the condition is rarely recognized as a specific entity and often not separated from SJS/TEN, although it was distinguished from the latter already in 1971 (Kauppinen 1972). Although usually considered to be less severe, a case-control study comparing cases of GBFDE and cases of SJS/TEN with a comparable amount of skin detachment demonstrated that mortality was rather high in elderly patients (22%) (Lipowicz et al. 2013). Repeated episodes are common and may lead to more extensive skin involvement and finally to an increased risk of death.

1.3.3.3 DRESS

For decades, a wide variety of adverse reactions had been reported under the denomination of hypersensitivity syndrome (HSS), and no epidemiologic studies were performed on the disease until recently. That may explain why no reliable incidence data are available for what is nowadays called DRESS or DIHS. The published data suggest an incidence of "anticonvulsant HSS" that varies between 1 in 1000 and 1 in 10,000 exposed patients (Shear and Spielberg 1988).

Of the 201 potential DRESS cases collected within RegiSCAR, 117 were finally validated as "probable" and "definite." The female/male ratio was 66/51, and women were significantly younger than men with a median age of 41.5 years compared to 51 years of men. Generalized exanthema was present in all patients, and further main features were eosinophilia (95%), visceral involvement (91%) predominantly of the liver (75%), high fever (90%), atypical lymphocytes (67%), mild mucosal involvement (56%) and lymphadenopathy (54%).

The reaction lasted 3 weeks and longer in all except two patients. The death rate was far lower than the previously reported 10% with 2 deaths in 117 patients (Kardaun et al. 2007).

1.3.3.4 AGEP

The EuroSCAR study collected the largest validated cohort of patients with AGEP. Since the case-control study did not work on a population-based scale, the incidence of AGEP could only be roughly estimated as one to five cases per million inhabitants per year in Europe. Furthermore, it seems that AGEP is more frequent in some European countries than in others. A potential reason could be the availability of specific drugs with a high risk to induce AGEP.

Of the 150 potential AGEP cases collected within EuroSCAR, 97 were finally validated as "probable" and "definite." The majority of these cases (78/97) derived from France. The mean age was 56 years (range 4–91 years), and 80% of the patients were women. A death rate of almost 4% was calculated (Sidoroff et al. 2001).

1.3.4 Etiology of Cutaneous ADR

Numerous case reports and case series are published reporting a huge variety of drugs considered to be responsible for different types of cutaneous adverse reactions. In addition, one drug or drug group may induce clinically different reactions, whereas a specific adverse reaction may be caused by many different drugs (Bork 2009). Some drugs seem to have a high risk for cutaneous adverse reactions, especially if a viral infection is present in parallel, as stated before for aminopenicillins and EBV. In the epidemiological study from France mentioned above, beta-lactam antibiotics accounted for 21% of the cutaneous ADR (Fiszenson-Albala et al. 2003). In the study from Korea, antibiotics were thought to be responsible for 32% of the reactions, followed by 26% caused by contrast media (Park et al. 2008). In Singapore, antimicrobial and antiepileptic agents were the most common culprit drugs (75%), including penicillins (25%), cephalosporins (16%), co-trimoxazole (9%), phenytoin (8%), and carbamazepine (6%). Allopurinol (5.7%) was less frequently determined as etiologic factors. However, these percentages refer to various types of cutaneous adverse drug reactions of both delayed- and immediate-type hypersensitivities (63% MPE, 18% urticaria) (Thong et al. 2003). In a survey of cutaneous adverse reactions in Switzerland (comprehensive hospital drug monitoring, CHDM), which covers more than 20 years, penicillins were identified as the culprit drug in 8% and co-trimoxazole in 2.8% of the cases. In this study, more than 90% of the reactions were diagnosed as MPE, the remaining as urticaria (5.5%), vasculitis (1.4%), and FDE (0.5%) (Hunziker et al. 1997).

A histogram that can be prepared electronically, but also be drawn by hand, is most helpful to visualize the situation (Fig. 1.2).

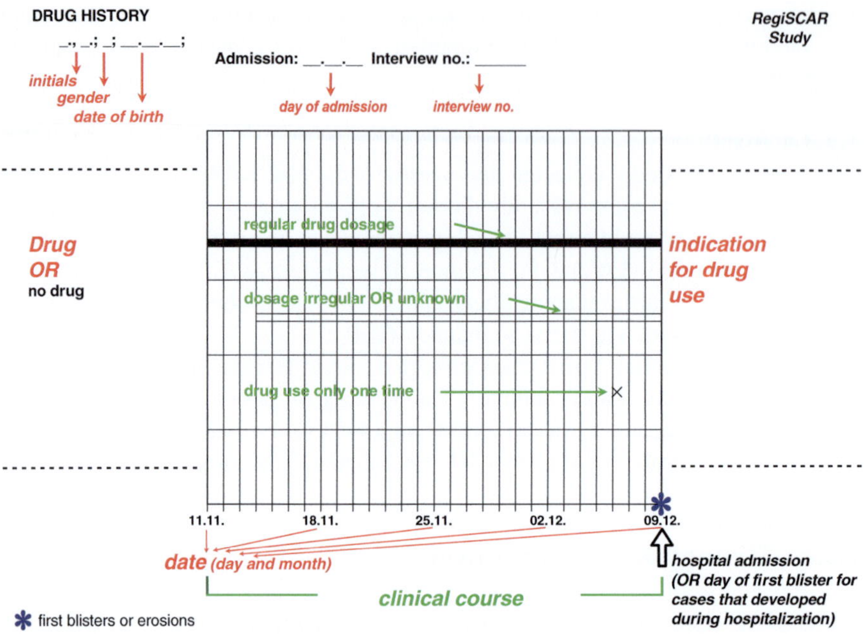

Fig. 1.2 Example of a histogram that can be used as an aide for a medication history

1.3.5 Etiology of Serious Cutaneous ADR

1.3.5.1 SJS/TEN

Most patients report drug use before the reaction began, but many medications were either taken for many years or very shortly before the reaction. Such medications are very unlikely the cause of SJS/TEN. Furthermore, medications that have been used before and been tolerated well are very unlikely causes of SJS/TEN, since the culprit drug is typically taken for the first time in consecutive use of 1–4 weeks. In some cases anti-infectives, antipyretics, and/or analgesics are taken to treat an infection that was present within 1 or 2 weeks before, which could be causal by itself (confounding by indication). Even more frequently, antipyretics, analgesics, and secretolytics are used to treat the first symptoms of the disease itself, which typically starts with prodromal symptoms mimicking an acute infection (protopathic bias) (Paulmann and Mockenhaupt 2017). Thus, the correct determination of the day of onset of the reaction (so-called index day) is crucial. This is typically not the appearance of blisters or erosions, often not even the first skin lesions, but unspecific symptoms preceding the objective signs for 1 day, e.g., fever, malaise, headache, and oronasal soreness (Paulmann and Mockenhaupt 2016, 2017; Mockenhaupt 2009).

Medications used after occurrence of such symptoms should not be considered to be responsible. As far as there is no reliable in vitro or in vivo test, the identification of the inducing agent relies on the time interval between the beginning of drug use and onset of SJS/TEN (Hernández-Salazar et al. 2006). With the help of two multinational case-control studies, which provided risk estimates for drugs, an algorithm for assessment of drug causality in SJS/TEN (ALDEN) was developed (Roujeau et al. 1995; Mockenhaupt et al. 2008; Sassolas et al. 2010). It provides structured help for identifying the most likely culprit drug and is based on the following criteria: time latency between the beginning of drug use and index day (i.e., onset of the adverse reaction), drug present in the body before index day (taking into account the drug's half-life as well as the patient's liver and kidney function), information on prechallenge/rechallenge and dechallenge (if available), type of drug/notoriety (based on drug lists that require a regular update), and alternative causes. Numerical score values lead to a causality assessment for each individual drug a patient has taken or was administered, ranging from "very unlikely," "unlikely," "possible," "probable" to "very probable" (Sassolas et al. 2010).

Causality assessment in the individual case is important for the affected patient, since otherwise there is huge uncertainty which medications can be taken safely in the future. Many patients and their physicians believe that all drugs with a risk for SJS/TEN should be avoided by a patient who had the reaction, but this is wrong. One patient only reacts to one drug or chemically closely related drug group, as pharmacogenetics investigations have shown (see Chap. 3). Further confusion is caused by the information leaflet in the drug package and in drug dictionaries (Haddad et al. 2013).

Drugs with a high risk to induce SJS/TEN are allopurinol, anti-infective sulfonamides, certain antiepileptic agents (carbamazepine, phenobarbital, phenytoin), and nonsteroidal anti-inflammatory drugs (NSAIDs) of the oxicam type (Table 1.2) (Mockenhaupt et al. 2008; Halevy et al. 2008). In 85–100% of the cases, such highly suspected drugs were started less than 8 weeks before the onset of these adverse reactions. The median time latency between the beginning of drug use and reactions onset (index day) in the more recent study was 20 days for allopurinol, 15 days for carbamazepine, and 24 days for phenytoin, and the overall time latency was less than 4 weeks. In contrast, for medications with no associated risk, the exposure period was much longer, e.g., more than 30 weeks for ACE inhibitors, calcium channel blockers, and valproic acid. Drug intake of more than 8 weeks was not associated with an increased risk to induce SCAR (Roujeau et al. 1995; Mockenhaupt et al. 2008). In the more recent study, there were two medications strongly associated with SJS/TEN: lamotrigine and nevirapine. They share the exposure pattern of strongly associated drugs (Mockenhaupt et al. 2008). It was thought that a slow titration of the dosage could prevent such adverse reactions, which is obviously not the case (Fagot et al. 2001; Mockenhaupt et al. 2008; Schlienger et al. 1998).

For safety reasons, oral provocation tests cannot be recommended to confirm the identification of the culprit drug, although the reaction may not occur again, as studies performed in Finland in the 1970s demonstrated (Kauppinen 1972). Patch tests with the potentially culprit drug often remain false negative (Barbaud et al. 2013).

In both case-control studies, approximately 65% of the cases were exposed to a strongly associated (55%) and/or associated (10%) drug. However, these studies focused on community acquired cases and did not include cases that developed in

Table 1.2 Drug causality in SJS/TEN (according to Mockenhaupt et al. (2008))

A. Drugs with a high risk to induce SJS/TEN Their use should be carefully weighed and they should be suspected promptly
Allopurinol
Carbamazepine
Co-trimoxazole (and other anti-infective sulfonamides and sulfasalazine)
Lamotrigine
Nevirapine
NSAIDs (oxicam type, e.g., meloxicam)
Phenobarbital
Phenytoin
An interval of 4–28 days between the beginning of drug use and onset of the adverse reaction is most suggestive of an association between the medication and SJS/TEN
When patients are exposed to several medications with high expected benefits, the timing of administration is important to determine which one(s) must be stopped and if some may be continued or reintroduced
The risks of various antibiotics to induce SJS/TEN are within the same order of magnitude, but substantially lower than the risk of anti-infective sulfonamides
Valproic acid does not seem to have an increased risk for SJS/TEN in contrast to other antiepileptics
Diuretics and oral antidiabetics with sulfonamide structure do not appear to be risk factors for SJS/TEN
B. Drugs with a moderate (significant but substantially lower) risk for SJS/TEN
Cephalosporins
Macrolides
Quinolones
Tetracyclines
NSAIDs (acetic acid type, e.g., diclofenac)
C. Drugs without increased risk for SJS/TEN
Beta-blockers
ACE inhibitors
Calcium channel blockers
Thiazide diuretics (with sulfonamide structure)
Sulfonylurea antidiabetics (with sulfonamide structure)
Insulin
NSAIDs (propionic acid type, e.g., ibuprofen)

the hospital setting. Some cases may be caused by new drugs, for which risk estimates do not yet exist (Valeyrie-Allanore et al. 2008), but no more than 75% of all SJS/TEN cases can be explained by drug intake. Although infections, e.g., upper respiratory tract infections due to *Mycoplasma pneumoniae* or virus- and influenza-like illness, have been reported as etiologic factor, in many of these cases, an infection may be clinically diagnosed, but no specific virus or bacterium can be determined (Paulmann and Mockenhaupt 2017; Grosber et al. 2006).

1.3.5.2 GBFDE

Although epidemiological studies have just started to investigate GBFDE, a number of medications have been observed by the German Registry to frequently induce this reaction. Among them are co-trimoxazole (sulfamethoxazole/trimethoprim) and metamizole, which are both frequently administered to elderly persons. Carbamazepine also induces bullous fixed drug eruptions, especially when given repeatedly for alcohol withdrawal (unpublished data of the German Registry). In contrast to SJS/TEN, there is usually a previous exposure to the drug that induced a sensitization. The time latency between the beginning of drug use and onset of the reaction is short with only a few days and even shorter in recurrent cases with sometimes just a few hours (Table 1.1). Patch tests have a good chance to confirm the culprit drug in GBFDE (see Chap. 18).

1.3.5.3 DRESS

Information on drugs inducing DRESS is mainly based on case reports and case series. Often, the reaction itself was named after the drug that was considered to be culprit, e.g., allopurinol HSS, dapsone syndrome, anticonvulsant syndrome, etc. (Shear and Spielberg 1988). Within the RegiSCAR study, drug exposure was analyzed in 117 validated cases of DRESS. A median of five (interquartile range 2–8) drugs were taken in the month before onset of the reaction. In 77% of the cases one and in 3% two equally (very) probable culprit drugs could be identified, whereas in 4% causality remained undetermined and in 7% unlikely. Antiepileptic drugs including carbamazepine, phenytoin, and lamotrigine were thought to be responsible in 36% of the cases, followed by allopurinol in 18%, and sulfonamides in 12%. Other previously reported drugs were found less frequently. The median time latency between the beginning of drug use and onset of DRESS was 28 (±17) days for all drugs with a "probable" or "very probable" causality assessment (Kardaun et al. 2007). The culprit drugs were also taken for the first time in consecutive use of 2–8 weeks before reaction onset.

Furthermore, viral reactivation and antiviral T-cell response are observed in DRESS, especially in cases with a prolonged course or flare-ups of the reaction (Shiohara et al. 2012; Mardivirin et al. 2010). Nevertheless, it is not clear whether the reactivation of HHV6 and other members of the human herpes virus family plays a role in the etiology of the disease, has to be considered as an epiphenomenon, or should be interpreted as a complication. In vitro tests such as lymphocyte transformation or stimulation test may be able to confirm the inducing agent, and patch tests have shown good results, when performed in the correct time period after the reaction resolved (Shiohara et al. 2012; Barbaud et al. 2013) (see Chap. 18).

1.3.5.4 AGEP

The EuroSCAR case-control study also provided risk estimates for AGEP. Thirteen of the 97 patients reported the use of a macrolide antibiotic in the week before onset of the skin reaction. Ten of these cases were associated with pristinamycin, a macrolide that was only marketed in France. Other macrolide antibiotics were also associated with a significant but lower risk, as were ampicillin and amoxicillin, both often reported causes of AGEP. The results were similar for quinolones. Further drugs with an increased risk for AGEP are chloroquine and hydroxychloroquine, anti-infective sulfonamides, terbinafine, and diltiazem. No other single calcium channel blocker was associated with a significant risk, and no patient exposed to diltiazem had been simultaneously exposed to another high-risk drug. The latter was also observed for the other agents listed above (Sidoroff et al. 2001).

In terms of the relevant exposure period for drugs with a high risk, two different patterns were observed, a very short one and a longer one. For all exposures to antibiotics (41 cases), including antibacterial sulfonamides, the median time of use was 1 day. In contrast, for all other associated drugs, the median was 11 days. Interestingly, medications with a longer exposure period were characterized by a longer half-life of their active ingredient, but the explanation of these observations still remains to be found (Sidoroff et al. 2001). In the German Registry and RegiSCAR project, aminopenicillins are the most frequent cause of AGEP.

Patch tests have shown good results to confirm the culprit drug in AGEP, when performed 2–6 months after the reaction resolved (Barbaud et al. 2013) (see Chap. 18).

References

Auquier-Dunant A, Mockenhaupt M, Naldi L et al (2002) Correlations between clinical patterns and causes of erythema multiforme majus, Stevens-Johnson syndrome, and toxic epidermal necrolysis: results of an international prospective study. Arch Dermatol 138:1019–1024

Barbaud A, Collet E, Milpied B et al (2013) A multicentre study to determine the value and safety of drug patch tests for the three main classes of severe cutaneous adverse drug reactions. Br J Dermatol 168:555–562. https://doi.org/10.1111/bjd.12125

Bastuji-Garin S, Rzany B, Stern RS et al (1993) Clinical classification of cases of toxic epidermal necrolysis, Stevens-Johnson syndrome, and erythema multiforme. Arch Dermatol 129: 92–96

Bocquet H, Bagot M, Roujeau JC (1996) Drug-induced pseudolymphoma and drug hypersensitivity syndrome (Drug Rash with Eosinophilia and Systemic Symptoms: DRESS). Semin Cutan Med Surg 15:250–257

Bork K (2009) Cutaneous adverse drug reactions. In: Burgdorf W, Plewig G, Wolff HH, Landthaler M (eds) Braun-Falco's dermatology, 3rd edn. Springer, Heidelberg, pp 456–472

Bouvy JC, De Bruin ML, Koopmanschap MA (2015) Epidemiology of adverse drug reactions in Europe: a review of recent observational studies. Drug Saf 38:437–453. https://doi.org/10.1007/s40264-015-0281-0

Fagot JP, Mockenhaupt M, Bouwes-Bavinck JN et al (2001) Nevirapine and the risk of Stevens-Johnson syndrome or toxic epidermal necrolysis. AIDS Lond Engl 15:1843–1848

Fiszenson-Albala F, Auzerie V, Mahe E et al (2003) A 6-month prospective survey of cutaneous drug reactions in a hospital setting. Br J Dermatol 149:1018–1022

Grosber M, Carsin H, Leclerc F (2006) Epidermal necrolysis in association with Mycoplasma pneumoniae infection. J Invest Dermatol 126:S3–S116. https://doi.org/10.1038/sj.jid.5700514

Haddad C, Sidoroff A, Kardaun SH et al (2013) Stevens-Johnson syndrome/toxic epidermal necrolysis: are drug dictionaries correctly informing physicians regarding the risk? Drug Saf 36:681–686. https://doi.org/10.1007/s40264-013-0070-6

Halevy S, Ghislain P-D, Mockenhaupt M et al (2008) Allopurinol is the most common cause of Stevens-Johnson syndrome and toxic epidermal necrolysis in Europe and Israel. J Am Acad Dermatol 58:25–32. https://doi.org/10.1016/j.jaad.2007.08.036

Hernández-Salazar A, Rosales SP-L, Rangel-Frausto S et al (2006) Epidemiology of adverse cutaneous drug reactions. A prospective study in hospitalized patients. Arch Med Res 37:899–902. https://doi.org/10.1016/j.arcmed.2006.03.010

Hunziker T, Künzi UP, Braunschweig S et al (1997) Comprehensive hospital drug monitoring (CHDM): adverse skin reactions, a 20-year survey. Allergy 52:388–393

Johansson SGO, Bieber T, Dahl R et al (2004) Revised nomenclature for allergy for global use: Report of the Nomenclature Review Committee of the World Allergy Organization, October 2003. J Allergy Clin Immunol 113:832–836. https://doi.org/10.1016/j.jaci.2003.12.591

Kardaun SH, Sidoroff A, Valeyrie-Allanore L et al (2007) Variability in the clinical pattern of cutaneous side-effects of drugs with systemic symptoms: does a DRESS syndrome really exist? Br J Dermatol 156:609–611. https://doi.org/10.1111/j.1365-2133.2006.07704.x

Kardaun SH, Sekula P, Valeyrie-Allanore L et al (2013) Drug reaction with eosinophilia and systemic symptoms (DRESS): an original multisystem adverse drug reaction. Results from the prospective RegiSCAR study. Br J Dermatol 169:1071–1080. https://doi.org/10.1111/bjd.12501

Kauppinen K (1972) Cutaneous reactions to drugs with special reference to severe bullous mucocutaneous eruptions and sulphonamides. Acta Derm Venereol Suppl (Stockh) 68:1–89

Lipowicz S, Sekula P, Ingen-Housz-Oro S et al (2013) Prognosis of generalized bullous fixed drug eruption: comparison with Stevens-Johnson syndrome and toxic epidermal necrolysis. Br J Dermatol 168:726–732. https://doi.org/10.1111/bjd.12133

Mardivirin L, Valeyrie-Allanore L, Branlant-Redon E et al (2010) Amoxicillin-induced flare in patients with DRESS (Drug Reaction with Eosinophilia and Systemic Symptoms): report of seven cases and demonstration of a direct effect of amoxicillin on Human Herpesvirus 6 replication in vitro. Eur J Dermatol 20:68–73. https://doi.org/10.1684/ejd.2010.0821

Mockenhaupt M (2009) Severe cutaneous adverse reactions. In: Burgdorf W, Plewig G, Wolff HH, Landthaler M (eds) Braun-Falco's dermatology, 3rd edn. Springer, Heidelberg, pp 473–484

Mockenhaupt M, Viboud C, Dunant A et al (2008) Stevens-Johnson syndrome and toxic epidermal necrolysis: assessment of medication risks with emphasis on recently marketed drugs. The EuroSCAR-study. J Invest Dermatol 128:35–44. https://doi.org/10.1038/sj.jid.5701033

Park CS, Kim T-B, Kim SL et al (2008) The use of an electronic medical record system for mandatory reporting of drug hypersensitivity reactions has been shown to improve the management of patients in the university hospital in Korea. Pharmacoepidemiol Drug Saf 17:919–925. https://doi.org/10.1002/pds.1612

Paulmann M, Mockenhaupt M (2016) Severe drug hypersensitivity reactions: clinical pattern, diagnosis, etiology and therapeutic options. Curr Pharm Des 22:6852–6861. https://doi.org/10.2174/1381612822666160928125152

Paulmann M, Mockenhaupt M (2017) Fever in Stevens-Johnson syndrome and toxic epidermal necrolysis in pediatric cases: laboratory work-up and antibiotic therapy. Pediatr Infect Dis J 36:513–515. https://doi.org/10.1097/INF.0000000000001571

Roujeau JC, Guillaume JC, Fabre JP et al (1990) Toxic epidermal necrolysis (Lyell syndrome). Incidence and drug etiology in France, 1981–1985. Arch Dermatol 126:37–42

Roujeau JC, Kelly JP, Naldi L et al (1995) Medication use and the risk of Stevens-Johnson syndrome or toxic epidermal necrolysis. N Engl J Med 333:1600–1607. https://doi.org/10.1056/NEJM199512143332404

Rzany B, Mockenhaupt M, Baur S et al (1996) Epidemiology of erythema exsudativum multiforme majus, Stevens-Johnson syndrome, and toxic epidermal necrolysis in Germany (1990–1992): structure and results of a population-based registry. J Clin Epidemiol 49:769–773

Salopek TG (1997) Nikolsky's sign: is it "dry" or is it "wet"? Br J Dermatol 136:762–767

Sassolas B, Haddad C, Mockenhaupt M et al (2010) ALDEN, an algorithm for assessment of drug causality in Stevens-Johnson syndrome and toxic epidermal necrolysis: comparison with case-control analysis. Clin Pharmacol Ther 88:60–68. https://doi.org/10.1038/clpt.2009.252

Schlienger RG, Shapiro LE, Shear NH (1998) Lamotrigine-induced severe cutaneous adverse reactions. Epilepsia 39(Suppl 7):S22–S26

Schöpf E, Stühmer A, Rzany B et al (1991) Toxic epidermal necrolysis and Stevens-Johnson syndrome. An epidemiologic study from West Germany. Arch Dermatol 127:839–842

Schröder W, Mockenhaupt M, Schlingmann J et al (1999) Clinical re-classification of severe skin reactions and evaluation of their etiology in a population-based registry. In: Victor N, Blettner M, Edler L et al (eds) Medical informatics, biostatistics and epidemiology for efficient health care and medical research: contributions from the 44th annual conference of the GMDS... Heidelberg, September 1999. Urban und Vogel, München, pp 107–110

Sekula P, Dunant A, Mockenhaupt M et al (2013) Comprehensive survival analysis of a cohort of patients with Stevens-Johnson syndrome and toxic epidermal necrolysis. J Invest Dermatol 133:1197–1204. https://doi.org/10.1038/jid.2012.510

Shear NH, Spielberg SP (1988) Anticonvulsant hypersensitivity syndrome. In vitro assessment of risk. J Clin Invest 82:1826–1832. https://doi.org/10.1172/JCI113798

Shiohara T, Kano Y, Takahashi R et al (2012) Drug-induced hypersensitivity syndrome: recent advances in the diagnosis, pathogenesis and management. Chem Immunol Allergy 97:122–138. https://doi.org/10.1159/000335624

Sidoroff A, Halevy S, Bavinck JN et al (2001) Acute generalized exanthematous pustulosis (AGEP)—a clinical reaction pattern. J Cutan Pathol 28:113–119

Sidoroff A, Dunant A, Viboud C et al (2007) Risk factors for acute generalized exanthematous pustulosis (AGEP)—results of a multinational case-control study (EuroSCAR). Br J Dermatol 157:989–996. https://doi.org/10.1111/j.1365-2133.2007.08156.x

Strom BL, Carson JL, Halpern AC et al (1991) A population-based study of Stevens-Johnson syndrome. Incidence and antecedent drug exposures. Arch Dermatol 127:831–838

Thong BY-H, Leong K-P, Tang C-Y, Chng H-H (2003) Drug allergy in a general hospital: Results of a novel prospective inpatient reporting system. Ann Allergy Asthma Immunol 90:342–347. https://doi.org/10.1016/S1081-1206(10)61804-2

Valeyrie-Allanore L, Poulalhon N, Fagot J-P et al (2008) Stevens-Johnson syndrome and toxic epidermal necrolysis induced by amifostine during head and neck radiotherapy. Radiother Oncol J Eur Soc Ther Radiol Oncol 87:300–303. https://doi.org/10.1016/j.radonc.2008.01.021

World Health Organization (1972) International drug monitoring: the role of national centres. Report of a WHO meeting. World Health Organ Tech Rep Ser 498, pp 1–25

Ziemer M, Mockenhaupt M (2011) Severe drug-induced skin reactions: clinical pattern, diagnostics and therapy. In: Khopkar U (ed) Skin biopsy—perspectives. InTech, Rijeka

Ziemer M, Wiesend CL, Vetter R et al (2007) Cutaneous adverse reactions to valdecoxib distinct from Stevens-Johnson syndrome and toxic epidermal necrolysis. Arch Dermatol 143:711–716. https://doi.org/10.1001/archderm.143.6.711

Part II

Pathomechanisms of Cutaneous Adverse Drug Reactions

Immunology of Cutaneous Adverse Drug Reactions

2

Chuang-Wei Wang and Shuen-Iu Hung

Abbreviations

ADR	Adverse drug reactions
AGEP	Acute generalized exanthematous pustulosis
APC	Antigen-presenting cells
BCL2L10	B-cell lymphoma/leukemia-2-like protein 10
cADR	Cutaneous adverse drug reactions
CBZ	Carbamazepine
CCR	C–C chemokine receptor
CTL	Cytotoxic T lymphocytes
CXCR	CX chemokine receptor
DRESS	Drug reactions with eosinophilia and systemic symptoms
FADD	Fas-associated death domain protein
FDE	Fixed drug eruption
FPR1	Formyl peptide receptor 1
GM-CSF	Granulocyte-macrophage colony-stimulating factor
GPP	Generalized pustular psoriasis
HHV-6	Human herpesvirus 6

C.-W. Wang
Department of Dermatology, Drug Hypersensitivity Clinical and Research Center, Chang Gung Memorial Hospital, Linko, Taiwan

S.-I. Hung (✉)
Department and Institute of Pharmacology, School of Medicine, National Yang-Ming University, Taipei, Taiwan
e-mail: sihung@ym.edu.tw

N. H. Shear, R. P. Dodiuk-Gad (eds.), *Advances in Diagnosis and Management of Cutaneous Adverse Drug Reactions*, https://doi.org/10.1007/978-981-13-1489-6_2

HLA	Human leukocyte antigens
IFN-γ	Interferon-γ
IL	Interleukin
IL-15	Interleukin-15
IL-2	Interleukin-2
IL-36Ra	IL-36 receptor antagonist
MPE	Maculopapular exanthema
NK	Natural killer
NK/NKT	Natural killer/natural killer T cells
NS	Not significant
PBMC	Peripheral mononuclear cells
SCAR	Severe cutaneous adverse reactions
sFasL	Soluble FasL
SJS	Stevens–Johnson syndrome
TARC	Thymus- and activation-regulated chemokine
TCR	T cell receptors
TEN	Toxic epidermal necrolysis
Th	T helper
TNF-α	Tumor necrosis factor-α

Key Points

- Cutaneous adverse drug reactions (cADR) usually present as type B reactions which are considered as unpredictable and dose-independent idiosyncratic response, carrying high morbidity and mortality.
- Drugs-induced cADR have shown strong genetic association with different human leukocyte antigens (HLA) alleles. Increasing evidence demonstrate that polymorphic HLA alleles play a crucial role in the recognition of drug antigens in the initial development of cADRs. HLA proteins may present the drugs/metabolites to T cell receptors (TCR), resulting in T cell activation.
- Upon activation of T lymphocytes, various cytotoxic proteins, including perforin/granzyme B and granulysin, are released, and they can cause skin rash or epidermal necrosis. The secretory form granulysin has been identified as the key mediator for disseminated keratinocyte death in SJS/TEN.
- Cytokines/chemokines, including TNF-α, IFN-γ, GM-CSF, TARC/CCL17, IL-6, IL-8, IL-15, and IL-36 signaling, are known to participate in the immune reactions of cADR. These immune mediators are responsible for the trafficking, proliferation, regulation, or activation of T lymphocytes and other leukocytes to manipulate the clinical presentations of cADR.

2.1 Introduction

2.1.1 Cutaneous Adverse Drug Reactions

Adverse drug reactions (ADR) are a major public health problem in the world and account for about 10–20% of all hospitalizations (Friedmann et al. 2003). According to the definition by the World Health Organization, "ADR" is "a response to a drug that is noxious and unintended and which occurs in doses normally used for the treatment, prophylaxis, or diagnosis of disease, or the modification of physiological function." The ADR can be categorized into type A and B reactions. The type A reactions are considered to be predictable and dose-dependent response, and associated with the pharmacological effect, constituting about 80% of ADR (Pirmohamed et al. 2002). By contrast, type B reactions are unpredictable and dose-independent adverse effects and carry high morbidity and mortality. Most of the type B ADR affect the skin, which are also known as cutaneous ADR (cADR). Cutaneous ADR range from mild maculopapular exanthema (MPE), fixed drug eruption (FDE), urticaria, morbilliform eruption, and purpura to life-threatening severe cutaneous adverse drug reactions (SCAR). SCAR include acute generalized exanthematous pustulosis (AGEP), drug reactions with eosinophilia and systemic symptoms (DRESS), Stevens–Johnson syndrome (SJS), and toxic epidermal necrolysis (TEN) (Mockenhaupt 2012).

2.1.2 Interaction of HLAs, Drug Antigens, and T Cell Receptors

Cutaneous ADR are considered to be elicited from the excessive or inappropriate activation of T lymphocytes. Drugs or the reactive metabolites could act as foreign antigens and be able to bind to the receptors to activate immune response. Human leukocyte antigens (HLA) are the main immune anchor for presenting the foreign antigens and play a crucial role in the pathogenesis of cADR (Chung et al. 2007). The highly polymorphic property of HLA molecules among individuals offers a diverse interaction toward different kinds of drug antigens. A specific kind of HLA protein may have higher affinity toward a drug/metabolite antigen and present it to the T cell receptors (TCR), resulting in T lymphocyte activation, clonal expansion, and extensive keratinocyte death. The discovery of strong genetic associations between HLA-B*15:02 and carbamazepine (CBZ)-induced SJS/TEN (Chung et al. 2004), HLA-B*58:01 and allopurinol-induced SCAR (Hung et al. 2005), as well as HLA-B*57:01 and abacavir hypersensitivity (Mallal et al. 2002) supports that the interaction of HLA-drug antigen-TCR is essential for the initiation of immune recognition and triggering the downstream inflammation in cADR (Fig. 2.1).

There are four hypotheses trying to explain the interaction between drug/metabolite antigens and immune receptors: (1) the "hapten/prohapten" theory, (2) the "p-i

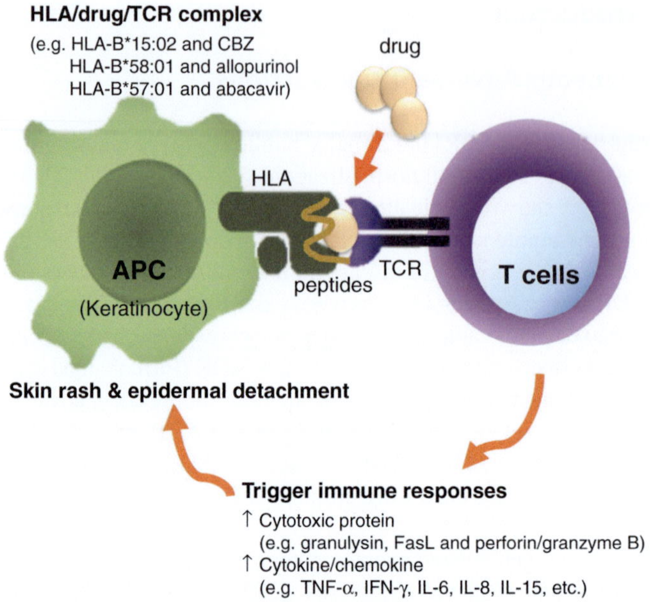

Fig. 2.1 Interaction of HLA/drug/TCR in the immune synapse of cADR. As illustrated, the immune response could be triggered by the binding of an antigenic drug to a specific HLA allele on an APC/keratinocyte in cADR. Then, specific TCR of the T cells recognizes the drug/HLA complex. Upon the activation, T cells produce the cytotoxic proteins as well as cytokines/chemokines and lead to skin rash or extensive epidermal detachment. Abbreviations: *APC* antigen-presenting cells, *CBZ* carbamazepine, *HLA* human leukocyte antigen, *TCR* T cell receptors, *TNF-α* tumor necrosis factor-α, *IFN-γ* interferon-γ

concept," (3) the "altered peptide repertoire" model, and (4) the "altered TCR repertoire" model (Chung et al. 2016).

First, the "hapten/prohapten" theory proposes that drugs or its reactive metabolites enable to covalently bind to the endogenous peptides to form an antigenic hapten-carrier complex. The hapten-carrier complex is presented to the HLA molecule and then recognized by TCR, resulting in the induction of drug–specific cellular or humoral immune responses. Haptens correspond to the chemically reactive small molecules which are able to bind covalently to peptides or larger proteins, whereas prohaptens originally are not reactive molecules, but become chemically active compounds after the metabolism in the human body. The theory of hapten/prohapten has been demonstrated in penicillin-induced cADR (Schneider and De Weck 1965).

Second, the "pharmacological interaction with immune receptors (p-i)" concept postulates that drugs/metabolites may directly, reversibly, and non-covalently bind to the HLA and/or TCR protein without a link to specific peptide ligands. In the "p-i" model, it is not essential to involve the antigenic peptide-processing pathway in the antigen-presenting cells (APC) (Pichler 2002). CBZ-induced SJS/TEN is one of the examples for the "p-i" model, in which CBZ was found to directly bind to the

HLA-B*15:02 protein without the involvement of antigen-processing pathway as the use of fixed APCs could still elicit the immune reaction upon drug stimulation (Wei et al. 2012).

Third, the "altered peptide repertoire" model proposes that drugs/metabolites could non-covalently and strongly bind to the binding pocket of HLA molecules and then alter the peptide repertoire of HLA. In this model, the drug doesn't directly interfere with HLA repertoire, but change the conformation or repertoire of peptides. Therefore, drugs serve as the initial antigens, change the binding cleft of HLA, cause the altered peptide repertoire, and therefore elicit T cell activation. One of the well-known examples of the altered peptide repertoire model is the interaction between abacavir and HLA-B*57:01, in which abacavir can trigger the conformational changes of endogenous peptides presented by HLA-B*57:01 (Illing et al. 2012).

Finally, the "altered TCR repertoire" model suggests that the drugs (e.g., sulfamethoxazole) bind to the specific TCR and alter the conformation of TCR, which is potential to bind HLA-self peptide complex to elicit immune reaction (Watkins and Pichler 2013). In this "altered TCR repertoire" model, drug antigens directly interact with TCR, but not the peptides or HLA molecules.

Taken together, the recent discovery of HLA genetic predisposition in cADR and the oligoclonal and clonotype-specific TCR usages in CBZ or allopurinol-induced SJS/TEN patients (Ko et al. 2011; Chung et al. 2015), supporting the concept that the immune synapse composed of HLA-drug-TCR, is the essential key for inducing cADR. The activation of drug-specific T lymphocytes which have preferential TCR against HLA/peptide/drug complex or recognizing drug antigen only leads to the downstream dysregulation of cytotoxic proteins, cytokines, and chemokines in cADR.

2.1.3 Cytotoxic Signals and Immune Molecules in cADR

The main concept to explain the pathomechanism of cADR is the cytotoxic T lymphocytes (CTL)-, natural killer (NK)/NKT cells-, and CD4 T helper (Th) cells-mediated immune reactions. Several cytotoxic proteins, cytokines, and chemokines are generally advocated for cADR (Fig. 2.2).

2.1.3.1 Fas–FasL Interaction

Fas–FasL interaction was first reported by Viard et al. in 1998 and suggested to be involved in the apoptosis of keratinocytes in SJS/TEN (Viard et al. 1998). Briefly, the activated Fas might serve as a death receptor upon FasL recognition. Fas-associated death domain protein (FADD) is recruited by Fas–FasL and binds to Fas–FasL complex and procaspase 8. The FADD recruits procaspase 8 and brings multiple copies of procaspase 8 together, which autoactivates to become caspase 8, triggering the caspase cascade and resulting in intracellular DNA degradation (Posadas et al. 2002). Viard et al. reported that FasL distributes on the keratinocyte cell surface, and soluble FasL (sFasL) presented with a high level in the serum of TEN patients (Viard et al. 1998). However, the proposed role of FasL in the

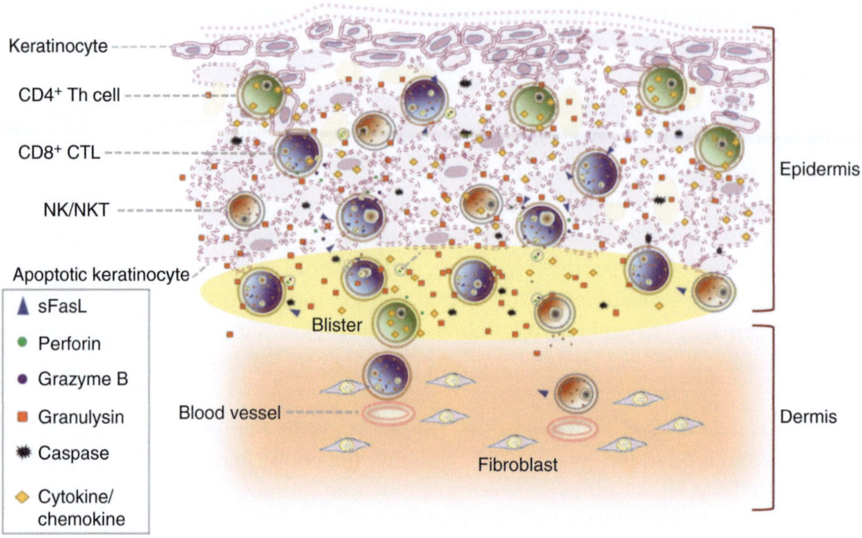

Fig. 2.2 Pathogenesis of skin rash and disseminated keratinocyte apoptosis in cADR. Due to the signals of immune synapse, the CD8⁺ CTL and NK/NKT cells as well as CD4⁺ Th cells immigrate to the epidermis of the skin. These immune cells produce a large amount of immune mediators (e.g., granulysin, perforin/granzyme B, sFasL, and cytokine/chemokine) into the extracellular space. In particular, secretory granulysin, expressed at a very high level in the skin lesions of SJS/TEN, is a main mediator of CTL, NK, and NKT cells, which attacks keratinocytes and results in extensive epidermal necrosis and blister formation. By comparison, granzyme B/perforin and Fas/FasL are produced via granule exocytosis upon cell-cell contact and present in lower concentrations than that of granulysin in the inflammatory skin lesions. After encountering the attacks of these cytotoxic proteins, keratinocytes are damaged, and then the caspase signaling pathway turns on, leading to the apoptosis progress. Abbreviations: *CTL* cytotoxic T lymphocytes, *NK/NKT* natural killer/natural killer T cells, *sFasL* soluble FasL

induction of keratinocyte apoptosis in SJS/TEN was challenged by later studies, and no difference of the levels of expression of membrane-bound FasL was noticed on the keratinocytes of TEN patients or the healthy individuals (Abe et al. 2003).

2.1.3.2 Perforin/Granzyme B Pathway

A controversial hypothesis to the Fas–FasL interaction suggests that the perforin/granzyme B plays an important role in the keratinocyte death in SJS/TEN (Nassif et al. 2002). Nassif et al. showed that the cytotoxic effect of the TEN blister lymphocytes toward keratinocytes could be attenuated by the inhibition of perforin/granzyme B expression, but not by the anti-Fas monoclonal antibody (Nassif et al. 2002). The activated CTL and NK cells produce perforin, which can bind and punch a channel to the target cell membrane and promote granzyme B to enter the keratinocytes. Once the granzyme B enters into the target cells, it activates the caspase cascade and the succeeding apoptosis (Voskoboinik et al. 2015). Increasing levels of perforin and granzyme B have been observed to be related to disease severity of cADRs, ranging from mild MPE to severe TEN (Posadas et al. 2002).

2.1.3.3 Granulysin

Granulysin is known as a cytotoxic protein for cell-mediated immunity. In 2008, Chung et al. have reported that 15-kDa granulysin is strongly expressed by the blister cells in the skin lesions and served as a key mediator for the widespread keratinocyte apoptosis in SJS/TEN (Chung et al. 2008). The 15-kDa granulysin, a cationic cytolytic protein, is secreted extracellularly by CTL and NK/NKT cells via a non-granule exocytotic pathway (Deng et al. 2005). The increased level of granulysin protein was found to be much higher than the other cytotoxic proteins, such as perforin, granzyme B, and sFasL, in the blister fluids of SJS/TEN patients (Chung et al. 2008). The finding could explain the histopathology observed in SJS/TEN, in which infiltration of sparse dermal mononuclear cells results in extensive epidermal necrosis. In addition, further studies demonstrated that the high levels of granulysin were found in patients with drug-induced SJS/TEN, DRESS, as well as FDE, but not MPE (Abe et al. 2009; Weinborn et al. 2016; Su et al. 2017).

Granulysin is not just a cytotoxic protein; it also serves as a chemoattractant for T lymphocytes, monocytes, and other inflammatory cells (Deng et al. 2005). It functions to activate the proinflammatory cytokines including RANTES (regulated upon activation, normal T cell expressed, and secreted), CCL (chemokine [C–C motif] ligand) 5, MCP (monocyte chemotactic protein)-1, MCP-3, MIP (macrophage inflammatory protein)-1a, CCL3, IL (interleukin)-1, IL-6, IL-10, and IFN (interferon)-α (Deng et al. 2005). In addition, the 15-kDa granulysin also has been shown to stimulate CCL20 expression in monocytes (Hogg et al. 2009), be capable of promoting APC (dendritic cells) and leukocyte recruitment, as well as act as an immune alarm to activate specific immune response (Tewary et al. 2010).

2.1.3.4 Other Cytotoxic Signals and Death-Mediated Molecules

A large proportion of NK or NKT cells were found in the blister fluid of the skin lesions of SJS/TEN patients (Chung et al. 2008). The high levels of granulysin secreted by NK/NKT cells, together with the expression of other cytotoxic proteins in blisters, suggested that NK/NKT cells are important immune effectors for epidermal detachment in SJS/TEN. When drug-specific T cells are activated through the interaction of HLA/drug/TCR, the induction of NK cells cytotoxicity is based on the balance between activating and inhibitory signals of NK receptors (Lanier 2005). It has been reported that the activating receptor CD94/NKG2C was found in NK cells as well as in CTL infiltrating the skin in SJS/TEN patients (Morel et al. 2010). Moreover, the nonclassical HLA molecule, soluble HLA-E (sHLA-E), is the ligand for CD94/NKG2C whose expression increased in the keratinocytes of the skin lesions of SJS/TEN patients (Morel et al. 2010). It is suggested that sHLA-E could enhance the cytotoxic activity of NKG2C^{+} NK cells thus contributing to keratinocyte apoptosis (Morel et al. 2010).

In addition to granulysin, FasL, and perforin/granzyme B, a recent study pointed out that annexin A1 plays a role in the keratinocyte death of SJS/TEN-like response of mouse model (Saito et al. 2014). Annexin A1 is upregulated in the supernatant of drug-stimulated peripheral mononuclear cells (PBMC) from the recovered SJS/TEN patients and acts through its receptor, the formyl peptide receptor 1 (FPR1), to trigger keratinocyte death (Saito et al. 2014). Furthermore, the anti-intrinsic apoptotic protein B-cell lymphoma/leukemia-2-like protein 10 (BCL2L10), which is downregulated by miR-18a-5p overexpression, was reported to be abnormally low in patients with TEN and results in inducing intrinsic keratinocyte apoptosis (Ichihara et al. 2014).

2.1.4 Cytokines/Chemokines and Other Signals Involved in cADR

There are many studies showing cytokines/chemokines involved in the immune reactions of cADR. These cytokines/chemokines are found to have increased expression levels in the skin lesions, blister fluids, blister cells, PBMC, or plasma of patients with cADR. These cytokines/chemokines may be responsible for the trafficking, proliferation, regulation, or activation of T cells and other leukocytes in cADR (Table 2.1).

2.1.4.1 IL-15, TNF-α, IFN-γ, and Other Cytokines/Chemokines in SJS/TEN

Interleukin-15 (IL-15), structural similarity to interleukin-2 (IL-2), can induce the proliferation of natural killer cells as well as other leukocytes. Through an initial screen of 28 serological factors, 5 immune mediators, including IL-6, IL-8, IL-15, tumor necrosis factor-α, and granulysin, showed increased expression in the patients with SJS/TEN (Su et al. 2017). After the further validation in 112 patients, the levels of IL-15 and granulysin showed significant correlation with the disease severity of SJS/TEN (Su et al. 2017). Furthermore, IL-15 was associated with mortality of SJS/TEN and shown to enhance cytotoxicity of cultured natural killer cells and blister cells from patients with TEN (Su et al. 2017).

Tumor necrosis factor-α (TNF-α) is a major proinflammatory cytokine involved in the inflammatory events of immune response, which can induce cell apoptosis, activation, differentiation, and inflammation (Liu 2005). The high levels of TNF-α was observed and suggested to be responsible for the extensive necrosis of skin lesions of TEN (Paquet et al. 1994; Paul et al. 1996). Interferon (IFN)-γ was also identified to be upregulated in SJS/TEN patients (Nassif et al. 2004). Viard-Leveugle et al. demonstrated that TNF-α and IFN-γ were two important cytokines in TEN (Viard-Leveugle et al. 2013). They found that TNF-α and IFN-γ increased iNOS and FasL expression and were associated with FasL-mediated cytotoxic activity in keratinocytes of TEN (Viard-Leveugle et al. 2013). In addition, there were studies reporting that other cytokines and chemokine receptors, including interleukins (IL-2, IL-5, IL-6, IL-8, IL-10, IL-12, IL-13, and IL-18), CCR3, CXCR3, CXCR4, and CCR10, were upregulated in the skin lesions, blister fluids, PBMC, or plasma of patients with SJS/TEN (Posadas et al. 2002; Su et al. 2017; Nassif et al. 2004; Tapia et al. 2004; Correia et al. 2002; Paquet et al. 2000; Caproni et al. 2006).

Table 2.1 cADR-related cytokines and chemokines

Cytokines/ chemokines	Phenotype	Functions	Skin tissue	Blister cell	Blister fluid	Plasma	PBMC	References
TNF-α	SJS/TEN	Proinflammatory cytokine, apoptosis	+	NS	+	+	+	Posadas et al. (2002), Su et al. (2017), Paul et al. (1996), Nassif et al. (2004), Viard-Leveugle et al. (2013), Caproni et al. (2006), Paquet and Pierard (1997)
	DRESS					+		Yoshikawa et al. (2006)
IFN-γ	SJS/TEN	Activation of immune cells	+	+	+		+	Posadas et al. (2002), Nassif et al. (2004), Viard-Leveugle et al. (2013), Caproni et al. (2006)
	DRESS		+			+	+	Beeler et al. (2006), Nishio et al. (2007), Hertl et al. (1993)
IL-2	SJS/TEN	All T cells growth	+	NS	NS		+	Posadas et al. (2002), Caproni et al. (2006)
	DRESS						+	Beeler et al. (2006)
IL-4	DRESS	Th cells growth					+	Beeler et al. (2006)
IL-5	SJS/TEN	Acute phase response, inflammation, eosinophil growth	+					Caproni et al. (2006)
	DRESS						+	Beeler et al. (2006)
IL-6	SJS/TEN	Acute phase response, proinflammatory cytokine	+			+	+	Su et al. (2017), Correia et al. (2002), Paquet et al. (2000), Caproni et al. (2006)
	DRESS					+		Yoshikawa et al. (2006)
IL-8/ CXCL8	SJS/TEN	Proinflammatory cytokine, proinflammatory cytokine				+		Su et al. (2017)
	AGEP	Neutrophils recruitment	+					Schaerli et al. (2004)
IL-10	SJS/TEN	Anti-inflammatory cytokine		NS	+	+	+	Nassif et al. (2004), Correia et al. (2002)
IL-12	SJS/TEN	Activation of NK and CTL			NS			Nassif et al. (2004)

(continued)

Table 2.1 (continued)

Cytokines/ chemokines	Phenotype	Functions	Skin tissue	Blister cell	Blister fluid	Plasma	PBMC	References
IL-13	SJS/TEN	Activation of NK and CTL	+					Caproni et al. (2006)
	DRESS						+	Beeler et al. (2006)
IL-15	SJS/TEN	Regulation of T and NK cell activation and proliferation			±	+		Su et al. (2017), Nassif et al. (2004)
	DRESS					+		Su et al. (2017)
IL-18	SJS/TEN	Stimulation of the growth of T lymphocytes			+			Nassif et al. (2004)
IL-36	AGEP	Proinflammatory cytokine	+					Navarini et al. (2013), Song et al. (2016)
GM-CSF	AGEP						+	Schaerli et al. (2004)
TARC/ CCL17	DRESS	Trafficking leukocytes				+		Ogawa et al. (2014)
CCR3	SJS/TEN	Binding chemokines (eotaxin, MCP-3, MCP-4, and RANTES)	+					Caproni et al. (2006)
CXCR3	SJS/TEN	Regulation of leukocyte trafficking	+					Caproni et al. (2006)
CXCR4	SJS/TEN	Chemotactic activity for lymphocytes	NS					Caproni et al. (2006)
CCR10	SJS/TEN	Trafficking leukocytes					+	Tapia et al. (2004)

Abbreviations: *CTL* cytotoxic T lymphocytes, *CCR* C–C chemokine receptor, *CXCR* CX chemokine receptor, *IFN-γ* interferon-γ, *IL* interleukin, *NK* natural killer cell, *NS* not significant, *TNF-α* tumor necrosis factor-α, + positive, – negative

2.1.4.2 Cytokines/Chemokines Involved in DRESS

DRESS is characterized by leukocytosis with atypical lymphocytosis or eosinophilia (Walsh and Creamer 2011). Eosinophilia can be observed in the range from 60% to 95% of the DRESS patients at the early stage of the illness (Kardaun et al. 2013). The elevation of eosinophil-associated cytokines (e.g., IL-4, IL-5, and IL-13), which are responsible for the maturation and differentiation of eosinophils, has been reported in drug-exposed PBMC isolated from DRESS patients (Beeler et al. 2006; Rozieres et al. 2009). In addition, the pathomechanism of DRESS has been suggested to involve T cell-mediated response. Approximately 90% of DRESS patients showed increased numbers of $CD4^+$ Th cells in the skin lesions during acute stage, and these T lymphocytes were associated with the severity of clinical symptoms, such as the extent of skin rash (Shiohara et al. 2010).

It has been reported that IFN-γ is the mainly upregulated cytokine in the DRESS patients during the acute phase (Nishio et al. 2007; Hertl et al. 1993). In addition, the levels of TNF-α and IL-6 also increased in the DRESS patients with human herpesvirus 6 (HHV-6) reactivation (Yoshikawa et al. 2006). Furthermore, thymus- and activation-regulated chemokine (TARC) was also found to be upregulated in DRESS patients with HHV-6 reactivation (Ogawa et al. 2014).

2.1.4.3 IL-8 and IL-36 in AGEP

The immune pathophysiology of AGEP has not been well understood. AGEP shows similar clinical, histological, and immunological features with generalized pustular psoriasis (GPP) (Whittam et al. 2000; Halevy 2009). AGEP has increased neutrophilic inflammatory processes regulated by T lymphocytes, which is important in the pathogenesis. High levels of IL-8 (also named CXCL8) production were noticed in AGEP patients, and the recruitment of neutrophils was observed in the skin lesions of the patients with the late phase of disease development (Halevy 2009; Schaerli et al. 2004). Drug-specific T cells isolated from AGEP patients could produce a large amount of granulocyte-macrophage colony-stimulating factor (GM-CSF), and the majority release immune mediators were IFN-γ and TNF-α (Schaerli et al. 2004). In addition, recent studies reported that mutations in the IL36RN gene encoding the IL-36 receptor antagonist (IL-36Ra) have been identified in fewer AGEP patients (Navarini et al. 2013; Song et al. 2016). The dysregulated IL-36 pathway may cause increased secretion of inflammatory cytokines, including IL-6, IL-8, and IL-1 (Onoufriadis et al. 2011), which may give rise to pustular eruptions in AGEP.

2.2 Conclusion

Increasing evidences have revealed that the immune receptors and mediators play important roles in cADR. In this chapter, we summarize the different hypotheses explaining the drug antigens interacting with HLA and TCR in cADR. The immunopathogenic mechanisms of cADR are complex, which involve drug antigen presentation to initiate the immune recognition, upregulated cytotoxic proteins to cause cell death, and dysregulated cytokines/chemokines to amplify the inflammatory reactions. Understanding the pathomechanism of cADR would facilitate the development of new approaches for the management of cADR patients, such as specific inhibitors for CTL or NK cell activation, neutralizing antibodies for major cytokines, chemokines, or cytotoxic proteins as well as inhibitors for apoptosis. Those translational studies give us better understanding of the immune mechanism, biomarkers for early diagnosis, and disease prevention as well as for developing therapeutic targets for the treatments of cADR.

References

Abe R, Shimizu T, Shibaki A, Nakamura H, Watanabe H, Shimizu H (2003) Toxic epidermal necrolysis and Stevens-Johnson syndrome are induced by soluble Fas ligand. Am J Pathol 162(5):1515–1520. https://doi.org/10.1016/S0002-9440(10)64284-8

Abe R, Yoshioka N, Murata J, Fujita Y, Shimizu H (2009) Granulysin as a marker for early diagnosis of the Stevens-Johnson syndrome. Ann Intern Med 151(7):514–515

Beeler A, Engler O, Gerber BO, Pichler WJ (2006) Long-lasting reactivity and high frequency of drug-specific T cells after severe systemic drug hypersensitivity reactions. J Allergy Clin Immunol 117(2):455–462. https://doi.org/10.1016/j.jaci.2005.10.030

Caproni M, Torchia D, Schincaglia E, Volpi W, Frezzolini A, Schena D, Marzano A, Quaglino P, De Simone C, Parodi A, Barletta E, Fabbri P (2006) Expression of cytokines and chemokine receptors in the cutaneous lesions of erythema multiforme and Stevens-Johnson syndrome/toxic epidermal necrolysis. Br J Dermatol 155(4):722–728. https://doi.org/10.1111/j.1365-2133.2006.07398.x

Chung WH, Hung SI, Hong HS, Hsih MS, Yang LC, Ho HC, Wu JY, Chen YT (2004) Medical genetics: a marker for Stevens-Johnson syndrome. Nature 428(6982):486. https://doi.org/10.1038/428486a

Chung WH, Hung SI, Chen YT (2007) Human leukocyte antigens and drug hypersensitivity. Curr Opin Allergy Clin Immunol 7(4):317–323. https://doi.org/10.1097/ACI.0b013e3282370c5f

Chung WH, Hung SI, Yang JY, Su SC, Huang SP, Wei CY, Chin SW, Chiou CC, Chu SC, Ho HC, Yang CH, Lu CF, Wu JY, Liao YD, Chen YT (2008) Granulysin is a key mediator for disseminated keratinocyte death in Stevens-Johnson syndrome and toxic epidermal necrolysis. Nat Med 14(12):1343–1350. https://doi.org/10.1038/nm.1884

Chung WH, Pan RY, Chu MT, Chin SW, Huang YL, Wang WC, Chang JY, Hung SI (2015) Oxypurinol-specific T cells possess preferential TCR clonotypes and express granulysin in allopurinol-induced severe cutaneous adverse reactions. J Invest Dermatol 135(9):2237–2248. https://doi.org/10.1038/jid.2015.165

Chung WH, Wang CW, Dao RL (2016) Severe cutaneous adverse drug reactions. J Dermatol 43(7):758–766. https://doi.org/10.1111/1346-8138.13430

Correia O, Delgado L, Barbosa IL, Campilho F, Fleming-Torrinha J (2002) Increased interleukin 10, tumor necrosis factor alpha, and interleukin 6 levels in blister fluid of toxic epidermal necrolysis. J Am Acad Dermatol 47(1):58–62

Deng A, Chen S, Li Q, Lyu SC, Clayberger C, Krensky AM (2005) Granulysin, a cytolytic molecule, is also a chemoattractant and proinflammatory activator. J Immunol 174(9):5243–5248

Friedmann PS, Lee MS, Friedmann AC, Barnetson RS (2003) Mechanisms in cutaneous drug hypersensitivity reactions. Clin Exp Allergy 33(7):861–872

Halevy S (2009) Acute generalized exanthematous pustulosis. Curr Opin Allergy Clin Immunol 9(4):322–328. https://doi.org/10.1097/ACI.0b013e32832cf64e

Hertl M, Bohlen H, Jugert F, Boecker C, Knaup R, Merk HF (1993) Predominance of epidermal CD8+ T lymphocytes in bullous cutaneous reactions caused by beta-lactam antibiotics. J Invest Dermatol 101(6):794–799

Hogg AE, Bowick GC, Herzog NK, Cloyd MW, Endsley JJ (2009) Induction of granulysin in CD8+ T cells by IL-21 and IL-15 is suppressed by human immunodeficiency virus-1. J Leukoc Biol 86(5):1191–1203. https://doi.org/10.1189/jlb.0409222

Hung SI, Chung WH, Liou LB, Chu CC, Lin M, Huang HP, Lin YL, Lan JL, Yang LC, Hong HS, Chen MJ, Lai PC, Wu MS, Chu CY, Wang KH, Chen CH, Fann CS, Wu JY, Chen YT (2005) HLA-B*5801 allele as a genetic marker for severe cutaneous adverse reactions caused by allopurinol. Proc Natl Acad Sci U S A 102(11):4134–4139. https://doi.org/10.1073/pnas.0409500102

Ichihara A, Wang Z, Jinnin M, Izuno Y, Shimozono N, Yamane K, Fujisawa A, Moriya C, Fukushima S, Inoue Y, Ihn H (2014) Upregulation of miR-18a-5p contributes to epidermal necrolysis in severe drug eruptions. J Allergy Clin Immunol 133(4):1065–1074. https://doi.org/10.1016/j.jaci.2013.09.019

Illing PT, Vivian JP, Dudek NL, Kostenko L, Chen Z, Bharadwaj M, Miles JJ, Kjer-Nielsen L, Gras S, Williamson NA, Burrows SR, Purcell AW, Rossjohn J, McCluskey J (2012) Immune self-reactivity triggered by drug-modified HLA-peptide repertoire. Nature 486(7404):554–558. https://doi.org/10.1038/nature11147

Kardaun SH, Sekula P, Valeyrie-Allanore L, Liss Y, Chu CY, Creamer D, Sidoroff A, Naldi L, Mockenhaupt M, Roujeau JC, RegiSCAR Study Group (2013) Drug reaction with eosinophilia and systemic symptoms (DRESS): an original multisystem adverse drug reaction. Results from the prospective RegiSCAR study. Br J Dermatol 169(5):1071–1080. https://doi.org/10.1111/bjd.12501

Ko TM, Chung WH, Wei CY, Shih HY, Chen JK, Lin CH, Chen YT, Hung SI (2011) Shared and restricted T-cell receptor use is crucial for carbamazepine-induced Stevens-Johnson syndrome. J Allergy Clin Immunol 128(6):1266–1276, e1211. https://doi.org/10.1016/j.jaci.2011.08.013

Lanier LL (2005) NK cell recognition. Annu Rev Immunol 23:225–274. https://doi.org/10.1146/annurev.immunol.23.021704.115526

Liu ZG (2005) Molecular mechanism of TNF signaling and beyond. Cell Res 15(1):24–27. https://doi.org/10.1038/sj.cr.7290259

Mallal S, Nolan D, Witt C, Masel G, Martin AM, Moore C, Sayer D, Castley A, Mamotte C, Maxwell D, James I, Christiansen FT (2002) Association between presence of HLA-B*5701, HLA-DR7, and HLA-DQ3 and hypersensitivity to HIV-1 reverse-transcriptase inhibitor abacavir. Lancet 359(9308):727–732

Mockenhaupt M (2012) Epidemiology of cutaneous adverse drug reactions. Chem Immunol Allergy 97:1–17. https://doi.org/10.1159/000335612

Morel E, Escamochero S, Cabanas R, Diaz R, Fiandor A, Bellon T (2010) CD94/NKG2C is a killer effector molecule in patients with Stevens-Johnson syndrome and toxic epidermal necrolysis. J Allergy Clin Immunol 125(3):703–710, 710.e701–710.e708. https://doi.org/10.1016/j.jaci.2009.10.030

Nassif A, Bensussan A, Dorothee G, Mami-Chouaib F, Bachot N, Bagot M, Boumsell L, Roujeau JC (2002) Drug specific cytotoxic T-cells in the skin lesions of a patient with toxic epidermal necrolysis. J Invest Dermatol 118(4):728–733. https://doi.org/10.1046/j.1523-1747.2002.01622.x

Nassif A, Moslehi H, Le Gouvello S, Bagot M, Lyonnet L, Michel L, Boumsell L, Bensussan A, Roujeau JC (2004) Evaluation of the potential role of cytokines in toxic epidermal necrolysis. J Invest Dermatol 123(5):850–855. https://doi.org/10.1111/j.0022-202X.2004.23439.x

Navarini AA, Valeyrie-Allanore L, Setta-Kaffetzi N, Barker JN, Capon F, Creamer D, Roujeau JC, Sekula P, Simpson MA, Trembath RC, Mockenhaupt M, Smith CH (2013) Rare variations in IL36RN in severe adverse drug reactions manifesting as acute generalized exanthematous pustulosis. J Invest Dermatol 133(7):1904–1907. https://doi.org/10.1038/jid.2013.44

Nishio D, Izu K, Kabashima K, Tokura Y (2007) T cell populations propagating in the peripheral blood of patients with drug eruptions. J Dermatol Sci 48(1):25–33. https://doi.org/10.1016/j.jdermsci.2007.05.013

Ogawa K, Morito H, Hasegawa A, Miyagawa F, Kobayashi N, Watanabe H, Sueki H, Tohyama M, Hashimoto K, Kano Y, Shiohara T, Ito K, Fujita H, Aihara M, Asada H (2014) Elevated serum thymus and activation-regulated chemokine (TARC/CCL17) relates to reactivation of human herpesvirus 6 in drug reaction with eosinophilia and systemic symptoms (DRESS)/drug-induced hypersensitivity syndrome (DIHS). Br J Dermatol 171(2):425–427. https://doi.org/10.1111/bjd.12948

Onoufriadis A, Simpson MA, Pink AE, Di Meglio P, Smith CH, Pullabhatla V, Knight J, Spain SL, Nestle FO, Burden AD, Capon F, Trembath RC, Barker JN (2011) Mutations in IL36RN/IL1F5 are associated with the severe episodic inflammatory skin disease known as generalized pustular psoriasis. Am J Hum Genet 89(3):432–437. https://doi.org/10.1016/j.ajhg.2011.07.022

Paquet P, Pierard GE (1997) Erythema multiforme and toxic epidermal necrolysis: a comparative study. Am J Dermatopathol 19(2):127–132

Paquet P, Nikkels A, Arrese JE, Vanderkelen A, Pierard GE (1994) Macrophages and tumor necrosis factor alpha in toxic epidermal necrolysis. Arch Dermatol 130(5):605–608

Paquet P, Paquet F, Al Saleh W, Reper P, Vanderkelen A, Pierard GE (2000) Immunoregulatory effector cells in drug-induced toxic epidermal necrolysis. Am J Dermatopathol 22(5):413–417

Paul C, Wolkenstein P, Adle H, Wechsler J, Garchon HJ, Revuz J, Roujeau JC (1996) Apoptosis as a mechanism of keratinocyte death in toxic epidermal necrolysis. Br J Dermatol 134(4):710–714

Pichler WJ (2002) Pharmacological interaction of drugs with antigen-specific immune receptors: the p-i concept. Curr Opin Allergy Clin Immunol 2(4):301–305

Pirmohamed M, Naisbitt DJ, Gordon F, Park BK (2002) The danger hypothesis—potential role in idiosyncratic drug reactions. Toxicology 181–182:55–63

Posadas SJ, Padial A, Torres MJ, Mayorga C, Leyva L, Sanchez E, Alvarez J, Romano A, Juarez C, Blanca M (2002) Delayed reactions to drugs show levels of perforin, granzyme B, and Fas-L to be related to disease severity. J Allergy Clin Immunol 109(1):155–161

Rozieres A, Vocanson M, Said BB, Nosbaum A, Nicolas JF (2009) Role of T cells in nonimmediate allergic drug reactions. Curr Opin Allergy Clin Immunol 9(4):305–310. https://doi.org/10.1097/ACI.0b013e32832d565c

Saito N, Qiao H, Yanagi T, Shinkuma S, Nishimura K, Suto A, Fujita Y, Suzuki S, Nomura T, Nakamura H, Nagao K, Obuse C, Shimizu H, Abe R (2014) An annexin A1-FPR1 interaction contributes to necroptosis of keratinocytes in severe cutaneous adverse drug reactions. Sci Transl Med 6(245):245ra295. https://doi.org/10.1126/scitranslmed.3008227

Schaerli P, Britschgi M, Keller M, Steiner UC, Steinmann LS, Moser B, Pichler WJ (2004) Characterization of human T cells that regulate neutrophilic skin inflammation. J Immunol 173(3):2151–2158

Schneider CH, De Weck AL (1965) A new chemical spect of penicillin allergy: the direct reaction of penicillin with epsilon-amino-groups. Nature 208(5005):57–59

Shiohara T, Kurata M, Mizukawa Y, Kano Y (2010) Recognition of immune reconstitution syndrome necessary for better management of patients with severe drug eruptions and those under immunosuppressive therapy. Allergol Int 59(4):333–343. https://doi.org/10.2332/allergolint.10-RAI-0260

Song HS, Kim SJ, Park TI, Jang YH, Lee ES (2016) Immunohistochemical comparison of IL-36 and the IL-23/Th17 axis of generalized pustular psoriasis and acute generalized exanthematous pustulosis. Ann Dermatol 28(4):451–456. https://doi.org/10.5021/ad.2016.28.4.451

Su SC, Mockenhaupt M, Wolkenstein P, Dunant A, Le Gouvello S, Chen CB, Chosidow O, Valeyrie-Allanore L, Bellon T, Sekula P, Wang CW, Schumacher M, Kardaun SH, Hung SI, Roujeau JC, Chung WH (2017) Interleukin-15 is associated with severity and mortality in Stevens-Johnson syndrome/toxic epidermal necrolysis. J Invest Dermatol 137(5):1065–1073. https://doi.org/10.1016/j.jid.2016.11.034

Tapia B, Padial A, Sanchez-Sabate E, Alvarez-Ferreira J, Morel E, Blanca M, Bellon T (2004) Involvement of CCL27-CCR10 interactions in drug-induced cutaneous reactions. J Allergy Clin Immunol 114(2):335–340. https://doi.org/10.1016/j.jaci.2004.04.034

Tewary P, Yang D, de la Rosa G, Li Y, Finn MW, Krensky AM, Clayberger C, Oppenheim JJ (2010) Granulysin activates antigen-presenting cells through TLR4 and acts as an immune alarmin. Blood 116(18):3465–3474. https://doi.org/10.1182/blood-2010-03-273953

Viard I, Wehrli P, Bullani R, Schneider P, Holler N, Salomon D, Hunziker T, Saurat JH, Tschopp J, French LE (1998) Inhibition of toxic epidermal necrolysis by blockade of CD95 with human intravenous immunoglobulin. Science 282(5388):490–493

Viard-Leveugle I, Gaide O, Jankovic D, Feldmeyer L, Kerl K, Pickard C, Roques S, Friedmann PS, Contassot E, French LE (2013) TNF-alpha and IFN-gamma are potential inducers of Fas-mediated keratinocyte apoptosis through activation of inducible nitric oxide synthase in toxic epidermal necrolysis. J Invest Dermatol 133(2):489–498. https://doi.org/10.1038/jid.2012.330

Voskoboinik I, Whisstock JC, Trapani JA (2015) Perforin and granzymes: function, dysfunction and human pathology. Nat Rev Immunol 15(6):388–400. https://doi.org/10.1038/nri3839

Walsh SA, Creamer D (2011) Drug reaction with eosinophilia and systemic symptoms (DRESS): a clinical update and review of current thinking. Clin Exp Dermatol 36(1):6–11. https://doi.org/10.1111/j.1365-2230.2010.03967.x

Watkins S, Pichler WJ (2013) Sulfamethoxazole induces a switch mechanism in T cell receptors containing TCRVbeta20-1, altering pHLA recognition. PLoS One 8(10):e76211. https://doi.org/10.1371/journal.pone.0076211

Wei CY, Chung WH, Huang HW, Chen YT, Hung SI (2012) Direct interaction between HLA-B and carbamazepine activates T cells in patients with Stevens-Johnson syndrome. J Allergy Clin Immunol 129(6):1562–1569, e1565. https://doi.org/10.1016/j.jaci.2011.12.990

Weinborn M, Barbaud A, Truchetet F, Beurey P, Germain L, Cribier B (2016) Histopathological study of six types of adverse cutaneous drug reactions using granulysin expression. Int J Dermatol 55(11):1225–1233. https://doi.org/10.1111/ijd.13350

Whittam LR, Wakelin SH, Barker JN (2000) Generalized pustular psoriasis or drug-induced toxic pustuloderma? The use of patch testing. Clin Exp Dermatol 25(2):122–124

Yoshikawa T, Fujita A, Yagami A, Suzuki K, Matsunaga K, Ihira M, Asano Y (2006) Human herpesvirus 6 reactivation and inflammatory cytokine production in patients with drug-induced hypersensitivity syndrome. J Clin Virol 37(Suppl 1):S92–S96. https://doi.org/10.1016/S1386-6532(06)70019-1

3 Pharmacogenomics and Cutaneous Adverse Drug Reactions

Ren-You Pan, Chun-Bing Chen, and Wen-Hung Chung

Abbreviations

cADRs	Cutaneous adverse drug reactions
CBZ	Carbamazepine
CYP2C9*3	Cytochrome P450 family 2 subfamily C member 9*3
DRESS	Drug reaction with eosinophilia and systemic symptoms
HLA	Human leukocyte antigens
HSS	Hypersensitivity syndrome
LTG	Lamotrigine
MPE	Maculopapular exanthema
OXC	Oxcarbazepine
PHT	Phenytoin

R.-Y. Pan
Department of Dermatology, Drug Hypersensitivity Clinical and Research Center, Chang Gung Memorial Hospital, Linkou, Taipei, Keelung, Taiwan

Chang Gung Immunology Consortium, Chang Gung Memorial Hospital and Chang Gung University, Taoyuan, Taiwan

C.-B. Chen · W.-H. Chung (✉)
Department of Dermatology, Drug Hypersensitivity Clinical and Research Center, Chang Gung Memorial Hospital, Linkou, Taipei, Keelung, Taiwan

Chang Gung Immunology Consortium, Chang Gung Memorial Hospital and Chang Gung University, Taoyuan, Taiwan

Whole-Genome Research Core Laboratory of Human Diseases, Chang Gung Memorial Hospital, Keelung, Taiwan

Graduate Institute of Clinical Medical Sciences, College of Medicine, Chang Gung University, Taoyuan, Taiwan

Department of Dermatology, Xiamen Chang Gung Hospital, Xiamen, Fujian, China
e-mail: chung1@cgmh.org.tw

N. H. Shear, R. P. Dodiuk-Gad (eds.), *Advances in Diagnosis and Management of Cutaneous Adverse Drug Reactions*, https://doi.org/10.1007/978-981-13-1489-6_3

SCAR	Severe cutaneous adverse reactions
SJS	Stevens–Johnson syndrome
TCR	T cell receptors
TEN	Toxic epidermal necrolysis

Key Points

- Increasing pharmacogenomic studies showed that certain *HLA* alleles are strongly associated with cADRs related to specific drugs. Examples include the associations between *HLA-B*15:02* allele and CBZ-induced SJS/TEN, *HLA-B*58:01* allele and allopurinol-induced SCAR, and *HLA-B*57:01* allele and abacavir-induced hypersensitivity syndrome.
- The drug presentation models that explain how small drug antigens might interact with HLA and TCR molecules in cADRs include the hapten theory, the p-i model, and the altered peptide repertoire model.
- The genetic screening test for high-risk genes prior to drug commencement has become an effective predictor for protecting patients who are at-risk ancestries and reduced the incidence of cADRs. Pharmacogenomic tests could be applied in the clinical setting for improving the drug safety to achieve the goal of precision medicine in the near future.

3.1 Introduction

Cutaneous adverse drug reactions (cADRs) are induced by specific offending drugs which often trigger a serial of immune reactions. cADRs range from mild maculopapular exanthema (MPE) to life-threatening severe cutaneous adverse reactions (SCAR), including drug reaction with eosinophilia and systemic symptoms (DRESS), Stevens-Johnson syndrome (SJS), and toxic epidermal necrolysis (TEN). SJS and TEN are considered as the same disease spectrum with different severity. Although the incidence of SJS/TEN is low (0.4–2 cases/million per year in Europe; 2–8 cases/million per year in Asia), the lethality they have brought is high (Rzany et al. 1996; Chung et al. 2004; Choon and Lai 2012). The mortality rate is approximately 10% for SJS, 30% for SJS/TEN overlap, and 50% for TEN (Roujeau and Stern 1994; Roujeau et al. 1995).

3.2 The Pathogenic Mechanisms of cADRs

Immune reaction of cADRs is triggered by the binding between a causative drug and HLA with TCR. Generally, after an offending drug is taken, the drug or its metabolite binds to specific HLA of the antigen-presenting cells, and the HLA/drug complex is then recognized by the TCR of T cells to initiate a serial of T cell activation responses. In SJS/TEN, the activated T cells along with the natural killer cells then migrate to the epidermis and produce various cytotoxic cytokines or chemokines, such as soluble Fas ligand, perforin, granzyme B (Nassif et al. 2002; Lowin et al. 1995), and granulysin (Chung et al. 2008) to attack the keratinocytes, resulting in extensive

Table 3.1 The risk factors related to cADRs

Risk factors	Examples
Drug antigen	Aromatic anticonvulsants, e.g., carbamazepine, oxcarbazepine, lamotrigine, phenytoin, for anticonvulsants-SCAR
Drug binding peptides	1. The hapten theory 2. Altered peptide repertoire
HLA	1. *HLA-B*15:02* for CBZ-SJS 2. *HLA-B*58:01* for allopurinol-SCAR 3. *HLA-B*57:01* for abacavir hypersensitivity
T cell-mediated response	1. Drug-specific TCR clonotypes 2. Cytotoxic protein secretion
Metabolism	Inherited: Impaired drug clearance with *CYP2C9*3* for phenytoin-SCAR Acquired: Renal impairment for allopurinol-SCAR
Environmental factor	Viral infection: EBV, CMV, HHV-6 for DRESS

Abbreviations: *cADRs* cutaneous adverse drug reactions, *CYP2C9*3* cytochrome P450 family 2 subfamily C member 9**3*, *DRESS* drug reaction with eosinophilia and systemic symptoms, *HLA* human leukocyte antigen, *SCAR* severe cutaneous adverse reactions, *SJS* Stevens-Johnson syndrome, *TEN* toxic epidermal necrolysis

epidermal necrosis and blister formation. Granulysin is the key mediator responsible for the disseminated keratinocyte death in SJS/TEN (Chung et al. 2008).

Drug antigens presentation mechanisms, genetic and immune factors, and environmental or non-genetic factors are involved in the pathogenesis of cADRs (Table 3.1). The molecular mechanisms and checkpoints for cADRs include genetic polymorphisms, specific *HLA* loci (e.g., *HLA-B*15:02* for carbamazepine (CBZ)-induced SJS/TEN, *HLA-B*58:01* for allopurinol-induced SCAR, and *HLA-B*57:01* for abacavir-induced hypersensitivity reactions), drug-specific TCR clonotypes, T cell activation responses and cytotoxic proteins secretion (e.g., granulysin, interferon-γ, Fas ligand, perforin, and granzyme B), impaired drug metabolism or clearance (e.g., strong association of cytochrome P450 family 2 subfamily C member 9**3 (CYP2C9*3)* with phenytoin-induced SCAR and impaired renal function with allopurinol-induced SCAR), and cell death mechanisms (e.g., miR-18a-5p-induced apoptosis, annexin A1 and formyl peptide receptor 1-induced necroptosis in keratinocytes). In addition, environmental factors, autoimmune disorders, and patients with a prior medical history of viral infection have also been reported to be implicated in susceptibility to cADRs (Table 3.1).

3.3 Pharmacogenomics and HLA Association in Drug-Induced cADRs

The common offending drugs, such as aromatic anticonvulsants, allopurinol, abacavir, and antibiotics, have potential risk to cause cADRs. Increasing pharmacogenomic studies have showed that specific *HLA* alleles are highly associated with drug-induced cADRs (Table 3.2). These associations are usually phenotype- and ethnic-specific. The frequencies of the common risk *HLA* alleles for cADRs are different among various ethnic groups (Fig. 3.1), which may explain the different incidences of cADRs related to specific drugs in different populations. For example, *HLA-B*15:02* is strongly

Table 3.2 Ethnic-specific HLA-associated cADRs

Associated drug	HLA allele	cADRs	Ethnicity	References
Aromatic anticonvulsants				
Carbamazepine	*B*15:02*	SJS/TEN	Han Chinese, Thai, Indian, Malaysian, Vietnam, Singapore, Hong Kong	Chung et al. (2004), Man et al. (2007), Locharernkul et al. (2008), Mehta et al. (2009), Chang et al. (2011), Chong et al. (2014), Nguyen et al. (2015), Kwan et al. (2014)
	*A*31:01*	DRESS	Han Chinese, European, Spanish	Hung et al. (2006), Genin et al. (2014), Ramirez et al. (2017)
	*A*31:01*	DRESS/ SJS/TEN	Northern European, Japanese, Korean	Ozeki et al. (2011), Kim et al. (2011), McCormack et al. (2011)
	*B*15:11*	SJS/TEN	Han Chinese, Japanese, Korean	Kaniwa et al. (2010), Kim et al. (2011), Sun et al. (2014)
	*B*59:01*	SJS/TEN	Japanese	Ikeda et al. (2010)
	*B*38:01*	SJS/TEN	Spanish	Ramirez et al. (2017)
Oxcarbazepine	*B*15:02*	SJS/TEN	Han Chinese, Thai	Hung et al. (2010), Chen et al. (2016)
Phenytoin	*B*15:02*	SJS/TEN	Han Chinese, Thai	Hung et al. (2010), Locharernkul et al. (2008)
	*B*15:02, B*13:01, B*51:01*		Han Chinese, Japanese, Malaysian	Chung et al. (2014)
	*A*33:03, B*38:02, B*51:01, B*56:02, B*58:01, C*14:02*	SJS/TEN	Thai	Tassaneeyakul et al. (2016)
	*B*51:01*	DRESS	Thai	Tassaneeyakul et al. (2016)
	*B*15:13*	DRESS/ SJS/TEN	Malaysian	Chang et al. (2016)
	*CYP2C9*3*	DRESS/ SJS/TEN	Han Chinese, Japanese, Malaysian	Chung et al. (2014)
	*CYP2C9*3*	SJS/TEN	Thai	Tassaneeyakul et al. (2016)
Phenobarbital	*B*15:02*	SJS/TEN	Han Chinese	Hung et al. (2010), Zeng et al. (2015), Shi et al. (2011)
Lamotrigine	*B*38; B*58:01, A*68:01, Cw*07:18*	SJS/TEN	European	Lonjou et al. (2008), Kazeem et al. (2009)
	*B*38:01*	SJS/TEN	Spanish	Ramirez et al. (2017)

Table 3.2 (continued)

Associated drug	HLA allele	cADRs	Ethnicity	References
	*A*31:01*	SJS/TEN	Korean	Kim et al. (2017)
	*A*24:02*	DRESS/ SJS/TEN	Spanish	Ramirez et al. (2017)
Allopurinol	*B*58:01*	DRESS	Han Chinese, Thai, Japanese, Korean, European	Hung et al. (2005), Tassaneeyakul et al. (2009), Lonjou et al. (2008), Kang et al. (2011), Kaniwa et al. (2008)
Antiretroviral drugs				
Abacavir	*B*57:01*	HSS	European, African	Hetherington et al. (2002), Mallal et al. (2002)
Nevirapine	*DRB1*01:01*	DRESS	Australian	Martin et al. (2005)
	*B*35:05*	DRESS	Thai	Chantarangsu et al. (2009)
	*B*14:02, Cw*08:01, Cw*08:02*	HSS	Sardinian, Japanese	Littera et al. (2006), Gatanaga et al. (2007)
	*C*04:01*	DRESS/ SJS/TEN	Malawian	Carr et al. (2013)
Antibiotics				
Co-trimoxazole	*B*15:02, C*06:02, C*08:01*	SJS/TEN	Thai	Kongpan et al. (2015)
Dapsone	*B*13:01*	HSS	Han Chinese	Zhang et al. (2013)
Sulfamethoxazole	*B*38:02*	SJS/TEN	European	Lonjou et al. (2008)
Sulfonamide	*A*29, B*12, DR*7*	TEN	European	Revuz et al. (1987)
Other drugs				
Oxicam	*B*73:01*	SJS/TEN	European	Lonjou et al. (2008)
Methazolamide	*B*59:01, CW*01:02*	SJS/TEN	Korean, Japanese	Kim et al. (2010)

Abbreviations: *cADRs* cutaneous adverse drug reactions, *DRESS* drug reaction with eosinophilia and systemic symptoms, *HSS* hypersensitivity syndrome, *MPE* maculopapular exanthema, *SJS* Stevens–Johnson syndrome, *TEN* toxic epidermal necrolysis

associated with CBZ-induced SJS/TEN in Han Chinese and other Asian populations but not in Caucasians (Chung et al. 2004; Man et al. 2007; Locharernkul et al. 2008; Mehta et al. 2009; Chang et al. 2011; Chong et al. 2014; Nguyen et al. 2015; Kwan et al. 2014), which may be due to the presence of the *HLA-B*15:02* allele that is high in Han Chinese (6–10%) but low in Caucasians (1%) (Fig. 3.1).

3.3.1 Aromatic Anticonvulsants

Aromatic anticonvulsants, including CBZ, oxcarbazepine (OXC), phenytoin (PHT), and lamotrigine (LTG), have the common benzene ring structure and are known to have higher risk to induce cADRs. The incident rate of aromatic anticonvulsant-induced SCAR varies from 1/1000 to 1/10,000 (Knowles et al. 2012). Patients with aromatic anticonvulsant-induced SCAR show cross-reactivity to different

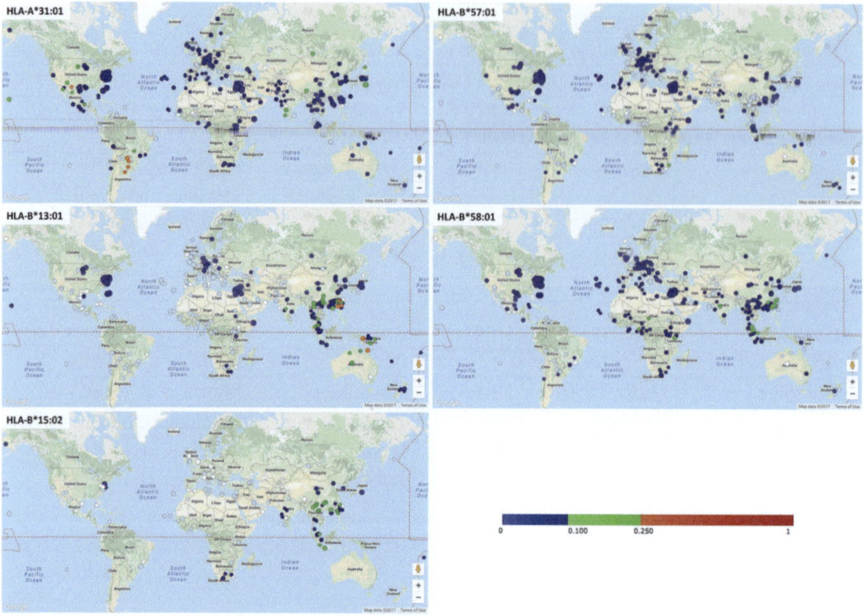

Fig. 3.1 The frequency of the common risk *HLA* alleles for cADRs in different ethnic groups. Data from allele frequency net database (http://www.allelefrequencies.net/) (Middleton et al. 2003)

anticonvulsants, which may explain their similar potential of pharmacogenomic associations. For example, the same *HLA-B*15:02* association in different aromatic anticonvulsant-induced SJS/TEN was reported. *HLA-B*15:02* allele is firstly identified as a genetic marker strongly associated with CBZ-induced SJS/TEN in Han Chinese (Chung et al. 2004), which has been validated in several Asian populations, including Taiwan, China, Hong Kong, India, Thailand, Malaysia, Singapore, and Vietnam (Man et al. 2007; Locharernkul et al. 2008; Mehta et al. 2009; Chang et al. 2011; Chong et al. 2014; Nguyen et al. 2015; Kwan et al. 2014). In addition, the association between *HLA* alleles and CBZ-induced hypersensitivity reaction is phenotype-specific and also ethnic-specific. Subsequent international cooperation study including patients with CBZ-SCAR in Europe and Asia revealed that *HLA-A*31:01* is a specific predictor of CBZ-induced DRESS (Hung et al. 2006; Genin et al. 2014). *HLA-A*31:01* was also reported to be associated with CBZ-DRESS/SJS/TEN in Northern Europeans, Japanese, and Koreans (Ozeki et al. 2011, McCormack et al. 2011, Kim et al. 2011). Other pharmacogenomic associations of CBZ-SCAR include *HLA-B*15:11* with CBZ-SJS/TEN in Han Chinese, Korean, and Japanese (Kaniwa et al. 2010, Kim et al. 2011, Sun et al. 2014), *HLA-B*59:01* with CBZ-SJS/TEN in Japanese (Ikeda et al. 2010), and *HLA-B*31:01* with CBZ-DRESS and *HLA-B*38:01* with CBZ-SJS/TEN in Spanish (Ramirez et al. 2017). In addition, OXC, a structural analogue of CBZ, could also induce SCAR though the severity and incidence of OXC-SJS/TEN are less than that of CBZ-SJS/TEN. A recent study also showed that *HLA-B*15:02* is significantly associated with OXC-SJS/TEN in Asian populations, including Han Chinese and Thai (Chen et al. 2016). *HLA-A*31:01* was not found to be associated with OXC-DRESS in this study. Moreover, *HLA-B*15:02* was associated with PHT-induced SJS/TEN in Southeast Asian populations (Man et al. 2007; Locharernkul et al. 2008). Other than *HLA-B*15:02*, *HLA-B*15:13* was also reported to be associated with PHT-DRESS/SJS/TEN in Malaysia (Chang et al. 2016). Recently, a genomic study in Spanish revealed *HLA-A*02:01/Cw*15:02* combination or *HLA-B*38:01* as risk factors for PHT-induced SJS/TEN and *HLA-A*11:01* for PHT-induced DRESS (Ramirez et al. 2017). A recent genome-wide association study showed a strong association of *CYP2C9*3* with PHT-induced SCAR, and it was further supported by the evidence of delayed clearance of plasma PHT in patients with PHT-induced SCAR from Taiwan, Japan, and Malaysia (Chung et al. 2014). Another study from Thai patients also validated the significance of the higher risk of *CYP2C9*3 in* PHT-induced SJS/TEN (Tassaneeyakul et al. 2016). For LTG, there has been reports with significant association of LTG-induced SJS/TEN with *HLA-B*15:02* in Han Chinese (Hung et al. 2010; Shi et al. 2011; Zeng et al. 2015); *HLA-B*38* (Lonjou et al. 2008) *or HLA-B*58:01*, *A*68:01*, and *Cw*07:18* in European (Kazeem et al. 2009); *HLA-A*31:01* in Korean (Kim et al. 2017); and *B*38:01* in Spanish (Ramirez et al. 2017) (Table 3.2).

3.3.2 Allopurinol

Allopurinol is a first-line drug used to treat gouty arthritis and urate nephropathy. In 2005, the strong pharmacogenomic association between *HLA-B*58:01* and allopurinol-SCAR in Han Chinese was reported (Hung et al. 2005), and this correlation was subsequently validated among different populations, including Asians and Europeans (Table 3.2) (Lonjou et al. 2008, Kaniwa et al. 2008, Tassaneeyakul et al. 2009, Kang et al. 2011). The strength of *HLA-B*58:01* association was correlated with disease severity of allopurinol-induced cADRs (OR = 44.0 for SCAR, OR = 8.5 for MPE), and the gene dosage effect of *HLA-B*58:01* also influenced the development of allopurinol-SCAR (OR = 15.25 for *HLA-B*58:01* heterozygotes and OR = 72.45 for homozygotes) (Ng et al. 2016). A recent showed that specific T cells with preferential TCR clonotypes also play crucial roles in allopurinol-SCAR (Chung et al. 2015b). In addition, other non-genetic factors, such as renal impairment correlated with high plasma levels of oxypurinol, have been reported to be important risk factors resulting in allopurinol-SCAR of greater severity and poorer prognosis (Chung et al. 2015a; Yang et al. 2015). Furthermore, an interaction between genetic and non-genetic factors in allopurinol-SCAR was also found. Another recent study further showed a coexistence of *HLA-B*58:01* and renal impairment increased the risk and predictive accuracy of allopurinol-SCAR (heterozygous *HLA-B*58:01* and normal renal function, OR = 15.25, specificity = 82%; homozygous *HLA-B*58:01* and severe renal impairment, OR = 1269.45, specificity = 100%) (Ng et al. 2016).

3.3.3 Antiretroviral Drugs, Antibiotics, and Other Drugs

Antiretroviral agents for human immunodeficiency virus-1 infections, including abacavir and nevirapine, have been shown to induce SCAR. Abacavir, a nucleoside reverse-transcriptase inhibitor, was demonstrated the significant association between the *HLA-B*57:01* and abacavir-induced hypersensitivity in 2002 in Caucasians (Hetherington et al. 2002; Mallal et al. 2002). However, the same genetic association with abacavir hypersensitivity has not been reported in Asian or African populations, which could be explained by that *HLA-B*57:01* allele frequency is almost absent in non-Caucasian populations (0–1%). A prospective study showed that *HLA-B*57:01* genetic screening could reduce the risk of hypersensitivity reactions to abacavir (Mallal et al. 2008). In addition, nevirapine-induced hypersensitivity or DRESS has been associated with *HLA-DRB1*01:01* in Western Australia (Martin et al. 2005), *HLA-B*35:05* in Thailand (Chantarangsu et al. 2009), and *HLA-B*14:02* and/or *HLA-Cw8* in Sardinia (Littera et al. 2006) and Japan (Gatanaga et al. 2007).

cADRs can also be induced by various types of antibiotics, such as sulfonamide-induced allergic reactions (Schnyder and Pichler 2013), dapsone-induced hypersensitivity syndrome (Zhang et al. 2013), penicillins, cephalosporins, quinolones, glycopeptides, trimethoprim-sulfamethoxazole, and other antibiotic-induced SJS, TEN, and DRESS (Lin et al. 2014). Though there has been a lot of antibiotic-induced SCAR cases reported, only few antibiotics with specific pharmacogenomic associations were found until now. The first association between *HLA* alleles and drug-induced SJS/TEN was demonstrated in cases of sulfonamide-induced TEN (*HLA-A29*, *B12*, and *DR7*) and oxicam-induced TEN (*HLA-A2* and *B12*) (Roujeau et al. 1987). Dapsone, an antibiotic and anti-inflammatory agent, is used to treat infectious diseases and was found to be associated with hypersensitivity syndrome in Chinese population presenting *HLA-B*13:01* (Zhang et al. 2013). Co-trimoxazole, a sulfonamide-containing antibiotic, is effective in the treatment of several infections and for prophylaxis of *Pneumocystis jiroveci pneumonia*. *HLA-B*15:02*, *HLA-C*06:02*, and *HLA-C*08:01* were significantly higher in the co-trimoxazole-induced SJS/TEN patients compared with controls (Kongpan et al. 2015). Table 3.2 summarizes the HLA association with drug-induced cADRs in different populations. In addition, some adverse events other than cADRs can be initiated by antibiotics and are associated with specific *HLA* alleles, such as *HLA-B*57:01* and flucloxacillin-induced liver injury (Monshi et al. 2013) and *HLA-A*02:01* and *HLA-DQB1*06:02* and amoxicillin-clavulanate hepatitis (Lucena et al. 2011).

3.4 The Interaction Between HLA, Drug Antigens, and T Cell Receptors in cADRs

The interactions of the immune synapse composed of specific HLA/drug/TCR molecules are complex. Three hypotheses of drug presentation mechanisms have been proposed to explain how small drug antigens might interact with HLA and TCR in cADRs: (1) the "hapten" theory, (2) the "pharmacological interaction with immune receptors" (p-i) concept, and (3) the "altered peptide repertoire" model (Fig. 3.2).

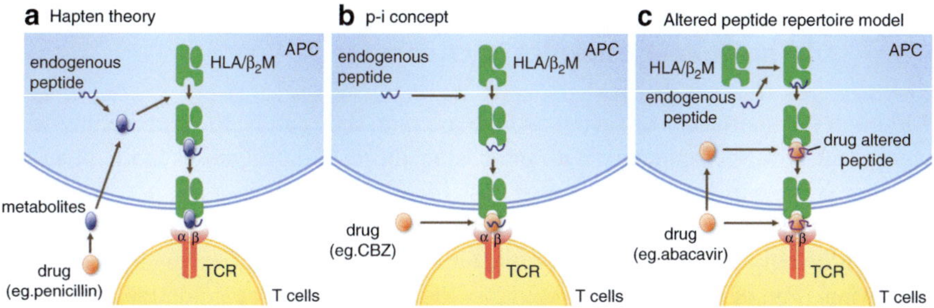

Fig. 3.2 Models of drug antigens presentation in cADRs. (**a**) The "hapten" theory. Drugs or metabolites serve as haptens to bind to the endogenous peptides to form the haptenated peptides. The drug/haptenated peptides are presented on HLA molecules, and the HLA/drug/peptide complex is recognized by TCR and then triggers T cell activation. (**b**) The "pharmacological interaction with immune receptors" (p-i) concept. Drugs directly bind to the HLA/peptide complex or TCR without intracellular processing and activate drug-specific T cells. (**c**) The "altered peptide repertoire" model. Drugs bind to specific HLA and alter the self-peptides repertoire, resulting in polyclonal T cell activation. *β2M* β-2 microglobulin, *CBZ* carbamazepine

The "hapten" theory states that the culprit drugs, such as penicillin or the reactive metabolites, are too small to be immunogenic on their own. They act like haptens and covalently bind to the endogenous peptides/proteins to form a drug/haptenated peptides complex presented on HLA molecules in the antigen-presenting cells. The HLA/drug/peptide complex is then recognized by TCR to trigger T cell activation resulting in drug-specific immune responses (Padovan et al. 1997). The "pharmacological interaction with immune receptors (p-i)" concept postulates that drugs may directly, reversibly, and non-covalently bind to the HLA and/or TCR protein. The classic antigen-processing pathway in antigen-presenting cells may be bypassed. For example, we previously found that CBZ/aromatic antiepileptic drugs can directly interact with HLA-B*15:02 protein (Wei et al. 2012). No intracellular antigen processing or drug metabolism was involved in the HLA-B*15:02 presentation of CBZ, and the appropriate endogenous peptides loading on HLA-B*15:02 was required for the stability of the HLA complex to present CBZ to T cells. Allopurinol is another example of p-i concept. A previous study reported that oxypurinol, the reactive metabolite of allopurinol, directly and immediately activates drug-specific T cells via the preferential use of HLA-B*58:01 without the intracellular processing (Yun et al. 2014). The "altered peptide repertoire" model states that the culprit drugs occupy the position in the peptide-binding groove of the HLA protein, changing the binding cleft and the peptide specificity of HLA binding. Abacavir is a well-known example of the "altered peptide repertoire" model. The crystal structure of HLA-B*57:01 in complex with abacavir and peptides has been reported (Illing et al. 2012; Ostrov et al. 2012). These studies showed that abacavir binds to the F-pocket of HLA-B*57:01 and alters the shape and chemistry of the antigen-binding cleft, thereby altering the repertoire of endogenous peptides and resulting in polyclonal T cell activation and autoimmune-like systemic reaction manifestations. Furthermore, viruses were proposed to be participated in the HLA/drug/TCR interactions in which they may provide exogenous peptides for drug presentation and play important roles in cADRs (White et al. 2015).

3.5 Clinical Applications and Progresses of Pharmacogenomics in cADRs

Although the incidences of severe cADRs are rare, they can be life-threatening with significant life-time sequelae. With increasing successful progresses in the pharmacogenomic researches, the screening test for high-risk genes prior to drug commencement has become an effective predictor for protecting patients who are first users of the culprit drugs or who are potential carriers with known ancestries of the risk genes (Pan et al. 2017). For example, the clinical practice guidelines have recommended the genetic testing for *HLA-B*15:02* should be mandatory before the first use of CBZ in Taiwan. Clinical trials of prospective screening for *HLA-B*15:02* have significantly reduced the risk of hypersensitivity reactions to CBZ. Pharmacogenomic tests are moving toward implementation for improving the drug safety to achieve the goal of precision medicine. Recent advances in pharmacogenomics will be widely applied into the clinic for prediction and prevention of cADRs related to high-risk drugs in the near future.

Acknowledgments *Source of Funding*: This work was supported in part by grants from the Ministry of Science and Technology, Taiwan (MOST 104-2314-B-182A-148-MY3, MOST 104-2325-B-182A-006, MOST 106-2314-B-182A-037-MY3), and Chang Gung Memorial Hospital (CLRPG2E0051~3, CORPG3F0041~2).

Conflict of Interest: The authors report no disclosures relevant to the manuscript.

References

Carr DF, Chaponda M, Jorgensen AL, Castro EC, Van Oosterhout JJ, Khoo SH, Lalloo DG, Heyderman RS, Alfirevic A, Pirmohamed M (2013) Association of human leukocyte antigen alleles and nevirapine hypersensitivity in a Malawian HIV-infected population. Clin Infect Dis 56:1330–1339

Chang CC, Ng CC, Too CL, Choon SE, Lee CK, Chung WH, Hussein SH, Lim KS, Murad S (2017) Association of HLA-B*15:13 and HLA-B*15:02 with phenytoin-induced severe cutaneous adverse reactions in a Malay population. Pharmacogenomics J 17(2):170–173

Chang CC, Too CL, Murad S, Hussein SH (2011) Association of HLA-B*1502 allele with carbamazepine-induced toxic epidermal necrolysis and Stevens-Johnson syndrome in the multi-ethnic Malaysian population. Int J Dermatol 50:221–224

Chantarangsu S, Mushiroda T, Mahasirimongkol S, Kiertiburanakul S, Sungkanuparph S, Manosuthi W, Tantisiriwat W, Charoenyingwattana A, Sura T, Chantratita W, Nakamura Y (2009) HLA-B*3505 allele is a strong predictor for nevirapine-induced skin adverse drug reactions in HIV-infected Thai patients. Pharmacogenet Genomics 19:139–146

Chen CB, Hsiao YH, Wu T, Hsih MS, Tassaneeyakul W, Jorns TP, Sukasem C, Hsu CN, Su SC, Chang WC, Hui RC, Chu CY, Chen YJ, Wu CY, Hsu CK, Chiu TM, Sun PL, Lee HE, Yang CY, Kao PH, Yang CH, Ho HC, Lin JY, Chang YC, Chen MJ, Lu CW, Ng CY, Kuo KL, Lin CY, Yang CS, Chen DP, Chang PY, Wu TL, Lin YJ, Weng YC, Kuo TT, Hung SI, Chung WH, Taiwan Severe Cutaneous Adverse Reaction Consortium (2017) Risk and association of HLA with oxcarbazepine-induced cutaneous adverse reactions in Asians. Neurology 88(1):78–86

Chong KW, Chan DW, Cheung YB, Ching LK, Hie SL, Thomas T, Ling S, Tan EC (2014) Association of carbamazepine-induced severe cutaneous drug reactions and HLA-B*1502 allele status, and dose and treatment duration in paediatric neurology patients in Singapore. Arch Dis Child 99:581–584

Choon SE, Lai NM (2012) An epidemiological and clinical analysis of cutaneous adverse drug reactions seen in a tertiary hospital in Johor, Malaysia. Indian J Dermatol Venereol Leprol 78:734–739

Chung WH, Chang WC, Lee YS, Wu YY, Yang CH, Ho HC, Chen MJ, Lin JY, Hui RC, Ho JC, Wu WM, Chen TJ, Wu T, Wu YR, Hsih MS, Tu PH, Chang CN, Hsu CN, Wu TL, Choon SE, Hsu CK, Chen DY, Liu CS, Lin CY, Kaniwa N, Saito Y, Takahashi Y, Nakamura R, Azukizawa H, Shi Y, Wang TH, Chuang SS, Tsai SF, Chang CJ, Chang YS, Hung SI (2014) Genetic variants associated with phenytoin-related severe cutaneous adverse reactions. JAMA 312:525–534

Chung WH, Chang WC, Stocker SL, Juo CG, Graham GG, Lee MH, Williams KM, Tian YC, Juan KC, Jan Wu YJ, Yang CH, Chang CJ, Lin YJ, Day RO, Hung SI (2015a) Insights into the poor prognosis of allopurinol-induced severe cutaneous adverse reactions: the impact of renal insufficiency, high plasma levels of oxypurinol and granulysin. Ann Rheum Dis 74: 2157–2164

Chung WH, Hung SI, Hong HS, Hsih MS, Yang LC, Ho HC, Wu JY, Chen YT (2004) Medical genetics: a marker for Stevens-Johnson syndrome. Nature 428:486

Chung WH, Hung SI, Yang JY, Su SC, Huang SP, Wei CY, Chin SW, Chiou CC, Chu SC, Ho HC, Yang CH, Lu CF, Wu JY, Liao YD, Chen YT (2008) Granulysin is a key mediator for disseminated keratinocyte death in Stevens-Johnson syndrome and toxic epidermal necrolysis. Nat Med 14:1343–1350

Chung WH, Pan RY, Chu MT, Chin SW, Huang YL, Wang WC, Chang JY, Hung SI (2015b) Oxypurinol-specific T cells possess preferential TCR clonotypes and express granulysin in allopurinol-induced severe cutaneous adverse reactions. J Invest Dermatol 135:2237–2248

Gatanaga H, Yazaki H, Tanuma J, Honda M, Genka I, Teruya K, Tachikawa N, Kikuchi Y, Oka S (2007) HLA-Cw8 primarily associated with hypersensitivity to nevirapine. AIDS 21:264–265

Genin E, Chen DP, Hung SI, Sekula P, Schumacher M, Chang PY, Tsai SH, Wu TL, Bellon T, Tamouza R, Fortier C, Toubert A, Charron D, Hovnanian A, Wolkenstein P, Chung WH, Mockenhaupt M, Roujeau JC (2014) HLA-A*31:01 and different types of carbamazepine-induced severe cutaneous adverse reactions: an international study and meta-analysis. Pharmacogenomics J 14:281–288

Hetherington S, Hughes AR, Mosteller M, Shortino D, Baker KL, Spreen W, Lai E, Davies K, Handley A, Dow DJ, Fling ME, Stocum M, Bowman C, Thurmond LM, Roses AD (2002) Genetic variations in HLA-B region and hypersensitivity reactions to abacavir. Lancet 359:1121–1122

Hung SI, Chung WH, Jee SH, Chen WC, Chang YT, Lee WR, Hu SL, Wu MT, Chen GS, Wong TW, Hsiao PF, Chen WH, Shih HY, Fang WH, Wei CY, Lou YH, Huang YL, Lin JJ, Chen YT (2006) Genetic susceptibility to carbamazepine-induced cutaneous adverse drug reactions. Pharmacogenet Genomics 16:297–306

Hung SI, Chung WH, Liou LB, Chu CC, Lin M, Huang HP, Lin YL, Lan JL, Yang LC, Hong HS, Chen MJ, Lai PC, Wu MS, Chu CY, Wang KH, Chen CH, Fann CS, Wu JY, Chen YT (2005) HLA-B*5801 allele as a genetic marker for severe cutaneous adverse reactions caused by allopurinol. Proc Natl Acad Sci U S A 102:4134–4139

Hung SI, Chung WH, Liu ZS, Chen CH, Hsih MS, Hui RC, Chu CY, Chen YT (2010) Common risk allele in aromatic antiepileptic-drug induced Stevens-Johnson syndrome and toxic epidermal necrolysis in Han Chinese. Pharmacogenomics 11:349–356

Ikeda H, Takahashi Y, Yamazaki E, Fujiwara T, Kaniwa N, Saito Y, Aihara M, Kashiwagi M, Muramatsu M (2010) HLA class I markers in Japanese patients with carbamazepine-induced cutaneous adverse reactions. Epilepsia 51:297–300

Illing PT, Vivian JP, Dudek NL, Kostenko L, Chen Z, Bharadwaj M, Miles JJ, Kjer-Nielsen L, Gras S, Williamson NA, Burrows SR, Purcell AW, Rossjohn J, McCluskey J (2012) Immune self-reactivity triggered by drug-modified HLA-peptide repertoire. Nature 486:554–558

Kang HR, Jee YK, Kim YS, Lee CH, Jung JW, Kim SH, Park HW, Chang YS, Jang IJ, Cho SH, Min KU, Kim SH, Lee KW, Adverse Drug Reaction Research Group in Korea (2011) Positive and negative associations of HLA class I alleles with allopurinol-induced SCARs in Koreans. Pharmacogenet Genomics 21:303–307

Kaniwa N, Saito Y, Aihara M, Matsunaga K, Tohkin M, Kurose K, Furuya H, Takahashi Y, Muramatsu M, Kinoshita S, Abe M, Ikeda H, Kashiwagi M, Song Y, Ueta M, Sotozono C, Ikezawa Z, Hasegawa R, JSAR Research Group (2010) HLA-B*1511 is a risk factor for carbamazepine-induced Stevens-Johnson syndrome and toxic epidermal necrolysis in Japanese patients. Epilepsia 51:2461–2465

Kaniwa N, Saito Y, Aihara M, Matsunaga K, Tohkin M, Kurose K, Sawada J, Furuya H, Takahashi Y, Muramatsu M, Kinoshita S, Abe M, Ikeda H, Kashiwagi M, Song Y, Ueta M, Sotozono C, Ikezawa Z, Hasegawa R, JSAR Research Group (2008) HLA-B locus in Japanese patients with anti-epileptics and allopurinol-related Stevens-Johnson syndrome and toxic epidermal necrolysis. Pharmacogenomics 9:1617–1622

Kazeem GR, Cox C, Aponte J, Messenheimer J, Brazell C, Nelsen AC, Nelson MR, Foot E (2009) High-resolution HLA genotyping and severe cutaneous adverse reactions in lamotrigine-treated patients. Pharmacogenet Genomics 19:661–665

Kim BK, Jung JW, Kim TB, Chang YS, Park HS, Moon J, Lee ST, Jung KH, Jung KY, Chu K, Lee SK, Kang HR, Park HW (2017) HLA-A*31:01 and lamotrigine-induced severe cutaneous adverse drug reactions in a Korean population. Ann Allergy Asthma Immunol 118(5): 629–630

Kim SH, Kim M, Lee KW, Kim SH, Kang HR, Park HW, Jee YK (2010) HLA-B*5901 is strongly associated with methazolamide-induced Stevens-Johnson syndrome/toxic epidermal necrolysis. Pharmacogenomics 11:879–884

Kim SH, Lee KW, Song WJ, Kim SH, Jee YK, Lee SM, Kang HR, Park HW, Cho SH, Park SH, Min KU, Chang YS, Adverse Drug Reaction Research Group in Korea (2011) Carbamazepine-induced severe cutaneous adverse reactions and HLA genotypes in Koreans. Epilepsy Res 97:190–197

Knowles SR, Dewhurst N, Shear NH (2012) Anticonvulsant hypersensitivity syndrome: an update. Expert Opin Drug Saf 11:767–778

Kongpan T, Mahasirimongkol S, Konyoung P, Kanjanawart S, Chumworathayi P, Wichukchinda N, Kidkeukarun R, Preechakul S, Khunarkornsiri U, Bamrungram W, Supharatwattanakun B, Mootsikapun P, Kwangsukstid S, Denjanta S, Vannaprasaht S, Rungapiromnan W, Suwankesawong W, Tassaneeyakul W, Tassaneeyakul W (2015) Candidate HLA genes for prediction of co-trimoxazole-induced severe cutaneous reactions. Pharmacogenet Genomics 25:402–411

Kwan PK, Ng MH, Lo SV (2014) Association between HLA-B*15:02 allele and antiepileptic drug-induced severe cutaneous reactions in Hong Kong Chinese: a population-based study. Hong Kong Med J 20(Suppl 7):16–18

Lin YF, Yang CH, Sindy H, Lin JY, Rosaline Hui CY, Tsai YC, Wu TS, Huang CT, Kao KC, Hu HC, Chiu CH, Hung SI, Chung WH (2014) Severe cutaneous adverse reactions related to systemic antibiotics. Clin Infect Dis 58:1377–1385

Littera R, Carcassi C, Masala A, Piano P, Serra P, Ortu F, Corso N, Casula B, La Nasa G, Contu L, Manconi PE (2006) HLA-dependent hypersensitivity to nevirapine in Sardinian HIV patients. AIDS 20:1621–1626

Locharernkul C, Loplumlert J, Limotai C, Korkij W, Desudchit T, Tongkobpetch S, Kangwanshiratada O, Hirankarn N, Suphapeetiporn K, Shotelersuk V (2008) Carbamazepine and phenytoin induced Stevens-Johnson syndrome is associated with HLA-B*1502 allele in Thai population. Epilepsia 49:2087–2091

Lonjou C, Borot N, Sekula P, Ledger N, Thomas L, Halevy S, Naldi L, Bouwes-Bavinck JN, Sidoroff A, De Toma C, Schumacher M, Roujeau JC, Hovnanian A, Mockenhaupt M, Regi SSG (2008) A European study of HLA-B in Stevens-Johnson syndrome and toxic epidermal necrolysis related to five high-risk drugs. Pharmacogenet Genomics 18:99–107

Lowin B, Peitsch MC, Tschopp J (1995) Perforin and granzymes: crucial effector molecules in cytolytic T lymphocyte and natural killer cell-mediated cytotoxicity. Curr Top Microbiol Immunol 198:1–24

Lucena MI, Molokhia M, Shen Y, Urban TJ, Aithal GP, Andrade RJ, Day CP, Ruiz-Cabello F, Donaldson PT, Stephens C, Pirmohamed M, Romero-Gomez M, Navarro JM, Fontana RJ, Miller M, Groome M, Bondon-Guitton E, Conforti A, Stricker BH, Carvajal A, Ibanez L, Yue

QY, Eichelbaum M, Floratos A, Pe'er I, Daly MJ, Goldstein DB, Dillon JF, Nelson MR, Watkins PB, Daly AK, Spanish DILI Registry, EUDRAGENE, DILIN, DILIGEN, International SAEC (2011) Susceptibility to amoxicillin-clavulanate-induced liver injury is influenced by multiple HLA class I and II alleles. Gastroenterology 141:338–347

Mallal S, Nolan D, Witt C, Masel G, Martin AM, Moore C, Sayer D, Castley A, Mamotte C, Maxwell D, James I, Christiansen FT (2002) Association between presence of HLA-B*5701, HLA-DR7, and HLA-DQ3 and hypersensitivity to HIV-1 reverse-transcriptase inhibitor abacavir. Lancet 359:727–732

Mallal S, Phillips E, Carosi G, Molina JM, Workman C, Tomazic J, Jagel-Guedes E, Rugina S, Kozyrev O, Cid JF, Hay P, Nolan D, Hughes S, Hughes A, Ryan S, Fitch N, Thorborn D, Benbow A, Team P-S (2008) HLA-B*5701 screening for hypersensitivity to abacavir. N Engl J Med 358:568–579

Man CB, Kwan P, Baum L, Yu E, Lau KM, Cheng AS, Ng MH (2007) Association between HLA-B*1502 allele and antiepileptic drug-induced cutaneous reactions in Han Chinese. Epilepsia 48:1015–1018

Martin AM, Nolan D, James I, Cameron P, Keller J, Moore C, Phillips E, Christiansen FT, Mallal S (2005) Predisposition to nevirapine hypersensitivity associated with HLA-DRB1*0101 and abrogated by low CD4 T-cell counts. AIDS 19:97–99

McCormack M, Alfirevic A, Bourgeois S, Farrell JJ, Kasperaviciute D, Carrington M, Sills GJ, Marson T, Jia X, de Bakker PI, Chinthapalli K, Molokhia M, Johnson MR, O'Connor GD, Chaila E, Alhusaini S, Shianna KV, Radtke RA, Heinzen EL, Walley N, Pandolfo M, Pichler W, Park BK, Depondt C, Sisodiya SM, Goldstein DB, Deloukas P, Delanty N, Cavalleri GL, Pirmohamed M (2011) HLA-A*3101 and carbamazepine-induced hypersensitivity reactions in Europeans. N Engl J Med 364:1134–1143

Mehta TY, Prajapati LM, Mittal B, Joshi CG, Sheth JJ, Patel DB, Dave DM, Goyal RK (2009) Association of HLA-B*1502 allele and carbamazepine-induced Stevens-Johnson syndrome among Indians. Indian J Dermatol Venereol Leprol 75:579–582

Middleton D, Menchaca L, Rood H, Komerofsky R (2003) New allele frequency database: http://www.allelefrequencies.net. Tissue Antigens 61:403–407

Monshi MM, Faulkner L, Gibson A, Jenkins RE, Farrell J, Earnshaw CJ, Alfirevic A, Cederbrant K, Daly AK, French N, Pirmohamed M, Park BK, Naisbitt DJ (2013) Human leukocyte antigen (HLA)-B*57:01-restricted activation of drug-specific T cells provides the immunological basis for flucloxacillin-induced liver injury. Hepatology 57:727–739

Nassif A, Bensussan A, Dorothee G, Mani-Chouaib F, Bachot N, Bagot M, Boumsell L, Roujeau JC (2002) Drug specific cytotoxic T-cells in the skin lesions of a patient with toxic epidermal necrolysis. J Invest Dermatol 118:728–733

Ng CY, Yeh YT, Wang CW, Hung SI, Yang CH, Chang YC, Chang WC, Lin YJ, Chang CJ, Su SC, Fan WL, Chen DY, Wu YJ, Tian YC, Hui RC, Chung WH, Taiwan Severe Cutaneous Adverse Reaction Consortium (2016) Impact of the HLA-B(*)58:01 allele and renal impairment on allopurinol-induced cutaneous adverse reactions. J Invest Dermatol 136:1373–1381

Nguyen DV, Chu HC, Nguyen DV, Phan MH, Craig T, Baumgart K, Van Nunen S (2015) HLA-B*1502 and carbamazepine-induced severe cutaneous adverse drug reactions in Vietnamese. Asia Pac Allergy 5:68–77

Ostrov DA, Grant BJ, Pompeu YA, Sidney J, Harndahl M, Southwood S, Oseroff C, Lu S, Jakoncic J, De Oliveira CA, Yang L, Mei H, Shi L, Shabanowitz J, English AM, Wriston A, Lucas A, Phillips E, Mallal S, Grey HM, Sette A, Hunt DF, Buus S, Peters B (2012) Drug hypersensitivity caused by alteration of the MHC-presented self-peptide repertoire. Proc Natl Acad Sci U S A 109:9959–9964

Ozeki T, Mushiroda T, Yowang A, Takahashi A, Kubo M, Shirakata Y, Ikezawa Z, Iijima M, Shiohara T, Hashimoto K, Kamatani N, Nakamura Y (2011) Genome-wide association study identifies HLA-A*3101 allele as a genetic risk factor for carbamazepine-induced cutaneous adverse drug reactions in Japanese population. Hum Mol Genet 20:1034–1041

Padovan E, Bauer T, Tongio MM, Kalbacher H, Weltzien HU (1997) Penicilloyl peptides are recognized as T cell antigenic determinants in penicillin allergy. Eur J Immunol 27: 1303–1307

Pan RY, Dao RL, Hung SI, Chung WH (2017) Pharmacogenomic advances in the prediction and prevention of cutaneous idiosyncratic drug reactions. Clin Pharmacol Ther. https://doi.org/10.1002/cpt.683

Ramirez E, Bellon T, Tong HY, Borobia AM, De Abajo FJ, Lerma V, Moreno Hidalgo MA, Castaner JL, Cabanas R, Fiandor A, Gonzalez-Ramos J, Herranz P, Cachafeiro L, Gonzalez-Herrada C, Gonzalez O, Aramburu JA, Laosa O, Hernandez R, Carcas AJ, Frias J (2017) Significant HLA class I type associations with aromatic antiepileptic drug (AED)-induced SJS/TEN are different from those found for the same AED-induced DRESS in the Spanish population. Pharmacol Res 115:168–178

Revuz J, Penso D, Roujeau JC, Guillaume JC, Payne CR, Wechsler J, Touraine R (1987) Toxic epidermal necrolysis. Clinical findings and prognosis factors in 87 patients. Arch Dermatol 123:1160–1165

Roujeau JC, Huynh TN, Bracq C, Guillaume JC, Revuz J, Touraine R (1987) Genetic susceptibility to toxic epidermal necrolysis. Arch Dermatol 123:1171–1173

Roujeau JC, Kelly JP, Naldi L, Rzany B, Stern RS, Anderson T, Auquier A, Bastuji-Garin S, Correia O, Locati F et al (1995) Medication use and the risk of Stevens-Johnson syndrome or toxic epidermal necrolysis. N Engl J Med 333:1600–1607

Roujeau JC, Stern RS (1994) Severe adverse cutaneous reactions to drugs. N Engl J Med 331:1272–1285

Rzany B, Mockenhaupt M, Baur S, Schroder W, Stocker U, Mueller J, Hollander N, Bruppacher R, Schopf E (1996) Epidemiology of erythema exsudativum multiforme majus, Stevens-Johnson syndrome, and toxic epidermal necrolysis in Germany (1990–1992): structure and results of a population-based registry. J Clin Epidemiol 49:769–773

Schnyder B, Pichler WJ (2013) Allergy to sulfonamides. J Allergy Clin Immunol 131(256-7):E1–E5

Shi YW, Min FL, Liu XR, Zan LX, Gao MM, Yu MJ, Liao WP (2011) Hla-B alleles and lamotrigine-induced cutaneous adverse drug reactions in the Han Chinese population. Basic Clin Pharmacol Toxicol 109:42–46

Sun D, Yu CH, Liu ZS, He XL, Hu JS, Wu GF, Mao B, Wu SH, Xiang HH (2014) Association of HLA-B*1502 and *1511 allele with antiepileptic drug-induced Stevens-Johnson syndrome in central China. J Huazhong Univ Sci Technol Med Sci 34:146–150

Tassaneeyakul W, Jantararoungtong T, Chen P, Lin PY, Tiamkao S, Khunarkornsiri U, Chucherd P, Konyoung P, Vannaprasaht S, Choonhakarn C, Pisuttimarn P, Sangviroon A, Tassaneeyakul W (2009) Strong association between HLA-B*5801 and allopurinol-induced Stevens-Johnson syndrome and toxic epidermal necrolysis in a Thai population. Pharmacogenet Genomics 19:704–709

Tassaneeyakul W, Prabmeechai N, Sukasem C, Kongpan T, Konyoung P, Chumworathayi P, Tiamkao S, Khunarkornsiri U, Kulkantrakorn K, Saksit N, Nakkam N, Satapornpong P, Vannaprasaht S, Sangviroon A, Mahasirimongkol S, Wichukchinda N, Rerkpattanapipat T, Tassaneeyakul W (2016) Associations between HLA class I and cytochrome P450 2C9 genetic polymorphisms and phenytoin-related severe cutaneous adverse reactions in a Thai population. Pharmacogenet Genomics 26:225–234

Wei CY, Chung WH, Huang HW, Chen YT, Hung SI (2012) Direct interaction between HLA-B and carbamazepine activates T cells in patients with Stevens-Johnson syndrome. J Allergy Clin Immunol 129:1562–1569.e5

White KD, Chung WH, Hung SI, Mallal S, Phillips EJ (2015) Evolving models of the immunopathogenesis of T cell-mediated drug allergy: the role of host, pathogens, and drug response. J Allergy Clin Immunol 136:219–234; quiz 235

Yang CY, Chen CH, Deng ST, Huang CS, Lin YJ, Chen YJ, Wu CY, Hung SI, Chung WH (2015) Allopurinol use and risk of fatal hypersensitivity reactions: a nationwide population-based study in Taiwan. JAMA Intern Med 175:1550–1557

Yun J, Marcaida MJ, Eriksson KK, Jamin H, Fontana S, Pichler WJ, Yerly D (2014) Oxypurinol directly and immediately activates the drug-specific T cells via the preferential use of HLA-B*58:01. J Immunol 192:2984–2993

Zeng T, Long YS, Min FL, Liao WP, Shi YW (2015) Association of HLA-B*1502 allele with lamotrigine-induced Stevens-Johnson syndrome and toxic epidermal necrolysis in Han Chinese subjects: a meta-analysis. Int J Dermatol 54:488–493

Zhang FR, Liu H, Irwanto A, Fu XA, Li Y, Yu GQ, Yu YX, Chen MF, Low HQ, Li JH, Bao FF, Foo JN, Bei JX, Jia XM, Liu J, Liany H, Wang N, Niu GY, Wang ZZ, Shi BQ, Tian HQ, Liu HX, Ma SS, Zhou Y, You JB, Yang Q, Wang C, Chu TS, Liu DC, Yu XL, Sun YH, Ning Y, Wei ZH, Chen SL, Chen XC, Zhang ZX, Liu YX, Pulit SL, Wu WB, Zheng ZY, Yang RD, Long H, Liu ZS, Wang JQ, Li M, Zhang LH, Wang H, Wang LM, Xiao P, Li JL, Huang ZM, Huang JX, Li Z, Liu J, Xiong L, Yang J, Wang XD, Yu DB, Lu XM, Zhou GZ, Yan LB, Shen JP, Zhang GC, Zeng YX, de Bakker PI, Chen SM, Liu JJ (2013) HLA-B*13:01 and the dapsone hypersensitivity syndrome. N Engl J Med 369:1620–1628

Viral Reactivation in Cutaneous Adverse Drug Reactions

4

Tetsuo Shiohara, Yoko Kano, Yoshiko Mizukawa, and Yumi Aoyama

Abbreviations

ADR	Adverse drug reactions
ART	Antiretroviral therapy
cADR	Cutaneous adverse drug reactions
cMOs	Classical monocytes
CMV	Cytomegalovirus
DiHS	Drug-induced hypersensitivity syndrome
DRESS	Drug reaction with eosinophilia and systemic symptoms
EBV	Epstein-Barr virus
GVHD	Graft-vs.-host disease
HHV-6	Human Herpesvirus 6
HLA	Human leukocyte antigens
IRIS	Immune reconstitution inflammatory syndrome
MOs	Monocytes
PV	Pemphigus vulgaris
SJS/TEN	Stevens–Johnson syndrome/Toxic epidermal necrolysis
VZV	Varicella zoster virus

T. Shiohara (✉) · Y. Kano · Y. Mizukawa
Department of Dermatology, Kyorin University School of Medicine, Mitaka, Tokyo, Japan
e-mail: tpshio@ks.kyorin-u.ac.jp

Y. Aoyama
Department of Dermatology, Kawasaki Medical School, Kurashiki, Okayama, Japan

N. H. Shear, R. P. Dodiuk-Gad (eds.), *Advances in Diagnosis and Management of Cutaneous Adverse Drug Reactions*, https://doi.org/10.1007/978-981-13-1489-6_4

Key Points

- It remains unknown whether viral reactivation could act as a trigger of cutaneous adverse drug reactions (cADRs) or represent the consequence of general immune dysregulation in cADRs.
- All patients with cADRs should be assessed for clinical signs suggestive of viral reactivations, because it is difficult to distinguish between viral reactivations and worsening of clinical symptoms of the disease.
- The shift from regulatory T cell to Th17 cell development occurring during the course of drug-induced hypersensitivity syndrome (DiHS)/drug reaction with eosinophilia and systemic symptoms (DRESS) would be mediated by the predominance of different subsets of monocytes.
- Because rapid and abrupt immune restoration after withdrawal or reduction of immunosuppressive agents has the potential to cause immune reconstitution inflammatory syndrome (IRIS), DiHS/DRESS patients treated with systemic corticosteroids are at greater risk of developing IRIS.
- Anti-inflammatory therapies for cADRs should be balanced with the need to prevent viral reactivation.

4.1 Introduction

Genetic factors predisposing to certain types of drug eruptions induced by limited drugs have been identified in several specific HLA alleles. However, given the low positive predictive value of HLA-B*58:01 carriage as a predictor of allopurinol-induced adverse drug reactions (ADRs), other environmental factors, such as viral infection status, likely contribute to the pathogenesis of ADRs (White et al. 2015). Because HLA alleles are also associated with an increasing number of viral infections (Iampietro et al. 2014), viral infections are very likely to act as inducible trigger of drug hypersensitivity in an HLA-associated manner. Indeed, several features of antiviral immune responses are strikingly similar to those displayed by T-cell-mediated ADRs, such as HLA allele association, drug-/virus-peptide MHC interaction, and $CD8^+$ T-cell-dominated responses (White et al. 2015). The most likely candidate involved in the development of drug eruptions is the family *Herpesviridae*, because these viruses have in common the ability to establish a latent state of infection with low levels of viral gene expression for the life of the host by establishing many means of evading or neutralizing the host's immune system. Because of these properties, they can induce and maintain potent-specific memory T-cell responses. Consistent with this view, the skin of healthy young and old subjects is abundantly populated by varicella zoster virus (VZV)-specific $CD4^+$ T cells, thereby providing efficient and rapid immunity in this tissue (Vukmanovic-Stejic et al. 2015). These T cells, unless stimulated, could be induced to persist as a stable, resident population in a quiescent state by tissue microenvironments in vivo: they are called as tissue-resident memory T (T_{RM}) cells. They have the ability to defend host tissue against attack from the wide microbial pathogens, because they are cross-reactive in nature (White et al. 2015). Once activated, however, they would serve to play an important role not only for tissue protection against invading pathogens but also collateral tissue damage.

The fundamental question of why certain individuals respond to specific drugs while many other individuals do not is still largely unresolved. According to the "danger" model (Matzinger 2007), danger signals possibly provided by damaged host cells would be needed to activate drug-antigen-specific T cells that are otherwise at the resting state under nonpathological conditions. Thus, we can assume that immune responses to otherwise "innocent" certain drugs can be initiated by such danger signals from virally infected injured cells and tissues. If so, as we initially predicted (Shiohara et al. 2006), T-cell responses to drugs may stem from cross-reactivities of T_{RM} cells generated primarily for their recognition of viral antigens during viral infection. In this review, we will discuss how underlying viral infection can have an impact on drug hypersensitivity.

4.2 *Human Herpesvirus 6* (HHV-6) and *Cytomegalovirus* (CMV) in Drug-Induced Hypersensitivity Syndrome (DiHS)/Drug Reaction with Eosinophilia and Systemic Symptoms (DRESS)

DiHS/DRESS is a life-threatening multi-organ system reaction induced by certain drugs with immunosuppressive potential, mainly anticonvulsants, and associated with sequential reactivations of herpesviruses (Shiohara et al. 2006; Shiohara and Kano 2017). This syndrome has several unique features, including delayed onset, paradoxical deterioration of clinical symptoms after withdrawal of the causative drug, and unexplained cross-reactivity to multiple drugs with different chemical features, thereby creating uncertainty over whether it represents true drug eruption (Shiohara and Kano 2017). Nineteen years ago, we (Suzuki et al. 1998) and Hashimoto's group (Tohyama et al. 1998) independently published landmark studies that sparked the current advances in our understanding of the role of viral infection in DiHS/DRESS. These studies detected HHV-6 DNA by PCR assay in blood and skin samples from patients with DiHS/DRESS. Because HHV-6 detection by PCR was largely limited to blood samples obtained at certain time points, usually 2–3 weeks after onset, the virus was initially regarded as being involved in acute exacerbation of the disease and representing a mere epiphenomenon; however, the retrospective nationwide survey of these patients who displayed typical clinical symptoms in Japan demonstrated that reactivations of HHV-6 as evidenced by a significant increase in serum HHV-6 IgG titers or detection of HHV-6 DNA in blood were observed in the vast majority of DiHS/DRESS patients, 2–3 weeks after onset, but not at onset.

Based on these findings, however, HHV-6 reactivations can be widely used as a specific and sensitive diagnostic marker in Japan (Suzuki et al. 1998; Tohyama et al. 1998; Kano et al. 2004, 2006) and EU (Descamps et al. 2013), although unfortunately these tests are not yet routinely available in other countries. Nevertheless, it remains unknown whether HHV-6 reactivation could represent a causal factor or consequences of inflammatory responses of DiHS/DRESS. In this regard, our recent studies have clearly demonstrated that HHV-6 reactivation would occur as part of an ordered cascade of viral reactivations, as shown in graft-vs.-host disease (GVHD): according to our sequential analyses of viral DNA loads in patients with DiHS/DRESS, the cascade of reactivation events is initiated by HHV-6 or Epstein-Barr virus (EBV) extends, with some delay, to HHV-7 as well and eventually to CMV (Kano et al. 2004, 2006) (Fig. 4.1), in obligate sequential order, as demonstrated in GVHD. This ordered sequence of reactivation events may occur well before patients become symptomatic, as demonstrated after onset. We therefore must recognize that clinically recognizable reactivations are just the tip of the iceberg although many clinicians believe that most of the reactivation events could be recognized as onset of clinical symptoms or worsening of laboratory findings. We also should recognize that viral DNA may no longer be detected after robust immune responses to the virus are generated: thus, no detection of viral DNA in the blood at onset should not be interpreted simply as evidence against viral involvement as triggers for DiHS/DRESS.

The pathogenic role of HHV-6 remains unknown, although some investigators suggested that liver dysfunction observed as an early or late event during the course of DiHS/DRESS could be caused by HHV-6 reactivation. Time course analyses of temporal relationship between HHV-6 reactivation and liver dysfunction revealed that liver dysfunction, either as early or late event, could

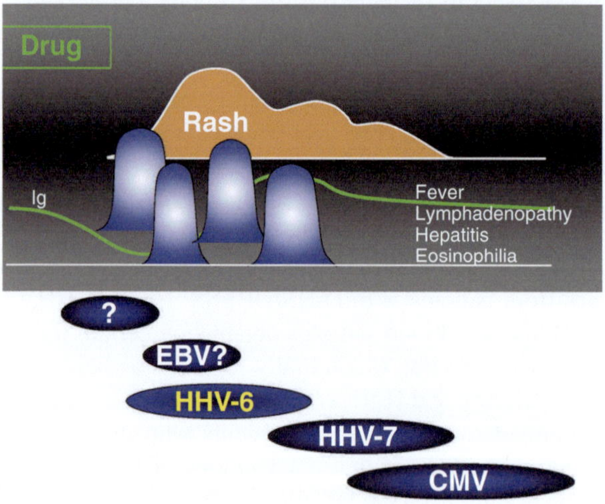

Fig. 4.1 The clinical course of DiHS/DRESS. This syndrome usually begins with a fever shortly followed by a maculopapular rash >3 weeks after starting therapy with a limited number of drugs, such as anticonvulsants. Patients usually develop two or three features of symptoms followed by a stepwise development of other symptoms. These symptoms continue to deteriorate, or several flare-ups can be seen even for weeks or months after stopping the offending drug. Serum Ig levels continue to decrease for a week after withdrawal of the drug. Despite such a wide variety of clinical symptoms, HHV-6 reactivation occurs 2–3 weeks after onset

be detected totally independently of HHV-6 reactivation. On the other hand, we described that HHV-6 DNA and antigens were successfully detected in the cellular infiltrates in the initial skin lesions despite their lack in the corresponding blood samples obtained at the same time as skin biopsy (Suzuki et al. 1998). So far, we have no satisfying explanation for this discrepancy; one possible explanation could be that the presence of viral DNA in the blood or skin is short-lived and becomes rapidly undetectable after generation of virus-specific immune responses. In support of this possibility, we previously reported that high levels of HSV DNA were detected in the saliva samples from 6 of 16 patients with pemphigus vulgaris (PV) with oral lesions at the earliest stage who had no episodes of herpes simplex, but HSV DNA was no longer detected in the saliva samples once antiviral immune responses became fully established (Kurata et al. 2014). Thus, the main difficulty in assigning a pathogenic role to any virus in any clinical symptoms of DiHS/DRESS is that during the prodromal period before the appearance of overt clinical and laboratory findings, the virus would have disappeared due to generation of antiviral immune responses, which make the detection of the virus at the onset of clinical symptoms almost impossible. Thus, great caution is needed in accepting a potential pathogen as cause of the disease simply because it is detected or its viral load significantly increases in many patients: the absence of viral DNA cannot be taken as evidence against causation of the disease. Consistent with this idea, Picard et al. demonstrated that cutaneous and visceral symptoms of DiHS/DRESS are mediated by activated $CD8^+$ effector T (Teff) cells which are largely directed against herpesviruses, such as EBV, and that the causative drug can reactivate herpesviruses in vitro (Picard et al. 2010). These results can be interpreted as indicating that both herpesvirus reactivations triggered by the causative drug and the subsequent generation of antiviral immune responses could have the pathogenic role in DiHS/DRESS, while the latter would serve to maintain tissue homeostasis in a physiologic naïve state.

The pathologic role of the sequential reactivation of other herpesviruses is debatable as only a portion of previous cases showed CMV disease leading to significant morbidity and mortality (Asano et al. 2009). CMV disease may aggravate the clinical course of DiHS/DRESS patients who either fail to respond or experience worsening of symptoms despite immunosuppressive therapy. The true incidence of CMV disease in DiHS/DRESS could be underestimated, because diagnostic examinations of CMV disease are not usually pursued in many patients with DiHS/DRESS presenting with pulmonary or gastrointestinal symptoms and DiHS/DRESS flares. Importantly, we reported that CMV disease occurring during the course of DiHS/DRESS can be predictable on the basis of our retrospective analysis: aged, particularly older than 60 years, patients with antecedent high HHV-6 DNA loads are at risk for subsequently developing CMV disease, irrespective of corticosteroid administration (Asano et al. 2009; Mizukawa et al. 2018); the timing of onset of CMV disease can be also predictable, given that CMV disease tended to occur 3–7 weeks after onset of DiHS/DRESS; and a rapid reduction in white blood cell and platelet counts may be an additional useful predictor of CMV disease. The diagnostic approach for CMV infection is to confirm the detection of CMV antigens or CMV DNA (by PCR) in blood and the presence of cytomegalic cells in histological analyses. A rise in anti-CMV IgG titers should not be regarded as a proof of CMV disease, because the significant rise can also be observed even in most DiHS/DRESS patients without overt CMV disease, particularly >1 month after onset.

4.3 Mechanisms Whereby Herpesvirus Reactivations Can Sequentially Occur in DiHS/DRESS

One of the most important questions raised by these data is why sequential reactivations of herpesviruses can be specifically observed in DiHS/DRESS. How do the observations described above fit with the scenario provided by the classical model of drug-specific effector T (Teff) cells in the development of drug eruptions?: according to the model, drug-specific Teff cells are thought to be major mediators involved in the development of not only SJS/TEN but also DiHS/DRESS. We previously demonstrated that Treg cells with suppressive function expanded during the acute stage (Shiohara et al. 2015; Takahashi et al. 2009) thereby causing the delayed onset of DiHS/DRESS (Shiohara et al. 2015; Takahashi et al. 2009) and possibly allowing sequential reactivations of herpesviruses. Contrary to the loss of Treg function, frequencies of Th17 cells were significantly increased after resolution of DiHS/DRESS (Ushigome et al. 2018). Such a dramatic increase in Th17 cells after resolution was never observed in other drug eruptions. These results suggest that clinical resolution of DiHS/DRESS may be accompanied by a shift from Treg development toward Th17 development. In this regard, recent studies have shown that Treg and Th17 cells are not at the final stage of their differentiation and have the potential to convert into Th17 cells and Treg cells, respectively, depending on cytokines and monocytes (Hoechst et al. 2011). These findings could be interpreted as suggesting that a gradual loss of Treg function occurring after clinical resolution of DiHS/DRESS may be secondary to the paucity/abundance of signals necessary for Treg/Th17 development, respectively. In view of recent studies indicating that Treg development can be differentially regulated by different subsets of monocytes (Zhong et al. 2012; Zhong and Yazdanbakhsh 2013), Treg expansions followed by a loss of their function could be secondary to alterations in monocyte subsets. Human blood monocytes (MOs) have been shown to be divided into distinct subsets: $CD14^{+}CD16^{-}$ classical monocytes (cMOs) and $CD14^{dim}CD16^{+}$ nonclassical pro-inflammatory (or patrolling) monocytes (pMOs) (Zhong et al. 2012; Zhong and Yazdanbakhsh 2013). pMOs have been reported to patrol the whole body for signs of infection (Cros et al. 2010; van de Veerdonk and Netea 2010) and control peripheral Treg development in immune thrombocytopenia (Zhong et al. 2012).

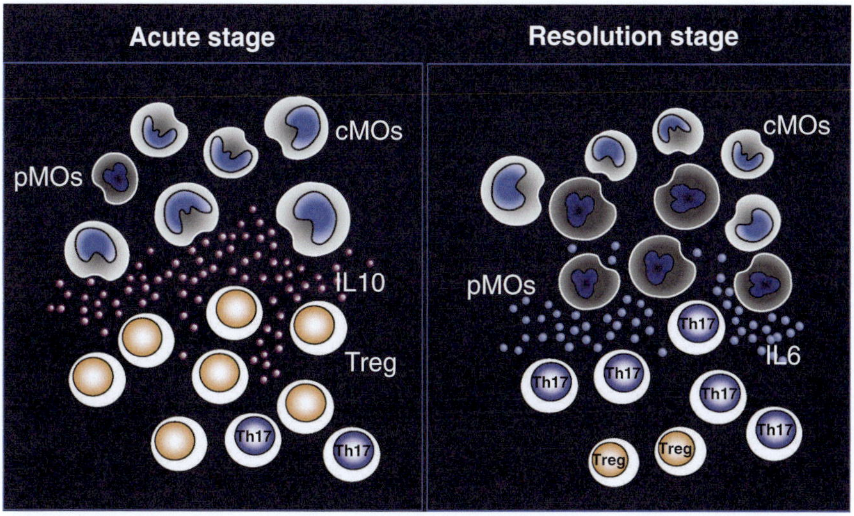

Fig. 4.2 The relative balance of the Treg/Th17 cells in different stages of DiHS/DRESS is determined by the predominance of different subsets of MOs, cMOs in the acute stage, and pMOs in the resolution stage, respectively. Upon selective depletion of "original" pMOs at the acute stage, "pathogenic" pMOs capable of producing IL-6 are alternatively recruited, thereby driving the shift from Treg to Th17 cells at the resolution stage

pMOs have been specifically depleted from the circulation at the acute stage of DiHS/DRESS (<10 days after onset). The dramatic change in the frequencies of Treg cells and MOs was observed during the subacute stage, day 11–36 after onset. The frequencies of pMOs returned to normal levels, while the expanded Treg cells were contracted during that time. The restoration in pMO frequency was negatively correlated with the decrease in Treg frequency and positively with the increase in Th17 frequencies. Overall, these findings highlight how MOs may have dramatic effects on the Treg/Th17 balance of the host, altering antiviral immune responses and resulting in reactivation of herpesviruses and the subsequent development of autoimmune diseases as a long-term sequela of DiHS/DRESS (Ushigome et al. 2015; Takehara et al. 2016). Our results clearly demonstrate that cMOs obtained at the acute stage, particularly when associated with selective depletion of pMOs, could serve to expand Tregs via the production of IL-10 (Fig. 4.2). However, pMOs alternatively recruited after selective depletion of "original" pMOs, however, had a potent ability to expand Th17 cells through the release of IL-6 (Fig. 4.2). Thus, different subsets of MOs, cMOs, or pMOs could determine, through their own unique pattern of cytokine production, whether immune responses will be dominated by Treg cells or Th17 cells. This scenario may explain why a variety of autoimmune responses and autoimmune diseases develop over prolonged periods of time after resolution of DiHS/DRESS.

4.4 Management of DiHS/DRESS-Associated Viral Reactivation

Although outcomes in infectious disease have long been regarded as damage caused by the pathogens themselves, immunologic responses to the pathogens are now believed to play a critical role in disease development (Sun 2011). Rapid and abrupt immune restoration during effective antimicrobial therapy and withdrawal of immunosuppression, therefore, has the potential to cause pathologic inflammatory responses, termed immune reconstitution inflammatory syndrome (IRIS) (Shelburne et al. 2002). The clinical symptoms of IRIS range from a self-limited mild disease to a severely ill, life-threatening disease. Although IRIS was originally defined as a paradoxical deterioration in clinical status attributable to the recovery of the immune response to pathogens following institution of antiretroviral therapy (ART), even in non-HIV setting, IRIS has been reported to develop on withdrawal of chemotherapy or reduction of immunosuppressive agents, such as prednisolone (Shiohara et al. 2010).

Based on the observations that paradoxical worsening of clinical symptoms associated with reduction in viral loads is typically observed after withdrawal of the causative drug with immunosuppressive potential in the acute phase of DiHS/DRESS, we propose that DiHS/DRESS is a manifestation of the newly described IRIS (Shiohara et al. 2010). Several unique clinical manifestations of DiHS/DRESS may be explained by assuming that the rapid restoration of pathogen-specific immune responses reduces viral loads at onset, thereby rendering them undetectable in the blood. The generally accepted diagnostic criteria for IRIS proposed by Shelburne et al. (2002) are as follows: (1) paradoxical deterioration of a preexisting, but previously unrecognized, infection, (2) a decrease in viral loads with or without an increase in $CD4^{+}$T-cell counts, (3) clinical symptoms not explained by a newly acquired infection, and (4) any event occurring after initiation of ART or after withdrawal or reduction of immunosuppressive agents including biologics.

Systemic corticosteroids have been the mainstay of treatment for DiHS/DRESS. However, because discontinuation or rapid tapering of prednisolone therapy as well as the withdrawal of the causative drugs may be a risk factor for the new development of IRIS, it should be recognized that DiHS/DRESS patients, particularly those treated with systemic corticosteroids, are at greater risk of developing IRIS, such as CMV disease (Fig. 4.3). In patients with severe forms of IRIS, anti-inflammatory therapies in addition to antimicrobial therapies are needed to ameliorate clinical symptoms due to robust immune recovery.

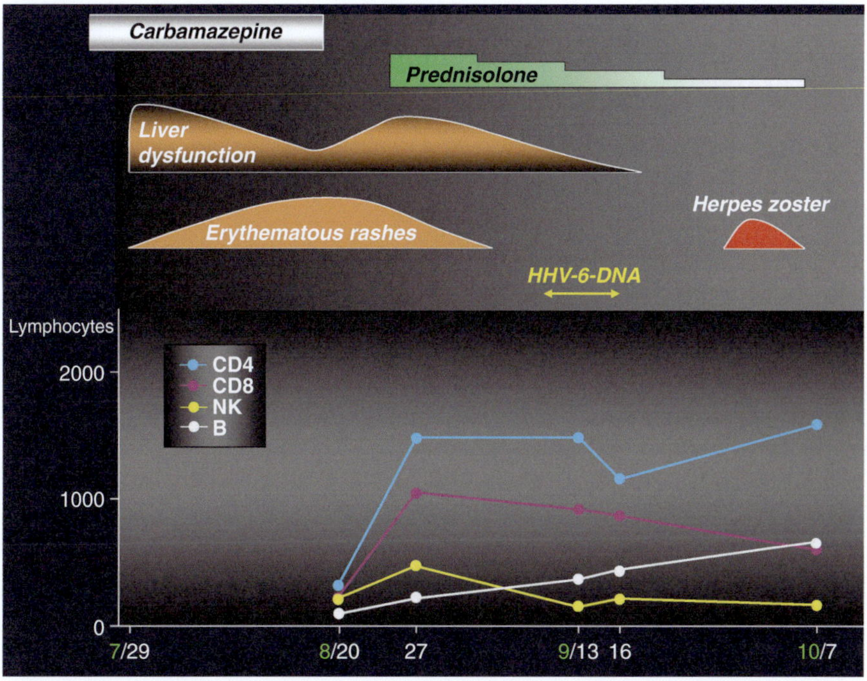

Fig. 4.3 The clinical course of a DiHS/DRESS patient representing typical IRIS. Liver dysfunction associated with a profound increase in the frequencies of these lymphocyte subsets was paradoxically induced immediately after withdrawal of the causative drug with immunosuppressive potential. Onset of herpes zoster was also coincident with the increase in the frequencies of $CD4^{+}$T cells, which appeared to be induced by the reduction of prednisolone doses

4.5 Conclusion

Most of the reactivations may be clinically unrecognized unless special attention is given. Reactivations of herpesviruses may be a causal factor in the pathogenesis of DiHS/DRESS; in many patients who develop DiHS/DRESS, there may indeed be preexisting underlying, but clinically unrecognized, sequential reactivations of herpesviruses: in other words, DiHS/DRESS may develop in the setting of antecedent or underlying viral reactivations. If viral reactivations are causal factors, the implications could open up new areas for potential therapeutic intervention in DiHS/DRESS or other severe drug eruptions: nevertheless, the desire to treat these patients with antivirals should be balanced with the need to ameliorate clinical symptoms by immunosuppressive agents. Confounding factors or reverse causality, however, offers alternative explanations for the association of DiHS/DRESS with sequential reactivations of herpesviruses, because causative drugs have been shown to reactivate herpesviruses (Asano et al. 2009).

From a broader perspective, the study of DiHS/DRESS provides a landmark example of how viral reactivations could contribute to the development of drug eruptions, vice versa. We recommend that all patients with drug eruptions be assessed for clinical signs and laboratory data suggestive of previously undiagnosed viral reactivations.

References

Asano Y, Kagawa H, Kano Y, Shiohara T (2009) Cytomegalovirus disease during severe drug eruption: report of 2 cases and retrospective study of 18 patients with drug-induced hypersensitivity syndrome. Arch Dermatol 145:1030–1036

Cros J, Cagnard N, Woollard K, Patey N, Zhang SY, Senechal B et al (2010) Human CD14dim monocytes patrol and sense nucleic acids and viruses via TLR7 and TLR8 receptors. Immunity 33:375–386

Descamps V, Avenel-Audran M, Valeyrie-Allanore L, Barbaud SA et al (2013) Saliva polymerase chain reaction assay for detection and follow-up of herpesvirus reactivation in patients with drug reaction with eosinophilia and systemic symptoms. JAMA Dermatol 149:565–569

Hoechst B, Gamrekelashvili J, Manns MP et al (2011) Plasticity of human Th17 cells and iTregs is orchestrated by different subsets of myeloid cells. Blood 117:6532–6541

Iampietro M, Morissette G, Gravel A, Dubuc I, Rousseau M, Hasan A, O'Reilly RJ, Flamand L (2014) Human herpes virus 6B immediate-early 1protein contains functional HLA-A*02, HLA-A*03, and HLA-B*07 class I restricted CD8+ T-cell epitopes. Eur J Immunol 44:3573–3584

Kano Y, Inaoka M, Shiohara T (2004) Association between anticonvulsant hypersensitivity syndrome and human herpesvirus 6 reactivation and hypogammaglobulinemia. Arch Dermatol 140:183–188

Kano Y, Hirahara K, Sakuma K et al (2006) Several herpesviruses can reactivate in a severe drug-induced multiorgan reaction in the same sequential order as in graft-versus-host disease. Br J Dermatol 155:301–306

Kurata M, Mizukawa Y, Aoyama Y, Shiohara T (2014) Herpes simplex virus reactivation as a trigger of mucous lesions in pemphigus vulgaris. Br J Dermatol 173:554–560

Matzinger P (2007) Friendly and dangerous signals: is the tissue in control? Nat Immunol 8:11–13

Mizukawa Y, Hirahara K, Kano Y, Shiohara T (2018) Drug-induced hypersensitivity syndrome (DiHS)/drug reaction with eosinophilia and systemic symptome (DRESS) severity score: a useful tool for assessing disease severity and predicting fatal cytomegalovirus disease. J Am Acad Dermatol. https://doi.org/10.1016/j.jaad.2018.08.052 (in press)

Picard D, Janela B, Descamps V et al (2010) Drug rash with eosinophilia and systemic symptoms (DRESS): a multiorgan antiviral T cell responses. Sci Transl Med 2:46ra62

Shelburne SA 3rd, Hamill RJ, Rodriguez-Barradas MC, Greenberg SB, Atmar RL, Musher DW, Gathe JC Jr, Visnegarwala F, Trautner BW (2002) Immune reconstitution inflammatory syndrome: emergence of a unique syndrome during highly active antiretroviral therapy. Medicine 81:213–227

Shiohara T, Kano Y (2017) Drug reaction with eosinophilia and systemic symptoms: incidence, pathogenesis and management. Expert Opin Drug Saf 16:139–147

Shiohara T, Inaoka M, Kano Y (2006) Drug-induced hypersensitivity syndrome (DiHS): a reaction induced by a complex interplay among herpesviruses and antiviral and antidrug immune responses. Allergol Int 55:1–8

Shiohara T, Kurata M, Mizukawa Y et al (2010) Recognition of immune reconstitution syndrome necessary for better management of patients with severe drug eruptions and those under immunosuppressive therapy. Allergol Int 59:333–343

Shiohara T, Ushigome Y, Kano Y, Takahashi R (2015) Crucial role of viral reactivation of severe drug eruption: a comprehensive review. Clin Rev Allergy Immunol 49:192–202

Sun HY, Singh N (2011) Opportunistic infection-associated immune reconstitution syndrome in transplant recipients. Clin Infect Dis 15:168–176

Suzuki Y, Inagi R, Aono T et al (1998) Human herpesvirus 6 infection as a risk factor for the development of severe drug-induced hypersensitivity syndrome. Arch Dermatol 134:1108–1112

Takahashi R, Kano Y, Yamazaki Y et al (2009) Defective regulatory T cells in patients with severe drug eruption: timing of the dysfunction is associated with the pathological phenotype and outcome. J Immunol 182:8071–8079

Takehara A, Aoyama Y, Kurosawa M et al (2016) Longitudinal analysis of antibody profiles against plakins in severe drug eruptions: emphasis on correlation with tissue damage in DiHS/DRESS. Br J Dermatol 175:944–952

Tohyama M, Yahata Y, Yasukawa M et al (1998) Severe hypersensitivity syndrome due to sulfasalazine associated with reactivation of human herpesvirus 6. Arch Dermatol 134:1113–1117

Ushigome Y, Kano Y, Ishida T et al (2015) Short- and long-term outcome of 34 patients with drug-induced hypersensitivity syndrome in a single institution. J Am Acad Dermatol 68:721–728

Ushigome Y, Mizukawa Y, Shiohara T et al (2018) Monocytes are involved in the balance between regulatory T cells and Th17cells in severe drug eruption. Clin Exp Allergy. https://doi.org/10.1111/cea.13252 (in press)

van de Veerdonk FL, Netea MG (2010) Diversity: a hallmark of monocyte society. Immunity 33:289–291

Vukmanovic-Stejic M, Sandhu D, Seidel JA, Patel N et al (2015) The characterization of varicella zoster virus-specific T cells in skin and blood during aging. J Invest Dermatol 135:1752–1762

White KD, Chung W-H, Hung S-I, Mallal S, Phillips EJ (2015) Evolving models of the immunopathogenesis of T-cell mediated drug allergy: the role of host, pathogens, and drug response. J Allergy Clin Immunol 136:219–234

Zhong H, Yazdanbakhsh K (2013) Differential control of Helios (+/−) Treg development by monocyte subsets through disparate inflammatory cytokines. Blood 121:2494–2502

Zhong H, Bao W, Li X, Miller A, Seery C, Haq N et al (2012) $CD16^+$ monocytes control T-cell subset development in immune thrombocytopenia. Blood 120:3326–3335

Using Technology to Learn About Immunology of Cutaneous Adverse Drug Reactions

5

Ryan J. Schutte and David A. Ostrov

Abbreviations

cADR Cutaneous adverse drug reactions
HLA Human leukocyte antigens
TCR T cell receptors

Key Points

- Biochemical assays can be used to measure effects of drugs on peptide/HLA interactions.
- Peptides eluted from HLA molecules isolated from drug-treated cells permit identification of immunologically relevant antigens.
- X-ray crystallography can reveal intermolecular contacts between drugs and off-targets such as HLA molecules.
- Molecular docking permits prediction of drug/HLA interactions.

5.1 Using Technology to Learn About Immunology of cADRs

Application of biochemical, biophysical, and structure-based molecular docking technologies has the potential to gain new insight into mechanisms of drug hypersensitivity (Table 5.1). Abacavir hypersensitivity syndrome is strongly associated

R. J. Schutte · D. A. Ostrov (✉)
Department of Pathology, Immunology and Laboratory Medicine, University of Florida College of Medicine, Gainesville, FL, USA
e-mail: ostroda@pathology.ufl.edu

N. H. Shear, R. P. Dodiuk-Gad (eds.), *Advances in Diagnosis and Management of Cutaneous Adverse Drug Reactions*, https://doi.org/10.1007/978-981-13-1489-6_5

Table 5.1 Technologies used to study immunological mechanisms underlying cADRs

Technology	Advantage	Limitation	References
Peptide/HLA binding assay	*In vitro* quantitative measurement of drug effects on peptide/HLA binding affinity	Dependent on established drug/HLA association, limited to drugs that bind the peptide binding cleft	Ostrov et al. (2012), Illing et al. (2012)
HLA-bound peptide elution assay	Permits characterization of HLA-bound peptides unique to drug-treated cells	HLA specificity dependent on cell lines expressing single HLA alleles or inferred from multiple HLA molecules	Ostrov et al. (2012), Illing et al. (2012)
X-ray crystallography	Permits definition of intermolecular drug contacts with off-targets (e.g., HLA)	Requires high-affinity drug binding to permit visibility of electron density	Ostrov et al. (2012), Illing et al. (2012)
Molecular docking	Permits *in silico* prediction of drug binding to specific HLA alleles, scalable	Requires experimental validation	Wei et al. (2012), Yun et al. (2014), Zhou et al. (2016)

with HLA-B*57:01 (Mallal et al. 2002; Phillips et al. 2005) and provides an example of how technology can provide evidence for mechanisms that promote immunologically mediated adverse events.

5.2 Peptide Binding Assays Show How Drugs Can Modulate Affinity of Peptide for HLA

HLA-B*57:01, but not closely related HLA alleles, is associated with abacavir hypersensitivity syndrome (Chessman et al. 2008). These data suggested that small differences between the risk allele and tolerant alleles were involved in the mechanism of drug recognition by T cells. HLA-B*57:01 is unique because it exhibits specific residues in the peptide binding cleft (Asp114 and Ser116 distinguish HLA-B*57:01 from the abacavir-insensitive allele HLA-B*57:03) (Ostrov et al. 2012). These data suggested a model in which the drug contacts the peptide binding cleft directly.

Peptide binding assays were utilized to determine if abacavir altered the affinity of peptides for HLA-B*57:01 (Ostrov et al. 2012). Using a positional scanning approach (Sidney et al. 2008), libraries of nonamer peptides were tested for their ability to compete with a high-affinity radiolabeled peptide for binding HLA-B*57:01 (in the presence and absence of abacavir). It was revealed that abacavir altered the preference for peptides capable of binding HLA-B*57:01. In the absence of abacavir, HLA-B*57:01 exhibited a preference for peptides with aromatic side chains at peptide position 9 (P9), such as Trp or Phe. In the presence of abacavir, HLA-B*57:01 exhibited a preference for peptides with aliphatic side chains (Val, Ala, Ile) (Ostrov et al. 2012; Illing et al. 2012). These data suggested a model in which the drug contacts HLA-B*57:01 in the P9 interaction site (referred to as the F pocket).

Positional scanning peptide binding assays have been used to measure the affinities of peptides complexed to HLA molecules implicated in cADRs. Peptide binding affinities to HLA-B*15:02 was not significantly altered in the presence of carbamazepine. Similarly, allopurinol did not significantly alter the affinity of peptides bound to HLA-B*58:01 (DAO unpublished). These data suggest that HLA associated cADRs result from T-cell recognition of distinct types of peptide/HLA complexes (with the drug bound in or outside the antigen binding cleft).

The positional scanning peptide binding approach permits measurement of drug effects on peptide/HLA affinity. However, it is dependent on, and limited by, the ability to assay peptide binding affinities for HLA molecules known to be associated with cADRs. This assay is informative for identifying drugs that contact the antigen binding cleft of HLA molecules associated with cADRs.

5.3 HLA Ligand Elution Assays Permit Identification of Peptides Recognized by T Cells from Hypersensitive Patients

Effects of drugs on HLA-bound ligands in cells can be determined (Ostrov et al. 2012; Illing et al. 2012). The process involves (1) purification of HLA molecules from drug-treated cells by immunoprecipitation, (2) elution of HLA-bound peptides, and (3) characterization of peptide ligands (Udeshi et al. 2008; Depontieu et al. 2009). There are established methods to conduct HLA elution studies using cell lines expressing a single HLA molecule (Shimizu and DeMars 1989), which is advantageous because it restricts analysis to the relevant HLA molecule.

For abacavir, a B-cell line expressing HLA-B*57:01 (and no other HLA molecule) was treated with the drug or vehicle control. HLA molecules from the cells were immunoprecipitated and peptides were eluted. Eluted peptides from drug-treated cells versus vehicle control were compared, revealing the sequences of self-peptides unique to drug-treated cells. A number of these self-peptides bound HLA-B*57:01 with higher affinity in the presence of abacavir. To determine which peptides were recognized by abacavir hypersensitivity syndrome patients, T-cell stimulation assays were used to identify a peptide derived from a translation elongation factor, VTTDIQKV (SPT51 976–984), as a self-peptide recognized in the context of abacavir and HLA-B*57:01 (Ostrov et al. 2012).

Similar experiments evaluated the effects of carbamazepine and allopurinol on the repertoires of peptides complexed to HLA-B*15:02 and HLA-B*58:01, respectively. Carbamazepine altered the repertoire of peptides bound to HLA-B*15:02, although the magnitude of the carbamazepine-induced repertoire shift was smaller than observed for abacavir (Illing et al. 2012). For allopurinol, peptides eluted from purified HLA-B*58:01 molecules in the presence and absence of drug were not significantly different (DAO, unpublished results). These data suggest that carbamazepine and allopurinol do not contact primary anchor positions in the associated HLA molecules. Carbamazepine and allopurinol may interact with subdominant anchor positions within the antigen binding cleft or at alternative sites including at the interface between TCR and HLA.

Technology in mass spectrometry has been improving to the degree in which it is possible to characterize HLA-bound ligands in cells expressing multiple HLA molecules (Bergseng et al. 2015). This represents a potentially important advance because analysis of different cell types would be useful for understanding presentation of cADR-causing drugs to pathogenic T cells. The cell types that present drugs to T cells are likely to be important in mechanisms of cADRs. Since cell lines expressing single HLA alleles are difficult to generate, and not necessarily relevant for disease pathology, HLA elution studies on keratinocytes (Chung et al. 2016), or other antigen presenting cells relevant to cADRs, would be expected to yield novel insights in understanding immunological mechanisms.

5.4 X-Ray Crystallography Permits Definition of Intermolecular Drug/HLA Interactions

Crystal structures of abacavir complexed to peptides and HLA-B*57:01 show the location of the drug (buried in the antigen binding cleft) and intermolecular contacts (Ostrov et al. 2012; Illing et al. 2012). The drug forms contacts (H bonds and van der Waals) with the HLA-B*57:01 at the P9 (F pocket) site and forms additional contacts to peptide directly and indirectly through water-mediated H bonds. The crystal structures explain why the drug alters the preference for P9 side chains: abacavir occupies the site where bulky P9 side chains normally protrude into the antigen binding cleft of HLA-B*57:01. Abacavir binding alters the shape of the HLA-B*57:01 binding cleft, permitting binding of peptides not normally presented by HLA-B*57:01. These data suggest a mechanism in which the drug permits presentation of peptides that are recognized as neoantigens (since the peptides do not bind HLA-B*57:01 with high affinity in the absence of drug) (Ostrov et al. 2012; Illing et al. 2012).

X-ray crystallography can answer important questions regarding drug/HLA interactions. Is the drug solvent exposed and available for T-cell recognition, or is it buried in the antigen binding cleft? Does the drug alter the conformation of HLA-bound peptides? There are technical challenges to crystallizing drug-bound HLA complexes, however. The visibility of experimental electron density for a small molecule drug depends on how tightly it is bound. For abacavir, the affinity of the drug for peptide and HLA-B*57:01 is high: the K_d for the complex of abacavir bound to VTTDIQKV (SPT51 976–984) and HLA-B*57:01 was estimated to be 0.2 nM (Pompeu et al. 2012), Fig. 5.1. Drugs that bind HLA with low affinity would be expected to result in limited visibility of electron density representing the drug from X-ray diffraction data. Comprehension of HLA-restricted drug presentation for cADRs may require analysis of multiple complexes of components involved in T-cell recognition: (1) drug/peptide/HLA and (2) drug/peptide/HLA-specific T-cell receptor (e.g., isolated from blister fluid (Chung et al. 2016; Chung et al. 2008)).

X-ray crystallography is a valuable technology that can provide unbiased experimental evidence supporting specific structural interactions between

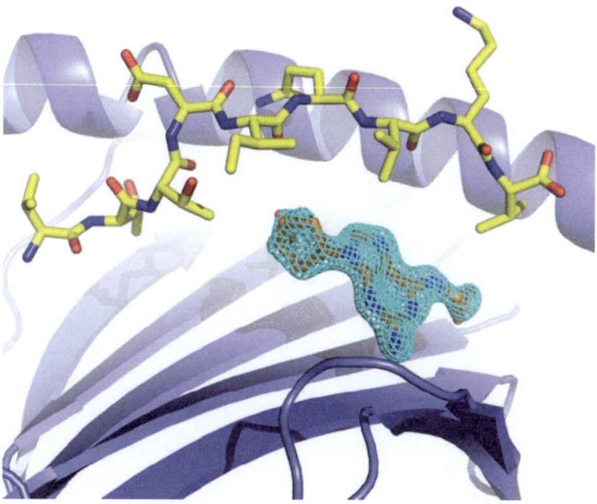

Fig. 5.1 X-ray crystallography permitted visibility of abacavir complexed to HLA-B*57:01 and a self-peptide. The crystal structure of abacavir complexed to VTTDIQKV (SPT51 976–984) and HLA-B*57:01 (PDB code 5U98) is shown. HLA-B*57:01 is shown as a ribbon diagram in violet, with the α2 helix omitted for clarity. VTTDIQKV (SPT51 976–984) is shown as sticks with yellow for carbon, blue for nitrogen, red for oxygen. An Fo-Fc difference electron density map is shown (as mesh in cyan) in which abacavir was omitted from the model

drugs and off-target proteins including HLA. It is necessary to understand the molecular components that form high-affinity complexes to generate crystals that yield interpretable X-ray diffraction data, thus limiting the scalability of this approach.

5.5 Molecular Docking Predicts HLA Interactions and Implicates Immunological Mechanisms for Specific Drugs

Since the crystal structure of abacavir complexed to HLA-B*57:01 showed that a small molecule can fit in the antigen binding cleft of a specific HLA allele, drugs and/or metabolites may be capable of binding specific HLA molecules that promote cADRs. One method to identify compounds capable of binding specific HLA alleles is molecular docking (Irwin et al. 2012; Morris et al. 2009). This computational structure-based method may be used to predict drug binding sites and affinities for any HLA molecule. Although there are important limitations to molecular docking, this method has a long history of utility in predicting small molecule interactions (Shoichet et al. 2002), including with HLA molecules (Michels et al. 2011).

Crystal structures have been solved for multiple alleles of HLA-A, HLA-B, HLA-C, HLA-DR, HLA-DQ and HLA-DP (Rudolph et al. 2006; Jones et al. 2006). Since individual sequences of HLA alleles are typically >90% identical to a solved structure, crystal structures provide the basis for the generation of high-confidence structural models. Structural models of HLA associated with cADRs have been generated and used as the basis for molecular docking with specific drugs to predict sites of interaction (PMID: 28819312).

Molecular docking of drugs to specific HLA antigen binding clefts can reveal clear predictions regarding binding. For example, small molecule drugs (mw < 500, e.g., abacavir 286.3 g/mol) have been predicted to bind HLA molecules with high affinity in the presence of peptide (Wei et al. 2012; Yun et al. 2014). Since abacavir alters the repertoire of peptides bound to HLA-B*57:01, other drugs may bind within the HLA peptide binding cleft and likewise result in presentation of neoantigens.

Prediction of carbamazepine interactions with HLA-B*15:02 suggest potential interactions in the central portion of the antigen binding cleft (in close proximity to the P4 peptide position) (Illing et al. 2012). However, carbamazepine binding within the antigen binding cleft has not been verified by X-ray crystallography or other methods. Allopurinol, and its immunogenic metabolite oxypurinol, was predicted to bind multiple sites within the antigen binding cleft of HLA-B*58:01, including the B pocket (accommodating peptide P2) and the F pocket (accommodating peptide P9). The small size of allopurinol (mw 136.1) permitted more than one drug molecule to be simultaneously modeled in the antigen binding cleft of HLA-B*58:01 (DAO, unpublished). Allopurinol (or oxypurinol) binding within the antigen binding cleft has not been verified by X-ray crystallography or other methods.

A significant limitation to molecular docking studies is the lack of information regarding the sequence of peptides relevant to cADRs. Nonetheless, molecular docking is scalable in that screening drugs/metabolites for their abilities to bind all HLA alleles is feasible. These predictions can be validated using HLA binding assays, peptide elution studies, and X-ray crystallography.

Short List of Amino Acid Side Chains

Table of amino acids and their abbreviations

Full name	Three letters	One letter
Alanine	Ala	A
Arginine	Arg	R
Asparagine	Asn	N
Aspartate	Asp	D
Cysteine	Cys	C
Glutamate	Glu	E
Glutamine	Gln	Q
Glycine	Gly	G
Histidine	His	H
Isoleucine	Ile	I
Leucine	Leu	L
Lysine	Lys	K
Methionine	Met	M

Full name	Three letters	One letter
Phenylalanine	Phe	F
Proline	Pro	P
Serine	Ser	S
Threonine	Thr	T
Tryptophan	Trp	W
Tyrosine	Tyr	Y
Valine	Val	V

References

Bergseng E, Dorum S, Arntzen MO, Nielsen M, Nygard S, Buus S et al (2015) Different binding motifs of the celiac disease-associated HLA molecules DQ2.5, DQ2.2, and DQ7.5 revealed by relative quantitative proteomics of endogenous peptide repertoires. Immunogenetics 67(2):73–84

Chessman D, Kostenko L, Lethborg T, Purcell AW, Williamson NA, Chen Z et al (2008) Human leukocyte antigen class I-restricted activation of CD8+ T cells provides the immunogenetic basis of a systemic drug hypersensitivity. Immunity 28(6):822–832

Chung WH, Hung SI, Yang JY, Su SC, Huang SP, Wei CY et al (2008) Granulysin is a key mediator for disseminated keratinocyte death in Stevens-Johnson syndrome and toxic epidermal necrolysis. Nat Med 14(12):1343–1350

Chung WH, Wang CW, Dao RL (2016) Severe cutaneous adverse drug reactions. J Dermatol 43(7):758–766

Depontieu FR, Qian J, Zarling AL, McMiller TL, Salay TM, Norris A et al (2009) Identification of tumor-associated, MHC class II-restricted phosphopeptides as targets for immunotherapy. Proc Natl Acad Sci U S A 106(29):12073–12078

Illing PT, Vivian JP, Dudek NL, Kostenko L, Chen Z, Bharadwaj M et al (2012) Immune self-reactivity triggered by drug-modified HLA-peptide repertoire. Nature 486(7404):554–558

Irwin JJ, Sterling T, Mysinger MM, Bolstad ES, Coleman RG (2012) ZINC: a free tool to discover chemistry for biology. J Chem Inf Model 52(7):1757–1768

Jones EY, Fugger L, Strominger JL, Siebold C (2006) MHC class II proteins and disease: a structural perspective. Nat Rev Immunol 6(4):271–282

Mallal S, Nolan D, Witt C, Masel G, Martin AM, Moore C et al (2002) Association between presence of HLA-B*5701, HLA-DR7, and HLA-DQ3 and hypersensitivity to HIV-1 reverse-transcriptase inhibitor abacavir. Lancet 359(9308):727–732

Michels AW, Ostrov DA, Zhang L, Nakayama M, Fuse M, McDaniel K et al (2011) Structure-based selection of small molecules to alter allele-specific MHC class II antigen presentation. J Immunol 187(11):5921–5930

Morris GM, Huey R, Lindstrom W, Sanner MF, Belew RK, Goodsell DS et al (2009) AutoDock4 and AutoDockTools4: automated docking with selective receptor flexibility. J Comput Chem 30(16):2785–2791

Ostrov DA, Grant BJ, Pompeu YA, Sidney J, Harndahl M, Southwood S et al (2012) Drug hypersensitivity caused by alteration of the MHC-presented self-peptide repertoire. Proc Natl Acad Sci U S A 109(25):9959–9964

Phillips EJ, Wong GA, Kaul R, Shahabi K, Nolan DA, Knowles SR et al (2005) Clinical and immunogenetic correlates of abacavir hypersensitivity. AIDS 19(9):979–981

Pompeu YA, Stewart JD, Mallal S, Phillips E, Peters B, Ostrov DA (2012) The structural basis of HLA-associated drug hypersensitivity syndromes. Immunol Rev 250(1):158–166

Rudolph MG, Stanfield RL, Wilson IA (2006) How TCRs bind MHCs, peptides, and coreceptors. Annu Rev Immunol 24:419–466

Shimizu Y, DeMars R (1989) Production of human cells expressing individual transferred HLA-A,-B,-C genes using an HLA-A,-B,-C null human cell line. J Immunol 142(9):3320–3328

Shoichet BK, McGovern SL, Wei B, Irwin JJ (2002) Lead discovery using molecular docking. Curr Opin Chem Biol 6(4):439–446

Sidney J, Assarsson E, Moore C, Ngo S, Pinilla C, Sette A et al (2008) Quantitative peptide binding motifs for 19 human and mouse MHC class I molecules derived using positional scanning combinatorial peptide libraries. Immunome Res 4:2

Udeshi ND, Compton PD, Shabanowitz J, Hunt DF, Rose KL (2008) Methods for analyzing peptides and proteins on a chromatographic timescale by electron-transfer dissociation mass spectrometry. Nat Protoc 3(11):1709–1717

Wei CY, Chung WH, Huang HW, Chen YT, Hung SI (2012) Direct interaction between HLA-B and carbamazepine activates T cells in patients with Stevens-Johnson syndrome. J Allergy Clin Immunol 129(6):1562–1569.e5

Yun J, Marcaida MJ, Eriksson KK, Jamin H, Fontana S, Pichler WJ et al (2014) Oxypurinol directly and immediately activates the drug-specific T cells via the preferential use of HLA-B*58:01. J Immunol 192(7):2984–2993

Zhou P, Zhang S, Wang Y, Yang C, Huang J (2016) Structural modeling of HLA-B*1502/peptide/carbamazepine/T-cell receptor complex architecture: implication for the molecular mechanism of carbamazepine-induced Stevens-Johnson syndrome/toxic epidermal necrolysis. J Biomol Struct Dyn 34(8):1806–1817

Part III

Clinical Perspectives of Cutaneous Adverse Drug Reactions

Stevens-Johnson Syndrome/Toxic Epidermal Necrolysis (Epithelial Necrolysis)

6

Jean-Claude Roujeau

Abbreviations

BSA	Body surface area
CI	Confidence interval
EN	Epithelial necrolysis
ICU	Intensive care unit
IVIg	Intravenous immunoglobulins
PNDS	Protocole National de Diagnostic et de Soins
PTSD	Post-traumatic stress disorder
SSSS	Staphylococcal Scalded Skin Syndrome
TEN	Toxic epidermal necrolysis

Key Points

SJS and TEN are severity variants of a similar process of widespread apoptosis and detachment of epithelium of the skin and mucous membranes, supporting a unifying denomination of epithelial necrolysis (EN).

- Discard so-called EM spectrum. Erythema multiforme has nothing to do with epithelial necrolysis in terms of demography, risk factors, clinical pattern, causes, prognosis, and treatment.
- Epithelial necrolysis most often (60–80% of cases) results from a *drug-specific* HLA class I restricted lymphocytotoxicity. Very rare cases can be attributed to infections (especially *Mycoplasma pneumoniae*). About 20% of cases are "idiopathic."

J.-C. Roujeau (✉)
Université Paris-Est-Créteil, Créteil, France

N. H. Shear, R. P. Dodiuk-Gad (eds.), *Advances in Diagnosis and Management of Cutaneous Adverse Drug Reactions*, https://doi.org/10.1007/978-981-13-1489-6_6

- Epithelial necrolysis is the most severe form of adverse drug reaction with high mortality in acute phase and high prevalence of severe and potentially worsening sequelae.
- Symptomatic measures in specialized hospital departments are essential for reducing mortality in acute stage. Cyclosporine A and etanercept improve survival. Follow-up is mandatory for detection and treatment of frequent sequelae, especially those affecting the eyes.

6.1 Introduction

Historically, dermatologists depended on the heritage of von Hebra (Vienna 1884): erythema exsudativum multiforme (EEM).

In 1956 Alan Lyell reported as "toxic epidermal necrolysis (TEN)" four cases of what we now recognize to be three different disorders (staphylococcal scalded skin syndrome (SSSS), generalized bullous fixed drug eruption, and "drug-induced TEN") (Lyell 1956). Earlier, two pediatricians from the United States had reported two cases of eruptive fever, stomatitis, and ophthalmia that they suspected to be infectious in the absence of medication (Stevens and Johnson 1922) (Stevens-Johnson syndrome).

After years of confusion "the waters were un-muddied" (Goldstein et al. 1987; Guillaume et al. 1987; Roujeau et al. 1987), especially by a large multinational prospective case-control study (Kelly et al. 1995). The results clearly showed that patients with SJS or TEN significantly differed from these with EEM in all aspects: age, ratio of gender, associated diseases, clinical presentations, prognosis, and causes. On the other hand, SJS differed from TEN only by the extent of cutaneous involvement (major prognosis factor) but neither by causes nor severity of mucosal lesions and sequelae (Auquier-Dunant et al. 2002). The quantification of EN (epithelial necrolysis) using the extent of lesions seems a better way to report such cases.

6.2 Clinical Presentation of Epithelial Necrolysis

6.2.1 Early Symptoms and Signs

At the very beginning, symptoms and signs are nonspecific (fever, pain, or redness of the mucous membrane, red spots on the skin). Classic characteristics are intense pain, concomitant systemic signs, rapid progression of rash, and appearance of blisters and erosions. Making a diagnosis earlier can be influenced if a high-risk medication (e.g., nevirapine) has been introduced 2–4 weeks before.

Retrospectively, the chronology of early manifestations must be carefully analyzed for determining the most probable onset ("index date"). A precise "index date" helps to avoid the frequent error of incriminating a trivial "painkiller" taken because of initial symptoms. As a protection against such bias, the "SCAR study" investigators determined the index dates blindly from information on drug exposures. In the author's opinion such bias on evaluation of causality explains the frequent implication of

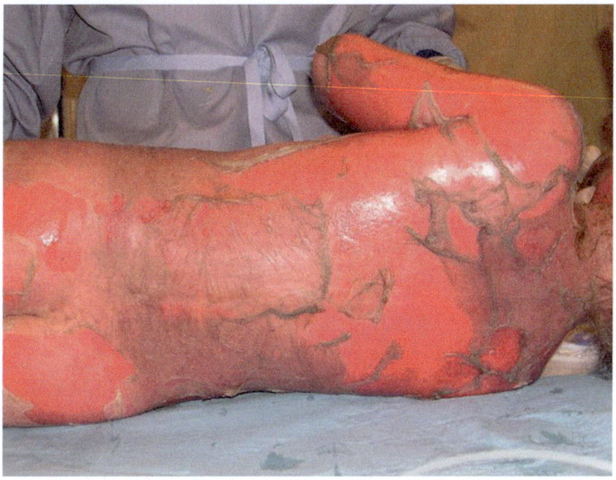

Fig. 6.1 Typical clinical pattern of skin lesions in EN

analgesics in many series and their absence or doubtful association in results from case-control analyses (Roujeau et al. 1995; Mockenhaupt et al. 2008) (Fig. 6.1).

6.2.2 On Hospital Admission

The prototypic patient with EN has a high fever, skin and mucosal tenderness and pain, blisters or erosions of the skin, Nikolsky's sign, dark purple coloration of isolated macules, inflammation, and erosions of mucosae. In the emergency department, one key decision is to determine if the patient needs an immediate transfer to a specialized department (ICU or Burn Unit).

A simple additive score (SCORTEN) has a proven prognostic value (Bastuji-Garin et al. 2000). A key part of evaluation is a correct estimation of the extent of detachable epidermis using burn tables and the "hand rule" (patient's hand = 1% of body surface area (BSA)).

Immediate transfer is recommended if the score is 2 or more and/or if more than 10% of BSA is involved (Protocole National de Diagnostic et de Soins (PNDS) n.d.; Creamer et al. 2016).

Even if a diagnosis is clinically obvious, a proper process for EN *requires documentation.*

The severity of lesions affecting mucous membranes must be evaluated, without forgetting genitalia and with a special focus on eyes that may need urgent specific intervention. The following simple grading of ocular lesions seems consensual (Sotozono et al. 2015): 0 = absence of lesions, 1 mild = conjunctival hyperemia, 2 severe = conjunctival epithelial defects OR pseudomembranes, and 3 very severe = conjunctival epithelial defects AND pseudomembranes.

Photographs of lesions help in the retrospective assessment of diagnosis and severity. A skin biopsy with direct immunofluorescence study is important for ruling out possible confounders (e.g., autoimmune blistering diseases, acute lupus erythematosus).

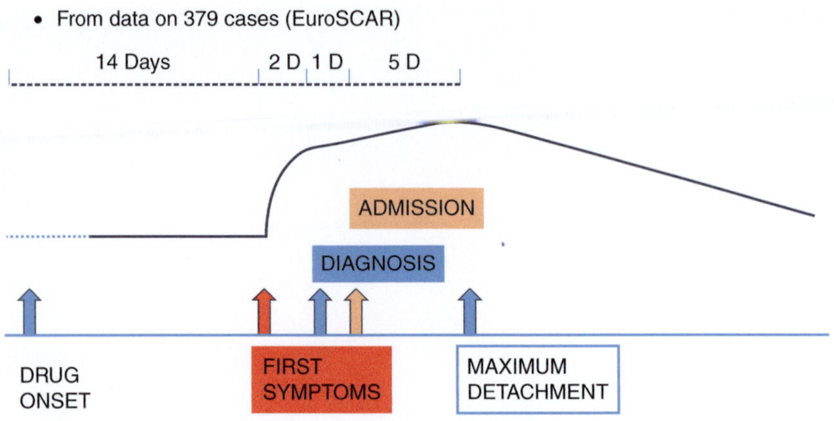

Fig. 6.2 Early events and progression in SJS/TEN

6.3 Spontaneous Evolution

EN generally has limited progression over 1 week followed by reepithelialization in 2–3 weeks if the patient survives life-threatening complications. That is essential to keep in mind before evaluating as "dramatic" the effect of any treatment in "stopping the progression."

In data obtained in 379 patients (EuroSCAR Study, Mockenhaupt et al. (2008), Fig. 6.2), the *mean* chronology was:

- From initial intake of suspected drug to first symptoms (index date): 14 days
- From index date to diagnosis: 2 days
- From diagnosis to hospitalization: 1 day
- From hospital admission to maximum progression: 5 days
- From index date to transfer to specialized settings: 5 days

Arrest in progression is not the end of the disease. Complete regrowth of normal epidermis will need at least 2–3 weeks with persistent risks for complications resulting from "skin failure" and/or infection.

6.4 Complications

Frequently they result from two different mechanisms:

1. Consequences of acute skin failure endanger life in the short term:
   (a) High losses of water, electrolytes, and proteins
   (b) Impaired thermoregulation
   (c) Colonization by pathogens and risk of sepsis

2. Direct effect of drug-specific cytotoxicity not only on epithelial cells of the skin and mucous membranes but also of the gut, bronchioles, gastrointestinal tract, bile ducts, kidney, and sweat glands. Potentially overlooked during the acute phase, such "internal lesions" may reveal as sequelae months later.

Ocular lesions are of major concern because of the high risk of progression and invalidating sequelae. Amniotic membrane transplantation (or application with a symblepharon ring) in acute phase likely decreases the severity of sequelae in case of conjunctival epithelial defects (Creamer et al. 2016).

6.5 Prognosis and Sequelae

1. *High mortality.*
2. The best overall evaluation of prognosis in "real life" was provided by a large *prospective cohort* of patients hospitalized in different wards, with different severity and treatments (Sekula et al. 2013).

   A common opinion that SJS has a benign course is erroneous and likely results from persisting confusion between EMM and SJS. In the RegiSCAR cohort, overall mortality rate was 23% (95% confidence interval (CI) 19–27%) at 6 weeks and 34% (95% CI 30–39%) at 1 year. When distinguishing by severity groups, mortality at 6 weeks was 12% (8–16%) for SJS, 29% (22–36%) for SJS/TEN overlap, and 46% (33–57%) for TEN. Corresponding numbers at 1 year were 24% (18–29%) for SJS, 43% (35–50%) for SJS/TEN overlap, and 49% (36–60%) for TEN (Sekula et al. 2013). These results evidenced a delayed mortality, suggesting the decompensation by acute EN of chronic underlying disorders.
3. *Frequent injurious and progressing sequelae*

   In the same RegiSCAR cohort (unpublished data) at 1 year after discharge, 93% of survivors complained of at least one abnormal symptom (and a mean of six different symptoms) affecting their skin, mucous membranes, hairs, nails, or even teeth. The most severe symptoms involved the eyes, including a few patients in whom no ocular involvement had been detected during acute phase. Several complaints were suggesting post-traumatic stress disorder. Daily life was considered as "severely affected" by 38% of survivors. SJS/TEN had a persisting impact on survivors' lives physically and psychologically long after the event, including a risk of post-traumatic stress disorder (PTSD) (Dodiuk-Gad et al. 2016; Lee et al. 2017; Olteanu et al. 2018).

6.6 Medications as the Cause of EN

It has been often stated that TEN is always drug-induced, while SJS was often related to infections. Both parts of the above statement are incorrect. When diagnoses are based on stringent criteria, the "etiologic fraction" of medication(s) are the same in SJS and TEN (64% vs. 65%) (Auquier-Dunant et al. 2002; Roujeau et al. 1995; Mockenhaupt et al. 2008; Sassolas et al. 2010), also indicating that up to one third of cases *in both severity variants* are likely provoked by "non-drug causes." *Mycoplasma pneumoniae* infections are a rare but definite cause of EN. Other infectious causes should be investigated.

Concerning medications, the ten "usual suspects" listed in Table 6.1 are responsible for one half of cases (i.e., the large majority of the 65% attributable to drugs). Despite this being emphasized in medical journals years ago (Mockenhaupt et al. 2008; Halevy et al. 2008), overprescription of these compounds, especially allopurinol, persists in Europe for asymptomatic hyperuricemia, leading to dozens of unacceptable deaths. With the current diversity of effective medications against AIDS, it is time to replace nevirapine with safer compounds (Table 6.2).

Table 6.1 Ten most usual culprits and ten frequently used and not associated to a measurable risk (Adapted from EuroSCAR (Protocole National de Diagnostic et de Soins (PNDS) n.d.))

Most common culprit drugs	Frequently used therapeutics with no measurable risk
• Allopurinol	• Acetylsalicylic acid (aspirin)
• Sulfamethoxazole	• Atenolol
• Lamotrigine	• Captopril
• Carbamazepine	• Digoxin
• Phenytoin	• Estradiol
• Phenobarbital	• Fenofibrate
• Nevirapine	• Hydrochlorothiazide
• Sulfasalazine	• Levothyroxine
• Oxicam NSAIDs	• Paroxetine
• Etoricoxib	• Spironolactone

Table 6.2 SCORTEN, death rate (Adapted from Bastuji-Garin et al. (2000)), and recommendations for transfer to a specialized center

Items	Items total number	Predicted mortality (%)
	0	1
Age above 40 years	1	4
Malignancy	2	12
Heart rate > 120/min	3	32
Detachment > 10% of BSA	4	62
Serum urea > 10 mMol/L	5	85
Serum glucose > 14 mMol/L	6	95
Serum bicarbonate < 20 mMol/L	7	99

Recommendation for transfer (Protocole National de Diagnostic et de Soins (PNDS) n.d.; Creamer et al. 2016): patients with detachment above 10% BSA and/or SCORTEN of 2 or more should be transferred to a specialized center (burn unit or specialized ICU). Early transfer is associated with improved survival

6.7 Mechanisms of Epithelial Necrolysis

It is now largely accepted that the acute and widespread destruction of epithelial cells results from a classical mechanism of drug-dependent, immune-mediated, delayed cytotoxicity. Effector cells are principally *drug-specific CD8 cytotoxic T cells and natural killer cells.*

Fas-ligand was proposed as a key mediator years ago to support the use of intravenous immunoglobulins (IVIg). Actually, blocking specifically Fas-ligand had no more effect on cytotoxicity in vitro (Chung et al. 2008) than high-dose IVIg in vivo on the death rate (Roujeau and Bastuji-Garin 2011). Best present evidence support granulysin and granzyme B as the main soluble mediators leading to drug-induced apoptosis of epithelial cells (Chung et al. 2008). This mechanism is quite similar to the rejection of allogenic skin graft or of the skin lesions of acute graft versus host disease.

6.8 Treatment of Acute Phase

1. *Withdrawal of suspected medication(s).* A retrospective analysis suggested that early discontinuation of the responsible medication is associated with a better prognosis. That should not lead to brutal interruption of all treatments, a possible source of rebound in basic illness. When an anticonvulsant is suspected, sodium valproate/VPA is usually considered as the safer alternative. If lamotrigine is suspected as the cause of EN, VPA is preferably withdrawn since VPA impairs the elimination of lamotrigine.
2. Recent recommendations insist *on the priority of symptomatic measures* (Protocole National de Diagnostic et de Soins (PNDS) n.d.; Creamer et al. 2016) *in specialized settings.* These measures should include a warm environment, perfect control of pain, adequate hydro-electrolytes equilibrium, continuous enteral feeding through nasogastric tube, protection of the skin with non-adhesive dressings, regular check of lesions of mucous membranes, and especially mandatory examination of the eyes by an *ophthalmologist expert in ocular lesions of EN* and of female genitalia by a gynecologist. Preservative-free corticosteroid eye drops are likely effective in decreasing the severity of ocular surface sequelae (Sotozono et al. 2015). Amniotic membrane grafts (or sutureless application with a symblepharon ring) may be necessary (Creamer et al. 2016).
3. Many *treatments* were proposed to block the progression of epithelial necrolysis, for example, high-dose corticosteroids, high-dose intravenous immunoglobulins, plasma exchanges, anti-TNF alpha, etc. *Cyclosporine A and etanercept are better options* (Gonzalez-Herrada et al. 2017; Roujeau et al. 2017; Wang et al. 2018).

6.9 Follow-Up

At discharge, the patient and family must be informed of the possible occurrence and progression of sequelae requesting follow-up at least at 6 months and 1 year and possibly further appointments.

During follow-up visits, symptoms and signs affecting the skin and mucous membranes must be assessed, especially dryness, inflammation, or pain. Patients with serious eye involvement during the acute phase must be closely followed by an ophthalmologist specialized in ocular surface disorders. Women require gynecologic examinations. In sum, the spectrum of chronic problems in patients who survive an episode of SJS/TEN necessitates multidisciplinary follow-up for assessing the physical and emotional complications (Dodiuk-Gad et al. 2016; Lee et al. 2017; Olteanu et al. 2018).

6.10 Future Use of Medicines

Identification of the inducing drug is critical for secondary prevention (occasionally also for primary prevention among first-degree family members especially if HLA associations are relevant). Drug patch tests and in vitro lymphocyte activation/proliferation tests may help, but their sensitivity is low in EN, meaning that a negative test is never enough to exclude the role of a medication clinically suspected. As long as many HLA associations are under investigation, I recommend avoidance of the suspected compound to all first-degree family members.

6.11 Primary Prevention

HLA class I associations have been observed in EN with a few inducing medications (carbamazepine and HLA-B*15:02, allopurinol and HLA-B*58:01) in specific ethnic groups (Halevy et al. 2008). Primary prevention by HLA class I testing proved cost-effective in populations where the prevalence of relevant alleles is high (Taiwan (Chen et al. 2011) and more generally Southeast Asia). But that cannot yet be generalized. Regulatory agencies indicated that patients originating from Southeast Asia should be tested for HLA-B*15:02 before prescription of carbamazepine.

References

Auquier-Dunant A et al (2002) Severe cutaneous adverse reactions. Correlations between clinical patterns and causes of erythema multiforme majus, Stevens-Johnson syndrome, and toxic epidermal necrolysis: results of an international prospective study. Arch Dermatol 138:1019–1024

Bastuji-Garin S et al (2000) SCORTEN: a severity-of-illness score for toxic epidermal necrolysis. J Invest Dermatol 115:149–153

Chen P et al (2011) Carbamazepine-induced toxic effects and HLA-B*1502 screening in Taiwan. N Engl J Med 364(12):1126–1133

Chung WH et al (2008) Granulysin is a key mediator for disseminated keratinocyte death in Stevens-Johnson syndrome and toxic epidermal necrolysis. Nat Med 14(12):1343–1350

Creamer D et al (2016) U.K. guidelines for the management of Stevens-Johnson syndrome/toxic epidermal necrolysis in adults 2016. Br J Dermatol 174:1194–1227. https://www.has-sante.fr

Dodiuk-Gad RP et al (2016) Major psychological complications and decreased health-related quality of life among survivors of Stevens-Johnson syndrome and toxic epidermal necrolysis. Br J Dermatol 175(2):422–424

Goldstein SM et al (1987) Toxic epidermal necrolysis. Unmuddying the waters. Arch Dermatol 123:1153–1156

Gonzalez-Herrada C et al (2017) Cyclosporine use in epidermal necrolysis is associated with an important mortality reduction: evidence from three different approaches. J Invest Dermatol 137:2092–2100

Guillaume JC et al (1987) The culprit drugs in 87 cases of toxic epidermal necrolysis (Lyell's syndrome). Arch Dermatol 123:1166–1170

Halevy S et al (2008) Allopurinol is the most common cause of Stevens-Johnson syndrome and toxic epidermal necrolysis in Europe and Israel. J Am Acad Dermatol 58(1):25–32

Kelly J et al (1995) An international collaborative case-control study of severe cutaneous adverse reactions (SCAR). Design and methods. J Clin Epidemiol 48:1099–1108

Lee HY et al (2017) Long term complications of Stevens-Johnson syndrome/toxic epidermal necrolysis: the spectrum of chronic problems in patients who survive an episode of SJS/TEN necessitates multi-disciplinary follow up. Br J Dermatol 177(4):924–937

Lyell A (1956) Toxic epidermal necrolysis: an eruption resembling scalding of the skin. Br J Dermatol 68:355–361

Mockenhaupt M et al (2008) Stevens-Johnson syndrome and toxic epidermal necrolysis: assessment of medication risks with emphasis on recently marketed drugs. The EuroSCAR-study. J Invest Dermatol 128:35–44

Olteanu C et al (2018) Severe physical complications among survivors of Stevens-Johnson syndrome and toxic epidermal necrolysis. Drug Saf 41(3):277–284. https://doi.org/10.1007/s40264-017-0608-0. [Epub ahead of print]

Protocole National de Diagnostic et de Soins (PNDS) (2009) French recommendations for treatment of EN (in French). Available at https://www.has-sante.fr

Roujeau JC, Bastuji-Garin S (2011) Systematic review of treatments for Stevens-Johnson syndrome and toxic epidermal necrolysis using the SCORTEN score as a tool for evaluating mortality. Ther Adv Drug Saf 2(3):87–94

Roujeau JC et al (1987) Genetic susceptibility to toxic epidermal necrolysis. Arch Dermatol 123:1171–1173

Roujeau JC et al (1995) Medication use and the risk of Stevens-Johnson syndrome or toxic epidermal necrolysis. N Engl J Med 333(24):1600–1607

Roujeau JC et al (2017) New evidence supporting cyclosporine efficacy in epidermal necrolysis. J Invest Dermatol 137:2047–2049

Sassolas B et al (2010) ALDEN, an algorithm for assessment of drug causality in Stevens-Johnson syndrome and toxic epidermal necrolysis: comparison with case-control analysis. Clin Pharmacol Ther 88(1):60–68

Sekula P et al (2013) Comprehensive survival analysis of a cohort of patients with Stevens-Johnson syndrome and toxic epidermal necrolysis. J Invest Dermatol 133:1197–1204

Sotozono C et al (2015) Predictive factors associated with acute ocular involvement in Stevens-Johnson syndrome and toxic epidermal necrolysis. Am J Ophthalmol 160:228–237

Stevens A, Johnson F (1922) A new eruptive fever associated with stomatitis and ophthalmia: report of two cases in children. Arch Pediatr Adolesc Med 24(6):526

Wang CW et al (2018) Randomized, controlled trial of TNF-α antagonist in CTL-mediated severe cutaneous adverse reactions. J Clin Invest 128(3):985–996

Drug Reaction with Eosinophilia and Systemic Symptoms (DRESS)

7

Sylvia H. Kardaun

Abbreviations

AED	Antiepileptic drugs
cADR	Cutaneous adverse drug reactions
CBZ	Carbamazepine
D(I)HS	Drug (induced) hypersensitivity syndrome
DRESS	Drug reaction with eosinophilia and systemic symptoms
HHV-6	Herpes virus type 6
LTA	Lymphocyte toxicity assay
LTT	Lymphocyte transformation test
MPE	Maculopapular exanthema

Key Points

- Compared to other drug reactions, DRESS is characterized by a relative long latency time, protracted course with relapses, and a great variability, also in time, of cutaneous and systemic signs and symptoms.
- Particularly in the early stage, DRESS may resemble other diseases and is a diagnosis by exclusion, necessitating appropriate further investigations, including laboratory examinations.
- The DRESS-score is aimed at a balanced validation of cutaneous, hematological, organ, and other features, including the course.

S. H. Kardaun (✉)
Department of Dermatology, University Medical Center Groningen, University of Groningen, Groningen, The Netherlands

N. H. Shear, R. P. Dodiuk-Gad (eds.), *Advances in Diagnosis and Management of Cutaneous Adverse Drug Reactions*, https://doi.org/10.1007/978-981-13-1489-6_7

- Although a causative role of herpes viruses in early DRESS has been speculated on, DRESS is primarily regarded an immune response to the drug, possessing an innate ability to stimulate T-cells.
- Early recognition, followed by prompt withdrawal of the culprit drug is the most decisive step to avoid disease progression, thus potentially resulting in less morbidity and mortality and restoring health.
- Mild organ involvement, pruritus, and skin inflammation can sufficiently be treated symptomatically, including supportive care, potent topical corticosteroids, and antihistamines. For severe cases with life-threatening organ involvement, especially with renal, lung, or central nervous system involvement, systemic corticosteroids can be used.

7.1 Introduction

A drug-induced clinical reaction pattern, originally noticed as the triad fever, rash, and lymphadenopathy, but later also associated with internal organ-involvement, has been described under a multitude of names, often referring to the drug involved, the most affected organ, or the disease mimicked (Chaiken et al. 1950; Kardaun et al. 1988; Prussick and Shear 1996; Lau et al. 2001; Michael and Mitch 1976; McMenamin et al. 1976; Gupta et al. 1992; Iwatsuki et al. 1984; Hicks et al. 1988; Shear and Spielberg 1988). Such ambiguity in nomenclature can be harmful for prompt recognition and treatment of this potential life-threatening but reversible pattern of drug hypersensitivity.

In 1996, the clinically relevant acronym DRESS was introduced to distinguish the syndrome from other cutaneous adverse drug reactions (cADR), not associated with systemic symptoms (Bocquet et al. 1996). In Asian countries, the acronym D(I)HS (drug (induced) hypersensitivity syndrome) was introduced for a similar syndrome. In 2007, the definition of both DRESS and DIHS was further specified and since then the acronym DRESS is gaining use (Kardaun et al. 2007; Shiohara et al. 2007). The incidence is difficult to define due to the rarity of epidemiologic studies on DRESS and inconsistencies in reporting, caused by the mentioned lack of consensus on nosology and case definition (Kardaun et al. 2007). It is estimated at over 1 per 10,000 exposers for phenytoin, carbamazepine (CBZ), and phenobarbital, and even higher for lamotrigine (Tennis and Stern 1997; Hirsch et al. 2006). Adults are more often affected and although no gender or age predilection has been observed in earlier reports, females were predominant and slightly younger, especially when related to antiepileptics and antibiotics, in a recent large multinational study (Vittorio and Muglia 1995; Kardaun et al. 2013; Cacoub et al. 2011).

7.2 Clinical Characteristics and Course

DRESS refers to a severe, idiosyncratic reaction, defined by a widespread, long-lasting edematous skin eruption, accompanied by fever, lymphadenopathy, hematological abnormalities, and visceral involvement (Bocquet et al. 1996; Kardaun et al. 2007; Kardaun et al. 2013; Cacoub et al. 2011; Knowles et al. 2000). Evolution of signs and symptoms is relatively slow and can present in haphazard combinations, also in time, resulting in an approach from different medical specialties and treatment of individual symptoms. Particularly when a single organ is dominant in its presentation, DRESS may go unrecognized as a syndrome.

DRESS commonly starts with a prodromal stage with flu-like symptoms. Fever, often accompanied by malaise or pharyngitis, cervical lymphadenopathy and "rash" are often the first symptoms (Prussick and Shear 1996; Bocquet et al. 1996; Vittorio and Muglia 1995; Kardaun et al. 2013; Knowles et al. 2000). Mild to high-grade spiking fever, ranging from 38 to over 40 °C, may persist for weeks, generating concern for an underlying infection; cultures however are negative (Kardaun et al. 2013).

The "rash" commonly starts with a morbilliform eruption on the face and upper trunk, initially often difficult to distinguish from benign drug eruptions or viral rashes. Later it extends and becomes burning/itching and erythroderma or exfoliative dermatitis may evolve (Bocquet et al. 1996; Vittorio and Muglia 1995). Reported reactions however vary and include maculopapular, urticarial, erythematous, exfoliative, lichenoid, purpuric, and eczematous eruptions (Vittorio and Muglia 1995; Kardaun et al. 2013; Cacoub et al. 2011). Blistering and sterile follicular and nonfollicular small pustules may occur, while (periorbital) facial edema presents a clue to diagnosis (Fig. 7.1a–d) (Prussick and Shear 1996; Bocquet et al. 1996; Vittorio

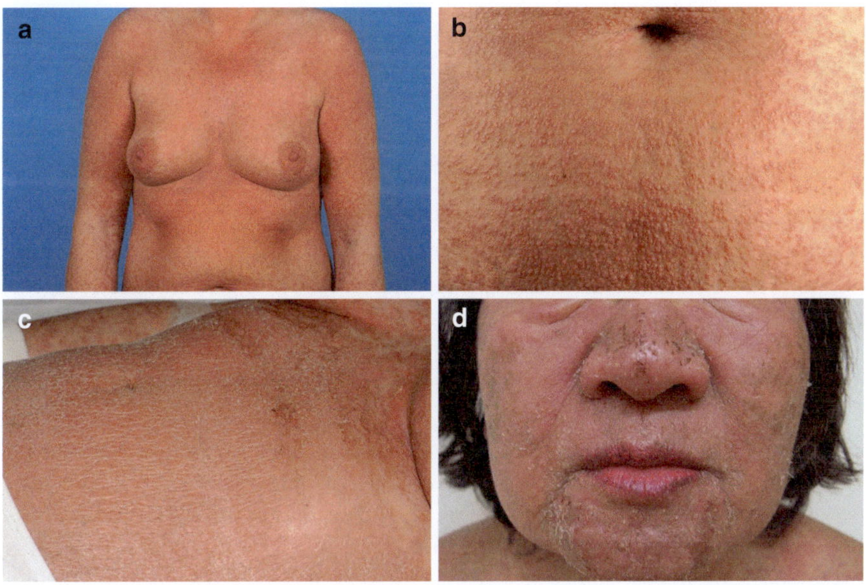

Fig. 7.1 Clinical manifestations of DRESS. (**a**) Extensive erythematous maculopapular rash with indurated papules. (**b**) Close-up of indurated papules on the abdomen. (**c**) Exfoliative dermatitis. (**d**) Facial and periorbital edema, scaling, and residual facial erythema and pustules

and Muglia 1995; Kardaun et al. 2013; Kleier et al. 1991). Enlarged, tender lymph nodes and splenomegaly are frequent (Vittorio and Muglia 1995; Kardaun et al. 2013; Cacoub et al. 2011).

Hematologic abnormalities concern leukocytosis, often with prominent eosinophilia (>700/μL), and mononucleosis-like atypical lymphocytes, predominantly consisting of CD8+ T cells (Shiohara et al. 2007; Vittorio and Muglia 1995; Kardaun et al. 2013; Knowles et al. 2000). Hyperleukocytosis can be considerable, sometimes >50,000/μL, and eosinophilia >1500/μL is regularly observed (Bocquet et al. 1996; Kardaun et al. 2013). Neutrophilia in the initial phase and monocytosis later on are frequent (Kardaun et al. 2013). Cytopenia, particularly thrombocytopenia and lymphopenia may occur, however less frequent than earlier presumed (Kardaun et al. 2013).

Visceral involvement can be extensive, most common of the liver (up to 75%), followed by kidney and lungs, whereas other organs are more rarely reported (Kardaun et al. 2013; Cacoub et al. 2011). Isolated elevated liver transaminases are common, but (acute) liver failure due to massive hepatocellular necrosis may occur, presenting a major cause of death (Chaiken et al. 1950; Lau et al. 2001; Kardaun et al. 2013; Cacoub et al. 2011; Knowles et al. 2000; Mennicke et al. 2009). After withdrawal of the culprit, paradoxical worsening of the symptoms often occurs. Particularly hepatitis, generally anicteric but sometimes presenting as hepatosplenomegaly, may worsen during weeks and may take months to resolve (Prussick and Shear 1996; Vittorio and Muglia 1995; Knowles et al. 2000). Other organ involvement includes (interstitial) nephritis or pneumonitis, heart failure (eosinophilic myocarditis), pericarditis, symptoms of the central nervous system (meningoencephalitis, sometimes complicated by SIADH), tonsillary pharyngitis, arthritis, myalgia, myositis, colitis, and sporadically thyreoiditis, cholangitis, diabetes, pancreatitis, and shock with respiratory distress and hypotension (Prussick and Shear 1996; Gupta et al. 1992; Bocquet et al. 1996; Vittorio and Muglia 1995; Kardaun et al. 2013; Knowles et al. 2000; Shaughnessy et al. 2010; Sakuma et al. 2008; Chiou et al. 2008).

Relapses of DRESS, related to viral reactivation, particularly of herpes viruses (HHV-6/7, EBV, CMV), have been described, often at a peak of 2–3 weeks after the onset of DRESS (Kano and Shiohara 2004; Tohyama et al. 2007). Relapses can also be observed after introduction of new drug(s), e.g., antibiotics for suspected bacterial infections, or rapid tapering of therapeutic systemic corticosteroids (Bocquet et al. 1996; Shiohara et al. 2007; Vittorio and Muglia 1995; Tas and Simonart 2003; Descamps et al. 2010).

The onset of DRESS is more delayed than that of other cADR, and often starts 2–6 weeks after initiating the inciting drug. Latency, however, can be shorter after previous use of the drug (Kardaun et al. 2013; Cacoub et al. 2011). Recovery is usual and total after drug withdrawal, although particularly the "rash" and hepatitis may persist for weeks, sometimes months; overall recovery has been reported at 6.4 ± 9.4 weeks (Cacoub et al. 2011). Long-term follow-up is indicated in view of reported long-term sequelae.

7.3 Prognosis/Sequelae

DRESS may cause considerable mortality and morbidity. Mortality, most often associated with older age, renal involvement, hepatitis with jaundice, and CMV reactivation, is generally estimated at up to 10% (Vittorio and Muglia 1995; Kardaun et al. 2013; Chiou et al. 2008; Tas and Simonart 2003; Ushigome et al. 2013). In particular, liver and renal involvement can be serious, sometimes necessitating transplantation or dialysis. The causative drug may also influence outcome. Allopurinol was associated with 1/3 of severe DRESS cases or a high death rate, and is regularly related to old age and poor renal function, because the kidney is important for excretion of its main metabolite oxypurinol, which has a long half-life (Cacoub et al. 2011; Peyrière et al. 2006; Eshki et al. 2009; Chung et al. 2015). Also minocycline might carry a worse prognosis (Eshki et al. 2009).

Besides post-traumatic stress, several case reports mention sequelae, months to years after resolution of DRESS: autoantibody production or autoimmune diseases, including (fulminant) type 1 diabetes mellitus, lupus erythematosus, Hashimoto's thyroiditis, Graves' disease, alopecia areata, hemolytic anemia, sclerodermiform lesions and bullous pemphigoid, particularly in those not treated with systemic corticosteroids, and end organ disease (generally renal failure) (Ushigome et al. 2013; Kano et al. 2010; Chiou et al. 2006; Chen et al. 2013). Contrarily, corticosteroids may promote HHV6, CMV, and other infections, e.g., pneumonia and sepsis, and worsening with secondary cutaneous and visceral lesions, but seem to protect against EBV reactivation and result in less autoantibody formation and autoimmunity (Ushigome et al. 2013; Ishida et al. 2014; Funck-Brentano et al. 2015).

Viral infection or reactivation and dysfunction of regulatory T cells (Tregs) during the resolution stage have been proposed to play a role in the development of autoimmune disease after DRESS (Kano et al. 2010; Shiohara et al. 2012; Picard et al. 2010).

Due to its variability, clinical markers for prognosis have not been sufficiently identified and a prognostic score for DRESS, such as the SCORTEN for SJS/TEN, could not yet be developed. However, some factors for poor prognosis have been suggested such as a high eosinophil count, multiple underlying diseases, early reactivation of HHV-6, and pancytopenia. Prognosis is generally worse in the elderly, while recovery is usually faster and complete in children (Eshki et al. 2009). Tachycardia, leukocytosis, tachypnea, coagulopathy, gastrointestinal bleeding, and SIRS were also associated with poor outcome (Wei et al. 2011).

7.4 Histopathology

Until recently, histopathology of the skin in DRESS was not extensively studied. Mainstay in the description was a substantial variability, often in parallel with the clinical appearance, with dense diffuse or superficial perivascular lymphocytic infiltrates with variable amounts of eosinophils, dermal edema, focal vacuolar degeneration of the basal layer, and occasionally band-like infiltrates, including atypical lymphocytes, and epidermotropia mimicking lymphoma (Kardaun et al. 1988; Bocquet et al. 1996; Vittorio and Muglia 1995). However, a histopathological diagnosis per se is not feasible, since the main features can generally be interpreted as a cADR nos.

Comparing patterns associated with DRESS and its severity with those in maculopapular exanthema (MPE), an erythema multiforme-like pattern is regularly found in DRESS, occasionally correlated with more severe hepatic involvement (Walsh et al. 2013). Others found severe epidermal dyskeratosis (correlated with more severe renal dysfunction), epidermal spongiosis, and severe vacuolization more prominent in DRESS (Chi et al. 2014). Recently, coexistence of several patterns and multiple changes in a single biopsy were observed in DRESS, compared to MPE; spongiosis was associated with a milder presentation, and a high number of changes and keratinocyte damage with severe DRESS (Skowron et al. 2015; Skowron et al. 2016). Another study also found coexisting inflammatory patterns, often including interface dermatitis, in a single biopsy of DRESS with many CD8+ granzenzyme B+ lymphocytes in severe eruptions (Ortonne et al. 2015).

Histopathology of lymph nodes generally shows features similar to viral lymphadenopathy or a pattern simulating lymphoma (Bocquet et al. 1996). Histopathology of other organs has rarely been reported.

7.5 Diagnosis

DRESS is a challenging diagnosis by exclusion, primarily made on clinical grounds. Complicating are its variable presentation, relatively late onset, gradual evolution, long duration, and regular relapses. Often, not all symptoms are present simultaneously and organ involvement can be asymptomatic. As a result, diagnosis can be delayed or go unrecognized as drug related.

In 2007, the RegiSCAR group proposed a validation scoring system for potential cases of DRESS. Simultaneously, the Japanese counterpart J-SCAR disseminated the criteria for DIHS (Kardaun et al. 2007; Shiohara et al. 2007). In both, validation is primarily established by clinical and laboratory abnormalities. Main difference is that for DIHS, all seven features, including reactivation of herpes viruses, are mandatory for qualifying as typical, and five for qualifying as atypical DIHS. On the other hand, according to the internal logic of the DRESS scoring system, all its features can contribute to the score, reflecting the variable character of DRESS. The DRESS-score is aimed at a balanced validation of cutaneous, hematological, organ, and other features, including the course. Features are only positively scored, when a relation to DRESS is suspected and alternative explanations, e.g., infection, are ruled out. The ultimate end score qualifies a case as definite, probable, possible, or as no case (Table 7.1). The specifics for evaluating if a parameter suggests involvement in DRESS have been disseminated in a separate document in which some rules have been agreed on, such as the minimal degree of deviation from reference values (Kardaun et al. 2013; Kardaun et al. 2014). Some state that DRESS may represent a milder form of DIHS because herpes reactivation is not a prerequisite for

Table 7.1 RegiSCAR DRESS validation score (Kardaun et al. 2007)

Score	−1	0	1	2	min	max
Fever ≥38.5 °C	No/U	Yes			−1	0
Enlarged lymph nodes		No/U	Yes		0	1
Eosinophilia		No/U			0	2
Eosinophils Eosinophils, if leukocytes <4000			700–1499/μL 10–19.9%	≥1500/μL ≥20%		
Atypical lymphocytes		No/U	Yes		0	1
Skin involvement					−2	2
Rash extent (>50% BSA)		No/U	Yes			
Rash suggesting DRESS	No	U	Yes			
Biopsy suggesting DRESS	No	Yes/U				
Organ involvement[a]					0	2
Liver		No/U	Yes			
Kidney		No/U	Yes			
Lung		No/U	Yes			
Muscle/heart		No/U	Yes			
Pancreas		No/U	Yes			
Other organ(s)		No/U	Yes			
Resolution ≥15 days	No/U	Yes			−1	0
Evaluation other potential causes					0	1
ANA						
Blood culture						
Serology for HVA/HVB/HVC						
Chlamydia-/Mycoplasma pneumoniae						
Other serology/PCR						
If none positive and ≥3 of above negative			Yes			
Total Score					−4	9

[a]After exclusion of other explanations: 1 = 1 organ, 2 = ≥2 organs
Final score <2: No case
Final score 2–3: Possible case
Final score 4–5: Probable case
Final score >5: Definite case
U unknown/unclassifiable

(continued)

Table 7.1 (continued)

Score	–1	0	1	2	min	max

Comments on Table 7.1:

Specifics for evaluation of diagnostic features in DRESS

Fever (−1, 0)

If core temperature is <38.5 °C (Fahrenheit 101.3): deduction of 1 point

Lymphadenopathy (0, 1)

Tender enlarged lymph nodes (>1 cm) at least at two different anatomic locations: 1 point

Peripheral blood:

Eosinophilia: (0, 1,2)

- Absolute eosinophilia of 700–1500 10^9E/l:1 point, if ≥ 1500 10^9E/l: 2 points
- If leukocyte count is <4000 10^9E/l: % eosinophils ≥10–19.9%: 1 point, eosinophils ≥20%: 2 points

Atypical lymphocytes: (0, 1)

If present: 1 point

Skin reaction (extent, morphology) **(−2, −1, 0, 1, 2)**

a. ***Extent rash (0, 1)*** If morphology is compatible with DRESS and extent eruption >50% body surface area (BSA): 1 point

b. ***Morphology rash (−1, 0, 1):*** If morphology is suggestive for DRESS: 1 point; if suggestive for a different type of reaction: deduction of 1 point, otherwise 0 points.

Morphology is considered suggestive for DRESS at presence of ≥2 of following criteria:

- Scaling/desquamation, e.g., exfoliative dermatitis
- Edema, especially facial edema (excluding lower leg edema)
- Purpura (excluding lower leg)
- Infiltration

c. ***Histology (−1, 0)*:**

When histology is compatible with DRESS: 0 points, when suggestive for another diagnosis: deduction 1 point;

Involvement internal organs: (0, 1, 2) For acute involvement of each organ, 1 point is given, with a maximum of 2 points. Organ involvement is based on history, clinical investigation, medical imaging, biopsy, or other tissue/fluid investigation. Organ involvement is also calculated at presence of the following abnormal laboratory values:

Liver (0, 1)

- ALAT >2 times upper normal limit (*UNL) on at least 2 successive dates **or**
- conjugated bilirubin >2* UNL on at least 2 successive dates **or**
- ASAT, total bilirubin, alkaline phosphatase (AP) all >2* UNL at least

Table 7.1 (continued)

Score	−1	0	1	2	min	max

Kidney (0, 1)

Serum creatinine more than 1.5 times above the base value for the patient on at least two successive dates, and/or proteinuria above 1 g/day, haematuria, decreased creatinine clearance, decreased GFR

Lungs (0, 1)

Cough and/or dyspnoea in conjunction with

- Evidence of interstitial involvement on imaging and/or
- Abnormal broncho-alveolar lavage fluid, or biopsy and/or
- Abnormal blood gasses

Muscle, heart: (0, 1)

- Muscle pain and/or—weakness, myocarditis (often nonspecific symptoms: hypotension, fatigue, chest pain, dyspnoea, malaise, palpitations, tachycardia, cardiac dysfunction, cardiomegaly, sudden cardiac death), with
- Raised serum creatine phosphokinase (CPK) >2*UNL
- Raised isoenzymes: CPK-3/CPK-MM (indicative for skeletal muscle), raised CPK-2/MB fraction (indicative for heart muscle involvement).
- Serum troponin T >0.01 μg/L
- Abnormal imaging: chest X-ray/ECHO/CT/MRI/EMG including ECG: ST-T electrocardiogram abnormalities or conduction defects (ST-segment depression, T-wave inversions or nondiagnostic ECG changes (paced or bundle branch block)).
- Endomyocardial biopsy.

Pancreas (0, 1):

Amylase and/or lipase ≥2*UNL

Other organs: spleen, thyroid gland, central nervous system, gastrointestinal tract

- Clinical symptoms and additional investigations: enlargement/imaging, including EEG
- Abnormal lab values: TSH, FT4, FT3.
- Biopsy

Duration: (−1, 0)

If the total duration of the reaction is ≤15 days or unknown: deduction 1 point

Exclusion of other causes, e.g., infections, virus (re)activation: (0, 1)

- *Hepatitis A/B/C*
- *Mycoplasma-/Chlamydia pneumoniae*
- *Blood cultures ≤3 days of index date*
- *Other (infections): serology, PCR, microbiological cultures*
- *ANA*

In case of a positive result for any of these, organ involvement is re-evaluated for a possible alternative cause. If ≥3 mentioned groups are investigated and no positive result is found, an extra point is given to express thorough investigation for alternative causes.

Viral (re)activation of EBV, CMV, and HHV6/7 are also recorded; results however do not influence the score.

diagnosis (Shiohara and Kano 2017). However, the DRESS score is not aimed at severity but at the degree of likelihood of the diagnosis.

The DRESS-score is nowadays frequently used as a diagnostic score (Kardaun et al. 2014). The score serves as a guideline for features to be investigated during the disease and can ascertain diagnosis retrospectively. However, because the signs and symptoms often emerge consecutively, no scoring system is suitable for early diagnosis.

7.6 Differential Diagnoses

Particularly in the early stage, DRESS may resemble other diseases and is a diagnosis by exclusion, necessitating appropriate further investigations, including laboratory examinations (Kardaun et al. 2007; Kardaun et al. 2013; Tas and Simonart 2003). Differential diagnostically one might consider other cADR including AGEP and SJS/TEN, immunologic and neoplastic disorders, acute infections including bacterial sepsis, toxic shock syndrome, acute viral infections (Epstein-Barr, hepatitis, influenza, cytomegalo, and human immunodeficiency virus), Kawasaki syndrome, Still's disease, (pseudo)lymphoma, idiopathic hypereosinophilic syndrome, connective tissue diseases, hemophagocytic syndrome, and angioimmunoblastic lymphadenopathy (Kardaun et al. 1988; Hicks et al. 1988; Tas and Simonart 2003; Bernstein et al. 1983; Potter et al. 1994; Martel et al. 2000). In SJS/TEN with systemic involvement, most often of liver or lungs, overlap with DRESS may be suggested, however in SJS/TEN involvement is generally milder (Teraki et al. 2010). Also, blistering in DRESS might suggest such overlap, but in DRESS this is caused by dermal edema and more limited and tense instead of flaccid as in SJS/TEN. Moreover, mucosal involvement in DRESS is less prominent, generally mild and not hemorrhagic (Kardaun et al. 2013). Crucial for differentiation is strict application of the case definition of both conditions (Kardaun et al. 2007; Bastuji-Garin et al. 1993). Because DRESS may initially comprise papulovesicles or pustules it might resemble AGEP. However, in DRESS pustules are less prominent, often follicular, and limited to the face and upper thorax, while a prolonged course, differences in blood count abnormalities, and severity of visceral involvement also allows differentiation (Kardaun et al. 2013).

7.7 Diagnostic Tests

In vivo and in vitro testing with the suspected drug(s) is helpful to confirm diagnosis and assign the culprit. However, testing should only be performed after resolution of the reaction and sensitivity and specificity are variable, also depending on the drug involved (Nyfeler and Pichler 1997; Santiago et al. 2010; Barbaud et al. 2013). Positive patch reactions in DRESS have been described in 32.1%, most often for antiepileptic drugs (AED), especially CBZ, while a multicenter study reported 64%, including multiple sensitization to chemical or antigenic unrelated drugs (Santiago et al. 2010; Barbaud et al. 2013).

Although a positive lymphocyte transformation test (LTT) in DRESS is regularly reported, sensitivity has not yet been established in larger series (Pichler and Tilch 2004; Kano et al. 2007). Results are markedly influenced by their timing, positivity is mainly obtained more than 8 weeks after resolution of the reaction (Kano et al. 2007; Houwerzijl et al. 1977). More sensitive peripheral lymphocyte reactivity might be yielded by measuring inflammatory cytokines, especially IL-5, through flow cytometry, the ELISA test, or a combination of both (Pichler and Tilch 2004; Sachs et al. 2002; Martin et al. 2010). The in vitro lymphocyte toxicity assay (LTA) may increase the accuracy of causality and could be used for screening potential "cross-reacting" drugs (Shear and Spielberg 1988; Sullivan and Shear 2000).

Rechallenge with the suspected culprit, even a small test dose, may result in a quick recurrence and even near-fatal reactions and should not be performed in DRESS (Bocquet et al. 1996; Cacoub et al. 2011; Brown and Schubert 1986).

7.8 Pathogenesis

The precise pathogenesis of DRESS is unknown, but appears to be multifactorial, possibly the result of a cascade of successive events on a predisposed genetic background. There is an interplay involving immunological mechanisms, drug detoxification pathways, and a genetic predisposition (Shear and Spielberg 1988; Shiohara et al. 2012). Viral reactivation has been reported in up to 60% of patients with DRESS (Tohyama et al. 2007). Although a causative role of herpes viruses in early DRESS has been speculated on, DRESS is primarily regarded an immune response to the drug, possessing an innate ability to stimulate T-cells (Picard et al. 2010; Roujeau and Dupin 2017). As such, DRESS is regarded a drug-induced delayed type IVb, sometimes IVc, hypersensitivity reaction, in which eosinophils are prominent and CD8+ cytotoxic T-cells are important effector cells.

The number of most frequent causative drugs seems to be limited (Kardaun et al. 2013). Some drugs, e.g., CBZ, possess immunomodulatory actions producing hypogammaglobulinemia preceding the onset of DRESS (Knowles et al. 2000). Pharmacogenetic variations in drug metabolism and detoxification are important and slow acetylation is probably a risk factor (Bocquet et al. 1996; Shear et al. 1986; Rieder et al. 1989; Ohtani et al. 2003). A relation between DRESS and a genetic defect of enzymes involved in the metabolic cascade of AED or sulfonamides has been suggested since long (Shear et al. 1986; Spielberg et al. 1981). After bio-transformation by cytochrome P-450, insufficient detoxification can result in accumulation of reactive toxic metabolites, responsible for the reaction. These arene oxide intermediates can bind to tissue macromolecules and may cause cell damage or cell death, or act as a hapten and provoke an immune response. Insufficient detoxification has been suggested to be based on a genetic defect for the enzyme epoxide hydroxylase. This "toxic metabolite theory" can be substantiated by the LTA (Knowles et al. 2000; Rieder et al. 1989; Spielberg et al. 1981; Leeder et al. 1988; Elzagallaai et al. 2010). Organ specificity may be due to differences in expression of enzymes responsible for the detoxification of drugs or their metabolites, alternate pathways of metabolism or immunologic reactivity (Shear and Spielberg 1988). An absolute eosinophil count over 1500/μL, regularly encountered in DRESS, is toxic to endothelial cells and may lead to cardiac, gastrointestinal, central nervous system, pulmonary, and renal dysfunction, including coronary artery thrombosis and eosinophilic pneumonias (Bocquet et al. 1996; Vittorio and Muglia 1995; Fruchter and Laptook 1981; Mahatma et al. 1989).

Relapses with fever and rash, about 2–3 weeks after onset of DRESS, accompanied by increased HHV-6 DNA and followed by increased anti-HHV-6 IgG, are frequently reported. Sequential reactivation of several herpes viruses is a phenomenon that can also be seen in immunocompromised patients with graft-versus-host disease (Kano and Shiohara 2004; Kano et al. 2006; Seishima et al. 2006; Wade et al. 1998). Immune aspects in DRESS are distinct from other cADR due to dynamic changes in the immune response during its course. In early DRESS, a transient state of immune suppression can be found, with hypogammaglobulinemia and reduced peripheral B cells, probably related to the expansion of functional Tregs, thereby possibly reducing lesion severity. This clonal expansion appears to inhibit activation of antiviral T-cells, potentially eliciting sequential virus reactivation, particularly of herpes viruses and exacerbation of clinical symptoms (Shiohara et al. 2006). In the last stage, cytotoxic T-cells become prominent and CD4+ lymphocytes become intensely diminished and depleted over time. Reduced Tregs may increase the risk of subsequently developing autoimmunity (Kano et al. 2004; Takahashi et al. 2009; Tohyama and Hashimoto 2011).

HHV-6 reactivation has been proposed to worsen the clinical course with more severe organ involvement, relapses, and a prolonged course (Shiohara et al. 2007; Kano and Shiohara 2004; Tohyama et al. 2007; Kano et al. 2006; Seishima et al. 2006). Reactivation may also include lymphadenopathy, hepatosplenomegaly, encephalitis, and severe lymphopenia, sometimes severe hepatitis and hepatic failure. Tohyama reported 5 deaths and 10 renal failures in 62 cases with HHV6 reactivation (Tohyama et al. 2007). Moreover, multiple and sequential reactivation of various herpes viruses has regularly been observed, which might explain occurrence of relapses following discontinuation of the drug.

It is further hypothesized that viral infections may induce autoantibodies against cytochrome P-450 enzymes and that reactivation of human herpes virus type 6 (HHV-6) may have potentially serious interactions with enzymes that detoxify drugs, such as cytochrome P-450 (Manns and Obermayer-Straub 1997).

7.9 Risk Factors

By definition, DRESS is drug-induced and this type of reaction was first described after phenobarbital and phenytoin, and later also after some other AED (Chaiken et al. 1950). "Cross-sensitivity" between these older AED is frequent (Shear and Spielberg 1988; Bocquet et al. 1996). Later, DRESS was also associated with sulfonamides such as sulfasalazine and dapsone, allopurinol, minocycline, mexiletine, lamotrigine, vancomycine, nevirapine, and many other drugs, often reported only anecdotally (Kardaun et al. 1988; Bocquet et al. 1996; Kardaun et al. 2013; Cacoub et al. 2011; Tohyama et al. 2007; Roujeau and Stern 1994; Knowles et al. 1996). Compared to most other cADR, the number of implicated drugs seems rather limited, with AED, especially CBZ, allopurinol, and sulfonamides, as most notorious (Kardaun et al. 2013).

Since long it has been suspected that DRESS may have a genetic background, suggesting direct involvement of HLA in its pathogenesis when the HLA molecule presents the binding site for an antigenic drug, inducing T-cell activation. Recently it was found that the HLA-B*5801 allele presents an important genetic risk factor for allopurinol-induced DRESS, especially in Han Chinese, whereas only a moderate association was observed in Europeans and Japanese (Hung et al. 2005; Kano et al. 2008; Tassaneeyakul et al. 2009; Phillips et al. 2011). In Northern Europeans, the HLA-A*3101 allele with a prevalence of 2–5% is significantly associated with CBZ (McCormack et al. 2011).

Genetic polymorphisms also seem to be a significant risk factor for DRESS. Delayed clearance and accumulation of reactive metabolites caused by genetic variants of drug-metabolizing enzymes may be one factor, and immunogenicity, such as the presence of risk HLA alleles and specific T-cell receptor clonotypes or polymorphisms in, e.g., IL-1 and IL-10 another factor in susceptible individuals, facilitating the reaction (Chung et al. 2015; Barbaud et al. 2014; Chung et al. 2014).

7.10 Management and Therapy

Early recognition, followed by prompt withdrawal of the culprit drug is the most decisive step to avoid disease progression, thus potentially resulting in less morbidity and mortality and restoring health. Introduction of new drugs should be avoided, because of the risk of flare-up, sensitization, and "multiple drug allergy."

Until now, no randomized controlled trials or consensus exist on management and therapy. Because of its unpredictable course and severity, patients should preferentially be hospitalized for monitoring, multidisciplinary evaluation, and treatment.

Although efficacy of corticosteroids, including optimal dose and duration, is still not evidenced in DRESS, many clinicians start systemic prednisolone or its equivalents at a dose of 0.5–1.0 mg/kg/day, especially for treating visceral involvement, regardless its severity. However, mild organ involvement, pruritus, and skin inflammation can sufficiently be treated symptomatically, including supportive care, potent topical corticosteroids, and antihistamines (Bocquet et al. 1996; Vittorio and Muglia 1995; Descamps et al. 2010; Funck-Brentano et al. 2015; Ghislain and Roujeau 2002). For severe cases with life-threatening organ involvement, especially with renal, lung, or central nervous system involvement, systemic corticosteroids can be used (Funck-Brentano et al. 2015). Initial prednisolon 1–2 mg/kg/day, depending on severity and slowly tapered after start of remission, has been proposed

(Descamps et al. 2010). Efficacy of alternatives, e.g., antiviral treatment, including ganciclovir and intravenous immunoglobulins has not been demonstrated and may even be deleterious (Funck-Brentano et al. 2015). Anecdotally, other immunosuppressive agents (e.g., cyclophosphamide, cyclosporine) have been suggested in therapy resistant DRESS (Descamps et al. 2010; Zuliani et al. 2005).

To prevent recurrences, it is essential to avoid the suspected medication, including cross-reacting drugs. Because cross-reactions between the older AED are frequent, non-aromatic antiepileptic drugs such as valproate, gabapentin, or benzodiazepines are alternatives.

Crucial is education/counseling of the patient and first-degree family members, not only on the precise type of hypersensitivity and the generic name of the offending and cross-reacting drugs, but also on future use of medication, including adequate alternatives, preferentially documented in an allergy passport.

Because of the prolonged course and potential long-lasting sequelae, patients should be followed after the active stage.

Disclosure *Funding sources*: None
Conflict of interest: None

References

Barbaud A, Collet E, Milpied B et al (2013) A multicentre study to determine the value and safety of drug patch tests for the three main classes of severe cutaneous adverse drug reactions. Br J Dermatol 168:555–562

Barbaud A, Waton J, Herbeth B et al (2014) Comparison of cytokine gene polymorphism in drug-induced maculopapular eruption, urticaria and drug reaction with eosinophilia and systemic symptoms (DRESS). J Eur Acad Dermatol Venereol 28:491–499

Bastuji-Garin S, Rzany B, Stern RS et al (1993) Clinical classification of cases of toxic epidermal necrolysis, Stevens-Johnson syndrome, and erythema multiforme. Arch Dermatol 129:92–96

Bernstein DI, Carney J, Cherry JD (1983) Pseudo-toxic-shock syndrome due to a drug reaction. Clin Pediatr 22:524–525

Bocquet H, Bagot M, Roujeau JC (1996) Drug-induced pseudolymphoma and drug hypersensitivity syndrome (drug rash with eosinophilia and systemic symptoms: DRESS). Semin Cutan Med Surg 15:250–257

Brown M, Schubert T (1986) Phenytoin hypersensitivity hepatitis and mononucleosis syndrome. J Clin Gastroenterol 8:469–477

Cacoub P, Musette P, Descamps V et al (2011) The DRESS syndrome: a literature review. Am J Med 124:588–597

Chaiken BH, Goldberg BI, Segal JP (1950) Dilantin sensitivity; report of a case of hepatitis with jaundice, pyrexia and exfoliative dermatitis. N Engl J Med 242:897–898

Chen YC, Chang CY, Cho YT et al (2013) Long-term sequelae of drug reaction with eosinophilia and systemic symptoms: a retrospective cohort study from Taiwan. J Am Acad Dermatol 68:459–465

Chi MH, Hui RC, Yang CH et al (2014) Histopathological analysis and clinical correlation of drug reaction with eosinophilia and systemic symptoms (DRESS). Br J Dermatol 170:866–873

Chiou CC, Chung WH, Hung SI et al (2006) Fulminant type 1 diabetes mellitus caused by drug hypersensitivity syndrome with human herpesvirus 6 infection. J Am Acad Dermatol 54(2 Suppl):S14–S17

Chiou CC, Yang LC, Hung SI et al (2008) Clinicopathological features and prognosis of drug rash with eosinophilia and systemic symptoms: a study of 30 cases in Taiwan. J Eur Acad Dermatol Venereol 22:1044–1049

Chung WH, Chang WC, Lee YS et al (2014) Genetic variants associated with phenytoin-related severe cutaneous adverse reactions. JAMA 312:525–534

Chung WH, Chang WC, Stocker SL et al (2015) Insights into the poor prognosis of allopurinol-induced severe cutaneous adverse reactions: the impact of renal insufficiency, high plasma levels of oxypurinol and granulysin. Ann Rheum Dis 74:2157–2164

Descamps V, Ben Saïd B, Sassolas B et al (2010) Management of drug reaction with eosinophilia and systemic symptoms (DRESS). Ann Dermatol Venereol 137:703–708

Elzagallaai AA, Jahedmotlagh Z, Del Pozzo-Magaña BR et al (2010) Predictive value of the lymphocyte toxicity assay in the diagnosis of drug hypersensitivity syndrome. Mol Diagn Ther 14:317–322

Eshki M, Allanore L, Musette P et al (2009) Twelve-year analysis of severe cases of drug reaction with eosinophilia and systemic symptoms: a cause of unpredictable multiorgan failure. Arch Dermatol 145:67–72

Fruchter L, Laptook A (1981) Diphenylhydantoin hypersensitivity reaction associated with pulmonary infiltrates and hypereosinophilia. Ann Allergy 47:453–454

Funck-Brentano E, Duong TA, Bouvresse S (2015) Therapeutic management of DRESS: a retrospective study of 38 cases. J Am Acad Dermatol 72:246–252

Ghislain PD, Roujeau JC (2002) Treatment of severe drug reactions: Stevens-Johnson syndrome, toxic epidermal necrolysis and hypersensitivity syndrome. Dermatol Online J 8:5

Gupta A, Eggo MC, Uetrecht JP et al (1992) Drug-induced hypothyroidism: the thyroid as a target organ in hypersensitivity reactions to anticonvulsants and sulfonamides. Clin Pharmacol Ther 51:56–67

Hicks RA, Murphy JV, Jackson MA (1988) Kawasaki-like syndrome caused by carbamazepine. Pediatr Infect Dis J 7:525–526

Hirsch LJ, Weintraub DB, Buchsbaum R, Spencer HT, Straka T, Hager M, Resor SR Jr (2006) Predictors of Lamotrigine-associated rash. Epilepsia 47:318–322

Houwerzijl J, De Gast GC, Nater JP et al (1977) Lymphocyte-stimulation tests and patch tests to carbamazepine hypersensitivity. Clin Exp Immunol 29:272–277

Hung SI, Chung WH, Liou LB et al (2005) HLA-B*5801 allele as a genetic marker for severe cutaneous adverse reactions caused by allopurinol. Proc Natl Acad Sci U S A 15:4134–4139

Ishida T, Kano Y, Mizukawa Y, Shiohara T (2014) The dynamics of herpesvirus reactivations during and after severe drug eruptions: their relation to the clinical phenotype and therapeutic outcome. Allergy 69:798–805

Iwatsuki K, Tsugiki M, Tagami H, Yamada M (1984) Infectious mononucleosis-like manifestations. An adverse reaction to sulfasalazine. Arch Dermatol 120:964–965

Kano Y, Shiohara T (2004) Sequential reactivation of herpesvirus in drug-induced hypersensitivity syndrome. Acta Derm Venereol 84:484–485

Kano Y, Inaoka M, Shiohara T (2004) Association between anticonvulsant hypersensitivity syndrome and human herpesvirus 6 reactivation and hypogammaglobulinemia. Arch Dermatol 140:183–188

Kano Y, Hiraharas K, Sakuma K, Shiohara T (2006) Several herpesviruses can reactivate in a severe drug-induced multiorgan reaction in the same sequential order as in graft-versus-host disease. Br J Dermatol 155:301–306

Kano Y, Hirahara K, Mitsuyama Y et al (2007) Utility of the lymphocyte transformation test in the diagnosis of drug sensitivity: dependence on its timing and the type of drug eruption. Allergy 62:1439–1444

Kano Y, Hirahara K, Asano Y, Shiohara T (2008) HLA-B allele associations with certain drugs are not confirmed in japanese patients with severe cutaneous drug reactions. Acta Derm Venereol 88:616–618

Kano Y, Ishida T, Hirahara K, Shiohara T (2010) Visceral involvements and long-term sequelae in drug-induced hypersensitivity syndrome. Med Clin North Am 94:743–759

Kardaun SH, Scheffer E, Vermeer BJ (1988) Drug induced pseudolymphomatous skin reactions. Br J Dermatol 118:545–552

Kardaun SH, Sidoroff A, Valeyrie-Allanore L et al (2007) Variability in the clinical pattern of cutaneous side-effects of drugs with systemic symptoms: does a DRESS syndrome really exist? Br J Dermatol 156:609–611

Kardaun SH, Sekula P, Valeyrie-Allanore L et al (2013) Drug reaction with eosinophilia and systemic symptoms (DRESS): an original multisystem adverse drug reaction. Results from the prospective RegiSCAR study. Br J Dermatol 169:1071–1080

Kardaun SH, Mockenhaupt M, Roujeau JC (2014) Comments on: DRESS syndrome. J Am Acad Dermatol 71:1000–1000.e2

Kleier RS, Breneman DL, Boiko S (1991) Generalized pustulation as a manifestation of the anticonvulsant hypersensitivity syndrome. Arch Dermatol 127:1361–1364

Knowles S, Shapiro L, Shear N (1996) Serious adverse reactions induced by minocycline: a report of 13 patients and review of the literature. Arch Dermatol 132:934–939

Knowles SR, Uetrecht J, Shear NH (2000) Idiosyncratic drug reactions: the reactive metabolite syndromes. Lancet 356:1587–1591

Lau G, Kwan C, Chong SM (2001) The 3-week sulphasalazine syndrome strikes again. Forensic Sci Int 122:79–84

Leeder JS, Cannon M, Nakhooda A, Spielberg SP (1988) Drug metabolite toxicity assessed in human lymphocytes with a purified, reconstituted cytochrome P-450 system. J Pharmacol Exp Ther 245:956–962

Mahatma M, Haponik EK, Nelson S, Lopez A, Summer WR (1989) Phenytoin-induced acute respiratory failure with pulmonary eosinophilia. Am J Med 87:93–94

Manns MP, Obermayer-Straub P (1997) Cytochromes P450 and uridine triphosphate-glucuronosyltransferases: model autoantigens to study drug-induced, virus-induced, and autoimmune liver disease. Hepatology 26:1054–1066

Martel P, Laroche L, Courville P et al (2000) Cutaneous involvement in patients with angioimmunoblastic lymphadenopathy with dysproteinemia. Arch Dermatol 136:881–886

Martin M, Wurpts G, Ott H et al (2010) In vitro detection and characterization of drug hypersensitivity using flow cytometry. Allergy 65:32–39

McCormack M, Alfirevic A, Bourgeois S et al (2011) HLA-A*3101 and carbamazepine-induced hypersensitivity reactions in Europeans. N Engl J Med 364:1134–1143

McMenamin RA, Davies LM, Craswell PW (1976) Drug induced interstitial nephritis, hepatitis and exfoliative dermatitis. Aust NZ J Med 6:583–587

Mennicke M, Zawodniak A, Keller M et al (2009) Fulminant liver failure after vancomycin in a sulfasalazine-induced DRESS syndrome: fatal recurrence after liver transplantation. Am J Transplant 9:2197–2202

Michael JR, Mitch WE (1976) Reversible renal failure and myositis caused by phenytoin hypersensitivity. J Am Med Assoc 236:2773–2775

Nyfeler B, Pichler WJ (1997) The lymphocyte transformation test for the diagnosis of drug allergy: sensitivity and specificity. Clin Exp Allergy 27:175–181

Ohtani T, Hiroi A, Sakurane M, Furukawa F (2003) Slow acetylator genotypes as a possible risk factor for infectious mononucleosis-like syndrome induced by salazosulfapyridine. Br J Dermatol 148:1035–1039

Ortonne N, Valeyrie-Allanore L, Bastuji-Garin S et al (2015) Histopathology of drug rash with eosinophilia and systemic symptoms syndrome: a morphological and phenotypical study. Br J Dermatol 173:50–58

Peyrière H, Dereure O, Breton H et al (2006) Network of the French pharmacovigilance centers. Variability in the clinical pattern of cutaneous side-effects of drugs with systemic symptoms: does a DRESS syndrome really exist? Br J Dermatol 155:422–428

Phillips EJ, Chung WH, Mockenhaupt M et al (2011) Drug hypersensitivity: pharmacogenetics and clinical syndromes. J Allergy Clin Immunol 127:S60–S66

Picard D, Janela B, Descamps V et al (2010) Drug reaction with eosinophilia and systemic symptoms (DRESS): a multiorgan antiviral T cell response. Sci Transl Med 2:46ra62

Pichler WJ, Tilch J (2004) The lymphocyte transformation test in the diagnosis of drug hypersensitivity. Allergy 59:809–820
Potter T, DiGregorio F, Stiff M, Hashimoto K (1994) Dilantin hypersensitivity syndrome imitating staphylococcal toxic shock. Arch Dermatol 130:856–858
Prussick R, Shear NH (1996) Dapsone hypersensitivity syndrome. J Am Acad Dermatol 35:346–349
Rieder MJ, Uetrecht J, Shear N et al (1989) Diagnosis of sulfonamide hypersensitivity reactions by in-vitro "rechallenge" with hydroxylamine metabolites. Ann Intern Med 110:286–289
Roujeau JC, Dupin N (2017) Virus reactivation in drug reaction with eosinophilia and systemic symptoms (DRESS) results from a strong drug-specific immune response. J Allergy Clin Immunol Pract 5:811–812
Roujeau JC, Stern RS (1994) Severe adverse cutaneous reactions to drugs. N Engl J Med 331:1272–1285
Sachs B, Erdmann S, Malte Baron J et al (2002) Determination of interleukin-5 secretion from drug-specific activated ex vivo peripheral blood mononuclear cells as a test system for the in vitro detection of drug sensitisation. Clin Exp Allergy 32:736–744
Sakuma K, Kano Y, Fukuhara M, Shiohara T (2008) Syndrome of inappropriate secretion of antidiuretic hormone associated with limbic encephalitis in a patient with drug-induced hypersensitivity syndrome. Clin Exp Dermatol 33:287–290
Santiago F, Gonçalo M, Vieira R et al (2010) Epicutaneous patch testing in drug hypersensitivity syndrome (DRESS). Contact Dermatitis 62:47–53
Seishima M, Yamanaka S, Fujisawa T et al (2006) Reactivation of human herpesvirus (HHV) family members other than HHV-6 in drug-induced hypersensitivity syndrome. Br J Dermatol 155:344–349
Shaughnessy KK, Bouchard SM, Mohr MR et al (2010) Minocycline-induced drug reaction with eosinophilia and systemic symptoms (DRESS) syndrome with persistent myocarditis. J Am Acad Dermatol 62:315–318
Shear NH, Spielberg SP (1988) Anticonvulsant hypersensitivity syndrome. In vitro assessment of risk. J Clin Invest 82:1826–1832
Shear N, Spielberg S, Grant D et al (1986) Differences in metabolism of sulfonamides predisposing to idiosyncratic toxicity. Ann Intern Med 105:179–184
Shiohara T, Kano Y (2017) Drug reaction with eosinophilia and systemic symptoms (DRESS): incidence, pathogenesis and management. Expert Opin Drug Saf 16:139–147
Shiohara T, Inaoka M, Kano Y (2006) Drug-induced hypersensitivity syndrome (DIHS): a reaction induced by a complex interplay among herpesviruses and antiviral and antidrug immune responses. Allergol Int 55:1–8
Shiohara T, Iijima M, Ikezawa Z, Hashimoto K (2007) The diagnosis of a DRESS syndrome has been sufficiently established on the basis of typical clinical features and viral reactivations. Br J Dermatol 156:1083–1084
Shiohara T, Kano Y, Takahashi R et al (2012) Drug-induced hypersensitivity syndrome: recent advances in the diagnosis, pathogenesis and management. Chem Immunol Allergy 97:122–138
Skowron F, Bensaid B, Balme B et al (2015) Drug reaction with eosinophilia and systemic symptoms (DRESS): clinicopathological study of 45 cases. J Eur Acad Dermatol Venereol 29:2199–2205
Skowron F, Bensaid B, Balme B et al (2016) Comparative histological analysis of drug-induced maculopapular exanthema and DRESS. J Eur Acad Dermatol Venereol 30:2085–2090
Spielberg S, Gordon G, Blake D et al (1981) Anticonvulsant toxicity in vitro: possible role of arene oxides. J Pharmacol Exp Ther 217:386–389
Sullivan JR, Shear NH (2000) What are some of the lessons learnt from in vitro studies of severe unpredictable drug reactions? Br J Dermatol 142:205–207
Takahashi R, Kano Y, Yamazaki Y et al (2009) Defective regulatory T cells in patients with severe drug eruptions: timing of the dysfunction is associated with the pathological phenotype and outcome. J Immunol 182:8071–8079
Tas S, Simonart T (2003) Management of drug rash with eosinophilia and systemic symptoms (DRESS syndrome): an update. Dermatology 206:353–356

Tassaneeyakul W, Jantararoungtong T, Chen P et al (2009) Strong association between HLA-B*5801 and allopurinol-induced Stevens-Johnson syndrome and toxic epidermal necrolysis in a Thai population. Pharmacogenet Genomics 19:704–709

Tennis P, Stern R (1997) Risk of serious cutaneous disorders after initiation of use of phenytoin, carbamazepine, or sodium valproate: a record linkage study. Neurology 49:542–546

Teraki Y, Shibuya M, Izaki S (2010) Stevens-Johnson syndrome and toxic epidermal necrolysis due to anticonvulsants share certain clinical and laboratory features with drug-induced hypersensitivity syndrome, despite differences in cutaneous presentations. Clin Exp Dermatol 35:723–728

Tohyama M, Hashimoto K (2011) New aspects of drug-induced hypersensitivity syndrome. J Dermatol 38:222–228

Tohyama M, Hashimoto K, Yasukawa M et al (2007) Association of human herpesvirus 6 reactivation with the flaring and severity of drug-induced hypersensitivity syndrome. Br J Dermatol 157:934–940

Ushigome Y, Kano Y, Ishida T et al (2013) Short- and long-term outcomes of 34 patients with drug-induced hypersensitivity syndrome in a single institution. J Am Acad Dermatol 68:721–728

Vittorio CC, Muglia JJ (1995) Anticonvulsant hypersensitivity syndrome. Arch Intern Med 155:2285–2290

Wade AW, McDonald AT, Acott PD et al (1998) Human herpes virus-6 or Epstein-Barr virus infection and acute allograft rejection in pediatric kidney transplant recipients: greater risk for immunologically naive recipients. Transplant Proc 30:2091–2093

Walsh S, Diaz-Cano S, Higgins E et al (2013) Drug reaction with eosinophilia and systemic symptoms: is cutaneous phenotype a prognostic marker for outcome? A review of clinicopathological features of 27 cases. Br J Dermatol 168:391–401

Wei CH, Chung-Yee Hui R, Chang CJ et al (2011) Identifying prognostic factors for drug rash with eosinophilia and systemic symptoms (DRESS). Eur J Dermatol 21:930–937

Zuliani E, Zwahlen H, Gilliet F, Marone C (2005) Vancomycin-induced hypersensitivity reaction with acute renal failure: resolution following cyclosporine treatment. Clin Nephrol 64:155–158

Acute Generalized Exanthematous Pustulosis

8

Sima Halevy

Abbreviations

AGEP	Acute generalized exanthematous pustulosis
ALEP	Acute localized exanthematous pustulosis
DRESS	Drug reaction with eosinophilia and systemic symptoms
GPP	Generalized pustular psoriasis
HLA	Human leukocyte antigen
IL36-Ra	IL-36 receptor antagonist
NSAID	Non-steroidal anti-inflammatory drug
SCAR	Severe cutaneous adverse reaction
TEN	Toxic epidermal necrolysis

Key Points

Acute generalized exanthematous pustulosis (AGEP) is a rare, severe, pustular reaction pattern, attributed mainly to drugs. It is characterized by typical morphology, unique histology, and a rapid clinical course.

The skin manifestations in AGEP are usually associated with fever and leukocytosis, mostly due to elevated neutrophil count. Involvement of the internal organs is usually not found. In most cases AGEP has a favorable prognosis.

A remarkable clinical and histological similarity exists between AGEP and pustular psoriasis. The AGEP validation score (EuroSCAR group criteria) is a useful tool for establishing the diagnosis.

S. Halevy
Faculty of Health Sciences, Ben-Gurion University of the Negev, Beer-Sheva, Israel
e-mail: halevy@bgu.ac.il

N. H. Shear, R. P. Dodiuk-Gad (eds.), *Advances in Diagnosis and Management of Cutaneous Adverse Drug Reactions*, https://doi.org/10.1007/978-981-13-1489-6_8

AGEP is mediated by drug-specific T-cells (CD4+ and CD8+) that may orchestrate a neutrophil-mediated inflammatory reaction in the skin due to massive release of additional inflammatory cytokines/chemokines and by drug-specific cytotoxicity.

8.1 Introduction

Acute generalized exanthematous pustulosis (AGEP) is a rare pustular severe cutaneous adverse reaction (SCAR), attributed mainly to drugs, although other trigger factors have been implicated (Roujeau et al. 1991; Sidoroff et al. 2001).

The term AGEP was introduced into the literature by Beylot et al. in (1980). Pustular rashes, similar or identical clinically to AGEP, have been described previously in the literature as toxic pustuloderma or generalized pustular drug rash/eruption (Macmillan 1973; Staughton et al. 1984; Bissonnette et al. 1992; Lazarov et al. 1998).

8.2 Epidemiology

8.2.1 Incidence

The estimated incidence of AGEP is 1–5 cases per million per year (Sidoroff et al. 2001).

8.2.2 Age

AGEP can occur at any age (Sidoroff et al. 2001). The mean age ranges between 37.6 (±19.4) and 56 years (Davidovici et al. 2008; Chang et al. 2008; Choi et al. 2010; Alniemi et al. 2017; Sidoroff et al. 2007).

8.2.3 Gender

Female predominance was documented in various studies of AGEP (Davidovici et al. 2008; Chang et al. 2008; Choi et al. 2010; Alniemi et al. 2017; Sidoroff et al. 2007; Tamir et al. 2006; Halevy 2009). The reported ratio of male/female was 0.8 (Sidoroff et al. 2007), 0.89 (Choi et al. 2010), and 0.36 (Halevy 2009).

8.2.4 Seasonality

A trend for seasonality has been suggested in a small series, but further studies are needed (Davidovici et al. 2008).

8.3 Clinical and Laboratory Findings

8.3.1 Morphology

The typical morphology of AGEP consists of the acute appearance of edematous erythema, followed by dozens of small, superficial, non-follicular, sterile pustules with a predilection for the big folds or with widespread distribution (Fig. 8.1). Involvement of mucous membranes may be present in about 20% of the cases. Mucous membrane involvement is mostly mild and nonerosive and is limited to one region (mostly oral). Uncommon findings such as face edema, purpura, "atypical" target lesions, and blisters may occur (Roujeau et al. 1991; Sidoroff et al. 2001; Beylot et al. 1996).

Such atypical findings may be responsible for the rare occurrence of overlap cases between AGEP and toxic epidermal necrolysis (TEN) or hypersensitivity syndrome/drug reaction with eosinophilia and systemic symptoms (DRESS) (Cohen et al. 2001; Goh et al. 2008; Meiss et al. 2007; Son et al. 2008; Lateef et al. 2009; Bouvresse et al. 2012). Acute *localized* exanthematous pustulosis (ALEP) has been described, but its relation to AGEP is not clear (Rastogi et al. 2009; Betto et al. 2008).

8.3.2 Systemic Symptoms and Laboratory Findings

The skin manifestations in AGEP are usually associated with systemic symptoms, mainly fever (above 38 °C). A burning or itching sensation (Roujeau et al. 1991; Sidoroff et al. 2001) and lymphadenopathy (Eeckhout et al. 1997; Syrigou et al. 2015) may be present. The clinical manifestations are usually associated with leukocytosis (>10,000/μL) mostly due to elevated neutrophil count (>7000/μL) (Goh et al. 2008; Meiss et al. 2007; Son et al. 2008). Mild eosinophilia can be present in

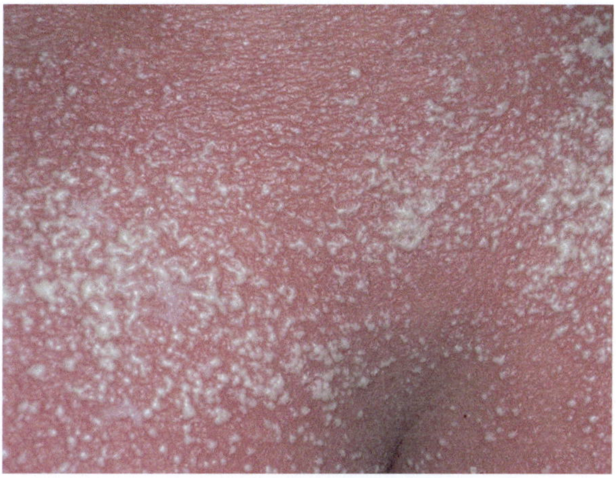

Fig. 8.1 Diffuse erythema and dozens of pustules on the trunk

about one third of the cases (Roujeau et al. 1991). High levels of C-reactive protein (Chang et al. 2008; Choi et al. 2010; Hotz et al. 2013) and hypocalcemia (probably due to hypoalbuminemia) (Roujeau et al. 1991; Hotz et al. 2013) have been recorded. Other deviations in laboratory tests include a slight reduction in creatinine clearance and a mild elevation of aminotransferases (Roujeau et al. 1991; Sidoroff et al. 2001).

Involvement of the internal organs is usually not found. However, two studies revealed internal organ involvement in 17% and 75% of the patients, respectively, manifested by hepatic dysfunction, renal insufficiency, respiratory distress, and bone marrow involvement with agranulocytosis (Alniemi et al. 2017; Hotz et al. 2013).

8.3.3 Course

AGEP is characterized by a rapid clinical course with an acute onset of skin signs and spontaneous resolution within 15 days (after withdrawal of the culprit drugs). Resolution of pustules is typically followed by a characteristic post-pustular pinpoint desquamation (Roujeau et al. 1991; Sidoroff et al. 2001; Alniemi et al. 2017).

8.3.4 Prognosis

AGEP has a favorable prognosis and the reported mortality is 5% (Roujeau 2005). However, secondary infection and the occurrence of high fever might endanger patients in poor medical condition (Roujeau et al. 1991). A recurrence of AGEP can follow reintroduction of the causative drug (Belda and Ferrolla 2005; Bracke et al. 2009; Park et al. 2010). Generalized skin eruptions or dermatitis occurred in a few cases weeks to months after the resolution of AGEP (Alniemi et al. 2017).

8.4 Histopathology

A systematic description of the histopathological features in AGEP, based on a standardized grading system, was reported in a multinational histopathological study of 102 cases of AGEP (Halevy et al. 2010). The histopathological features of AGEP consisted of sub-/intracorneal (41%) and/or intraepidermal pustules (20%) or a combination of them. The pustules were usually large (>15 keratinocytes) and contained eosinophils. Spongiform features were less prominent in the sub-/intracorneal pustules compared with the intraepidermal pustules. The main epidermal features were necrotic keratinocytes (67%), including incidental segmental necrosis, and spongiosis (80%) with neutrophil exocytosis (77%). The main dermal features were papillary edema (88%) and mixed superficial (100%), interstitial (93%), and mid/deep-dermal infiltrates (95%) containing neutrophils (100%) and eosinophils (81%).

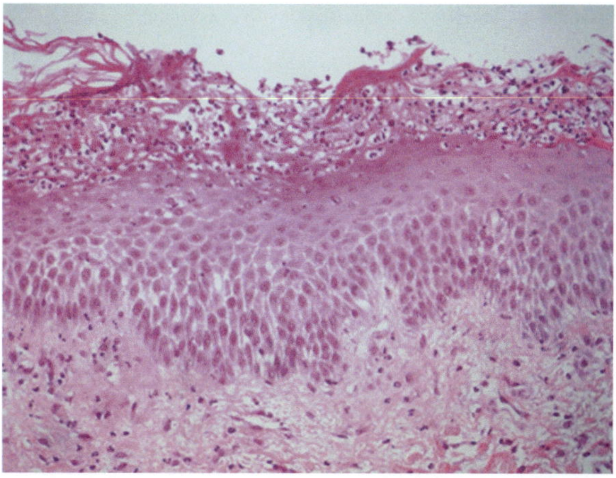

Fig. 8.2 A superficial intraepidermal spongiform pustule, slight spongiosis, and sparse eosinophils in the superficial dermis (hematoxylin-eosin stain) (Courtesy of Dr. Janine Wechsler, Henri-Mondor Hospital, Paris, France)

Classical features of plaque-type psoriasis were infrequent (up to 17% of the patients) and usually mild (Fig. 8.2).

Differentiating AGEP from generalized pustular psoriasis (GPP) histopathologically may be difficult. Proposed discriminating features in favor of AGEP include the presence of eosinophils, necrotic keratinocytes, a mixed interstitial and mid-dermal perivascular infiltrate, and the absence of tortuous or dilated blood vessels (Kardaun et al. 2010).

8.4.1 Immunohistochemical Studies

A comparison between AGEP and pustular psoriasis was done by immunohistochemical studies based on Ki-67 immunostaining (Chang et al. 2010) and on IL-36 and the IL-23/Th17 axis (Song et al. 2016). The results of these studies imply that common pathological mechanisms might exist in GPP and AGEP.

8.4.2 Diagnosis: The AGEP Validation Score

The AGEP validation score was developed by the EuroSCAR study group (Sidoroff et al. 2001) and has become an accepted tool for the diagnosis of AGEP (Halevy 2009). It is a standardized scoring system based on the morphology of the skin lesions, the course of the disease, and the histopathology. The score enables determination of the diagnosis on the following scale: no AGEP, possible AGEP, probable AGEP, and definite AGEP (Sidoroff et al. 2001) (Table 8.1).

Table 8.1 The AGEP validation score developed by the EuroSCAR study group (Sidoroff et al. 2001)

Morphology		
Pustules	Typical	+2
	Compatible	+1
	Insufficient	0
Erythema	Typical	+2
	Compatible	+1
	Insufficient	0
Distribution/pattern	Typical	+2
	Compatible	+1
	Insufficient	0
Post-pustular desquamation	Yes	+1
	No/insufficient	0
Morphology score: 0 to +7		
Course		
Mucosal involvement	Yes	−2
	No	0
Acute onset (≤10 days)	Yes	0
	No	−2
Resolution ≤ 15 days	Yes	0
	No	−4
Fever ≥38°C	Yes	+1
	No	0
Polymorphonuclear cells ≥ 7000/μL	Yes	+1
	No	0
Course score: −8 to +2		
Skin histology		
Other diseases		−10
Not representative/no histology		0
Exocytosis of polymorphonuclear cells		+1
Subcorneal and/or intraepidermal non-spongiform or NOS pustule(s) with papillary edema or subcorneal and/or intraepidermal spongiform or NOS pustule(s) without papillary edema		+2
Spongiform subcorneal and/or intraepidermal pustule(s) with papillary edema		+3
Skin histology score: −10 to +3		
Total score		
≤0: No AGEP		
1–4: Possible AGEP		
5–7: Probable AGEP		
8–12: Definite AGEP		

NOS not otherwise specified

8.5 Differential Diagnosis

The differential diagnosis of AGEP may include a large variety of rashes and skin diseases with sterile pustules, mainly non-follicular, such as pustular psoriasis, subcorneal pustular dermatosis (Sneddon-Wilkinson), pustular vasculitis, DRESS, and others.

8.5.1 AGEP and Pustular Psoriasis

Differentiation between AGEP and pustular psoriasis (von Zumbusch type) may be a challenge (Paradisi et al. 2008). The resemblance between these two entities has led some authors to classify AGEP as an exanthematic pustular psoriasis (a variant of GPP), triggered by drugs or infections (Baker and Ryan 1968; Burrows and Russell Jones 1993; Spencer et al. 1994).

Clinically, both AGEP and GPP are characterized by dozens of pustules, which are usually small, superficial, sterile, non-follicular, and located on edematous erythema and show widespread distribution. However, the short course of AGEP (less than 15 days) as opposed to GPP is a major clue to the differential diagnosis (Sidoroff et al. 2001).

The histopathology of AGEP and GPP is often indistinguishable (Roujeau et al. 1991; Beylot et al. 1996). Histopathological clues in favor of AGEP have been proposed (Halevy et al. 2010; Kardaun et al. 2010). Currently, there is support for the concept that AGEP and GPP are two distinct entities and the resemblance between the two may ensue from a common pathogenesis associated with neutrophil-attracting mechanisms.

8.6 Etiology

AGEP is attributed mainly to the ingestion of drugs (90% of the cases), although the role of other causes has been reported (Roujeau et al. 1991; Chang et al. 2008).

8.6.1 Drugs

Based on case reports or small series, a large variety of drugs, both systemic and topical, were associated with AGEP. The main culprit drugs were antibacterial, mostly β-lactam and macrolide antimicrobials (Roujeau et al. 1991; Sidoroff et al. 2001; Alniemi et al. 2017; Beylot et al. 1996; Paradisi et al. 2008; Smeets et al. 2016).

The causative role of corticosteroids also has been reported (Bar et al. 2008; Buettiker et al. 2006). Strong evidence for the role of drugs in AGEP was derived from the results of a large-scale multinational case-control study (the EuroSCAR study), comprised of 97 validated AGEP cases and 1509 controls. Highly suspected drugs for AGEP were prestinomycin, ampicillin/amoxicillin, quinolones, (hydroxy)chloroquine, anti-infective sulfonamides, terbinafine, and diltiazem. Other drugs with less strong associations with AGEP were corticosteroids, macrolides, oxicam non-steroidal anti-inflammatory drugs (NSAIDs), and antiepileptic drugs (Sidoroff et al. 2007).

Other culprit drugs include terazosin hydrochloride, omeprazole, sennoside, imatinib (Speck et al. 2008; Nantes Castillejo et al. 2008; Sugita et al. 2008), herbal medications (Choi et al. 2010; Pennisi 2006), lacquers (Choi et al. 2010; Park and Kang 2008), radiocontrast media (Choi et al. 2010), dihydrocodeine phosphate (Nakai et al. 2015), and fluconazole (Di Lernia and Ricci 2015).

The latency period (the time interval from drug intake to the appearance of a drug reaction) in most reported cases of AGEP was short: 2–3 days or 1–5 days (Roujeau et al. 1991; Sidoroff et al. 2001; Sidoroff et al. 2007; Beylot et al. 1996). The EuroSCAR study showed that the latency period can vary for different drugs. A short latency period of 1 day (median) was recorded for antibiotics, including sulphonamides, whereas for other drugs the latency period was 11 days (Sidoroff et al. 2007). The presence of an underlying malignancy may increase the latency period in AGEP for up to 1–3 months or 1 year (Sugita et al. 2008; Schwarz et al. 2002).

8.6.2 Contact Sensitivity

Hypersensitivity to mercury was reported (Roujeau et al. 1991; Sidoroff et al. 2001; Lerch and Bircher 2004) and supported by positive patch test reactions to mercury (Belhadjali et al. 2008).

The role of contact sensitivity to bufexamac as a cause of AGEP was supported by a positive withdrawal test and a positive patch test (Belhadjali et al. 2008). It appears that contact sensitivity to topical agents does play an etiological role in AGEP, but the evidence is scarce.

8.6.3 Infections

The role of infections in the induction of AGEP has been implied in case reports. The following pathogens were reported: Coxsackie B4 (Feio et al. 1997), cytomegalovirus (Haro-Gabaldon et al. 1996), parvovirus B19 (Lee et al. 2014; Ofuji and Yamamoto 2007), mycoplasma pneumonia (Lim and Lim 2009; Taguchi et al. 2016), chlamydia (Manzano et al. 2006), *Escherichia coli* (Klein et al. 2009), and echinococcus (Cannistraci et al. 2003).

On the other hand, based on the EuroSCAR study, infection was not a significant risk factor in AGEP (Sidoroff et al. 2007). One publication reported a combined etiology manifested by reactivation of parvovirus B19 infection and intake of drug (amoxicillin) in the induction of AGEP (Calistru et al. 2012).

8.6.4 Spider Bite

The role of spider bite as a new etiology of AGEP was reported in a series of three definite AGEP cases from Israel (Davidovici et al. 2006). The latency period for the appearance of AGEP following the spider bite was 24–48 h. It was hypothesized that sphingomyelinase in the spider venom stimulates the production of cytokines involved in the pathogenesis of AGEP (Davidovici et al. 2006; Hogan et al. 2004). After this report, another ten cases of AGEP triggered by a spider bite were reported in other countries, further supporting the role of spider bite in the etiology of AGEP (Makris et al. 2009; Ermertcan et al. 2010; Ben Said et al. 2010; Lane et al. 2011; Bhat et al. 2015; Milman Lde et al. 2016).

8.6.5 Psoriasis

A personal history or a family history of psoriasis has been recorded in a small percentage of AGEP cases, suggesting that AGEP is a reaction pattern that may be favored by a "psoriatic background" (Roujeau et al. 1991; Yamamoto and Minatohara 1997). However, the percentage of patients with a personal or family history of psoriasis did not differ significantly between AGEP cases and controls (Chang et al. 2008; Sidoroff et al. 2007). A common genetic background, related to neutrophil-attracting mechanisms, may explain the coexistence of AGEP and psoriasis.

8.6.6 Other Factors

There is a small amount of evidence in support of a causative role for an underlying malignancy (Bracke et al. 2009; Sugita et al. 2008; Schwarz et al. 2002; Scott et al. 2015), atopy (Belhadjali et al. 2008), and pregnancy (Matsumoto et al. 2008; Matsushita et al. 2012; De Cruz et al. 2015) in the induction of AGEP, although the most commonly incriminated agents were drugs.

Various systemic diseases and labors were recorded in 36 patients prior to the eruption of AGEP, but their role in its induction was not clear (Choi et al. 2010). In 36% of the patients, the etiology was reported as unknown (Choi et al. 2010).

8.7 Pathogenesis

8.7.1 Immune Mechanisms

AGEP is mediated by drug-specific T-cells (CD4+ and CD8+) that may orchestrate a neutrophil-mediated inflammatory reaction in the skin due to massive release of additional inflammatory cytokines/chemokines and by drug-specific cytotoxicity.

It has been shown that the production of interleukin-8 (IL-8, CXCL8), a potent neutrophil-attracting chemokine, by drug-specific T-cells is significantly increased in patients with AGEP. CXCL8/IL-8 plays a major rule in the formation of the sterile pustular eruption of AGEP by recruitment of neutrophils (Britschgi and Pichler 2002; Britschgi et al. 2001; Schmid et al. 2002; Schaerli et al. 2004; Padial et al. 2004; Kabashima et al. 2011).

Drug-specific CXCL8-producing T-cell clones obtained from AGEP patients displayed a Th1-type cytokine profile with high levels of interferon-gamma, granulocyte-macrophage colony-stimulating factor and various levels of tumor necrosis factors alpha. Rarely, high levels of Th2-type cytokines were recorded (Britschgi and Pichler 2002; Britschgi et al. 2001; Schmid et al. 2002).

Furthermore, Th17 cells and the cytokines IL-17 and IL-22 cooperatively stimulated keratinocytes to produce IL-8 (Kabashima et al. 2011).

A deficiency in the IL-36 receptor antagonist (IL36-Ra) recorded in some AGEP patients may lead to increased expression of various pro-inflammatory cytokines and chemokines and can further enhance neutrophilic recruitment and activation (Marrakchi et al. 2011; Gabay and Towne 2015; Navarini et al. 2013).

The possible role of granulysin, which is involved in the pathogenesis of TEN, has been proposed (Schlapbach et al. 2011).

8.7.2 Genetic Basis

Genetic predisposition manifested by a personal history of drug allergy prior to the appearance of AGEP was recorded in 8.3% (Choi et al. 2010) and 86% of patients (Alniemi et al. 2017).

Human leukocyte antigen (HLA) haplotypes B51, DR11, and DQ3 were more common in AGEP patients than in the general population (Bernard et al. 1995).

Recent research showed that mutations in the IL36RN gene may underlie pustular eruptions. IL-36RN mutations lead to uncontrolled IL-36 signaling and enhanced production of the cytokines IL-6, IL-8, IL-1α, and IL-1β (Gabay and Towne 2015; Onoufriadis et al. 2011). IL-36RN mutations already have been identified in GPP (Kanazawa et al. 2013; Song et al. 2014) and in four cases of AGEP (within a cohort study of 96 AGEP cases) without a previous history of psoriasis vulgaris (Navarini et al. 2013). The occurrence of drug-induced AGEP in a patient with psoriasis vulgaris and a heterozygous IL36RN mutation has been reported as well (Nakai et al. 2015).This suggests a possible genetic basis for a subset of AGEP patients and supports the idea of a common pathological mechanism between AGEP and GPP (Navarini et al. 2013).

8.8 Diagnostic Tests

In view of the immune pathogenesis of AGEP, in vivo and in vitro tests can serve as a diagnostic tool in AGEP.

8.8.1 Patch Tests

Positive patch test reactions have been recorded in AGEP for a variety of medications and chemicals, including antibiotics (i.e., amoxicillin, ampicillin, metronidazole, cefotaxime, ceftriaxone, ciprofloxacin), diltiazem, mercury, bufexamac, celecoxib, etoricoxibe, fluindione, prednisolone, tetrazepam (a benzodiazepine), hydroxychloroquine, and fluconazole (Di Lernia and Ricci 2015; Belhadjali et al. 2008; Belhadjali et al. 2008; Makela and Lammintausta 2008; Serrao et al. 2008; Chtioui et al. 2008; Girardi et al. 2005; Hausermann et al. 2005; Gensch et al. 2007; Thomas et al. 2008; Chaabane et al. 2010; Shin et al. 2011; Nacaroglu et al. 2014; Charfi et al. 2015).

Pustular patch tests reactions also have been observed with corticosteroids (Bar et al. 2008; Demitsu et al. 1996). The sensitivity of patch tests in AGEP ranges between 50% (Wolkenstein et al. 1996) and 58% (Barbaud et al. 2013).

A recent study showed that the reactivity of patch tests toward antibiotics in AGEP was only 18.1%, but the reactivity for dicloxacillin was 50% (Pinho et al. 2017).

Usually, the performance of patch testing in AGEP is considered safe. Yet, a case of AGEP-like systemic reaction (Mashiah and Brenner 2003) and a relapse of AGEP, requiring systemic corticosteroids, was observed following patch testing (Barbaud et al. 2013). A late positive patch test reaction was reported in a single case of tetrazepam-induced AGEP (Thomas et al. 2008) but was not observed in a larger study (Barbaud et al. 2013). An immunohistochemical analysis of positive patch test reactions in AGEP supported the role of IL-8 and drug-specific T-cells (Britschgi and Pichler 2002; Britschgi et al. 2001; Thomas et al. 2008).

In conclusion, patch tests are a useful and safe diagnostic tool in AGEP (Barbaud et al. 2013).

8.8.2 In Vitro Tests

The main reported in vitro test in AGEP is the lymphocyte proliferation test (Britschgi et al. 2001; Padial et al. 2004; Thomas et al. 2008; Kawaguchi et al. 1999; Noce et al. 2000; Anliker and Wuthrich 2003). In some cases the in vitro lymphocyte proliferation test responses were in agreement with the in vivo patch test responses (Girardi et al. 2005; Thomas et al. 2008).

The mast cell degranulation test and the release of the lymphokine macrophage migration inhibitory factor were used simultaneously to confirm the causative role of drugs in a series of patients with pustular drug eruptions, consistent with AGEP (Lazarov et al. 1998).

The diagnostic role of the in vitro drug-induced release of the Th1-type cytokine interferon-gamma was reported in a variety of drug eruptions, including AGEP (Halevy et al. 2000, 2005).

In view of the limited data concerning the diagnostic role of in vitro tests in AGEP, further studies are required.

8.9 Treatment

AGEP is a self-limited disease with a favorable prognosis in most cases. Usually no specific treatment is recommended other than withdrawal of the suspected drug and supportive care. Treatment may include topical steroids, antipyretics, and antihistamines. In severe cases systemic corticosteroids may be administered (Davidovici et al. 2008; Chang et al. 2008; Choi et al. 2010; Alniemi et al. 2017). However, in a retrospective analysis, there was no difference between various treatment regimens regarding the course of the disease (Chang et al. 2008).

8.10 Conclusion

AGEP is a rare severe pustular reaction attributed mainly to drugs. In view of the remarkable clinical and histological resemblance of this entity to pustular psoriasis, further investigation of the underlying pathological mechanism is needed.

References

Alniemi DT, Wetter DA, Bridges AG, El-Azhary RA, Davis MD, Camilleri MJ, McEvoy MT (2017) Acute generalized exanthematous pustulosis: clinical characteristics, etiologic associations, treatments, and outcomes in a series of 28 patients at Mayo Clinic, 1996–2013. Int J Dermatol 56:405. https://doi.org/10.1111/ijd.13434

Anliker MD, Wuthrich B (2003) Acute generalized exanthematous pustulosis due to sulfamethoxazole with positive lymphocyte transformation test (LTT). J Investig Allergol Clin Immunol 13:66–68

Baker H, Ryan TJ (1968) Generalized pustular psoriasis. A clinical and epidemiological study of 104 cases. Br J Dermatol 80:771–793

Bar M, John L, Wonschik S, Schmitt J, Kempter W, Bauer A, Meurer M (2008) Acute generalized exanthematous pustulosis induced by high-dose prednisolone in a young woman with optic neuritis owing to disseminated encephalomyelitis. Br J Dermatol 159:251–252. https://doi.org/10.1111/j.1365-2133.2008.08594.x

Barbaud A, Collet E, Milpied B, Assier H, Staumont D, Avenel-Audran M, Grange A, Amarger S, Girardin P, Guinnepain MT, Truchetet F, Lasek A, Waton J, Toxidermies group of the French Society of Dermatology (2013) A multicentre study to determine the value and safety of drug patch tests for the three main classes of severe cutaneous adverse drug reactions. Br J Dermatol 168:555–562. https://doi.org/10.1111/bjd.12125

Belda W, Ferrolla ACJ (2005) Acute generalized exanthematous pustulosis (AGEP). Case report. Rev Inst Med Trop S Paulo 47:171–176

Belhadjali H, Ghannouchi N, Njim L, Mohamed M, Moussa A, Bayou F, Chakroun M, Zakhama A, Zili J (2008) Acute generalized exanthematous pustulosis induced by bufexamac in an atopic girl. Contact Dermatitis 58(4):247–248. https://doi.org/10.1111/j.1600-0536.2007.01271.x

Belhadjali H, Mandhouj S, Moussa A, Njim L, Amri M, Zakhama A, Zili J (2008) Mercury-induced acute generalized exanthematous pustulosis misdiagnosed as a drug-related case. Contact Dermatitis 59:52–54. https://doi.org/10.1111/j.1600-0536.2007.01306.x

Ben Said Z, Saidi W, Boussofara L, Ghariani N, Belajouza C, Sriha B, Denguezli M, Nouira R (2010) Acute generalized exanthematous pustulosis following a spider bite: three cases from Tunisia. Ann Dermatol Venereol 137:813–818. https://doi.org/10.1016/j.annder.2010.06.015

Bernard P, Lizeaux-Parneix V, Miiossec V, Bonnetblanc JM (1995) HLA et predisposition genetique dans les pustuloses exanthematiques aigues generalisees (PEAG) et dans les exanthemes maculo-papuleux (EMP). Ann Dermatol Venereol 122(Suppl):S38–S39

Betto P, Germi L, Bonoldi E, Bertazzoni M (2008) Acute localized exanthematous pustulosis (ALEP) caused by amoxicillin-clavulanic acid. Int J Dermatol 47:295–296. https://doi.org/10.1111/j.1365-4632.2008.03477.x

Beylot C, Bioulac P, Doutre MS (1980) Acute generalized exanthematic pustuloses (four cases) (author's transl). Ann Dermatol Venereol 107:37–48

Beylot C, Doutre MS, Beylot-Barry M (1996) Acute generalized exanthematous pustulosis. Semin Cutan Med Surg 15:244–249

Bhat YJ, Hassan I, Sajad P, Yaseen A, Wani R (2015) Acute generalized exanthematous pustulosis due to insect bites? Indian J Dermatol 60:422. https://doi.org/10.4103/0019-5154.160529

Bissonnette R, Tousignant J, Allaire G (1992) Drug-induced toxic pustuloderma. Int J Dermatol 31:172–174

Bouvresse S, Valeyrie-Allanore L, Ortonne N, Konstantinou MP, Kardaun SH, Bagot M, Wolkenstein P, Roujeau JC (2012) Toxic epidermal necrolysis, DRESS, AGEP: do overlap cases exist? Orphanet J Rare Dis 7:72. https://doi.org/10.1186/1750-1172-7-72

Bracke A, Van Marck E, Lambert J (2009) Acute generalized exanthematous pustulosis after pemetrexed, and recurrence after re-introduction. Clin Exp Dermatol 34(3):337–339. https://doi.org/10.1111/j.1365-2230.2008.02902.x

Britschgi M, Pichler WJ (2002) Acute generalized exanthematous pustulosis, a clue to neutrophil-mediated inflammatory processes orchestrated by T cells. Curr Opin Allergy Clin Immunol 2:325–331

Britschgi M, Steiner UC, Schmid S, Depta JP, Senti G, Bircher A, Burkhart C, Yawalkar N, Pichler WJ (2001) T-cell involvement in drug-induced acute generalized exanthematous pustulosis. J Clin Invest 107:1433–1441. https://doi.org/10.1172/JCI12118

Buettiker U, Keller M, Pichler WJ, Braathen LR, Yawalkar N (2006) Oral prednisolone induced acute generalized exanthematous pustulosis due to corticosteroids of group A confirmed by epicutaneous testing and lymphocyte transformation tests. Dermatology 213:40–43. https://doi.org/10.1159/000092837

Burrows NP, Russell Jones RR (1993) Pustular drug eruptions: a histopathological spectrum. Histopathology 22:569–573

Calistru AM, Lisboa C, Cunha AP, Bettencourt H, Azevedo F (2012) Acute generalized exanthematous pustulosis to amoxicillin associated with parvovirus B19 reactivation. Cutan Ocul Toxicol 31:258–261. https://doi.org/10.3109/15569527.2011.645978

Cannistraci C, Parola IL, Rigan OR, Bassetti F, Ortona E, Santucci B, Picardo M, Siracusano S (2003) Acute generalized exanthematous pustulosis in cystic echinococcosis: immunological characterization. Br J Dermatol 148:1245–1249

Chaabane A, Aouam K, Gassab L, Njim L, Boughattas NA (2010) Acute generalized exanthematous pustulosis (AGEP) induced by cefotaxime. Fundam Clin Pharmacol 24:429–432. https://doi.org/10.1111/j.1472-8206.2009.00794.x

Chang SL, Hu S, Hung SI, Huang YL, Hsiao WC, Chung WH (2010) A comparison of Ki-67 antigen presentation in acute generalized exanthematous pustulosis and pustular psoriasis. Arch Dermatol Res 302:525–529. https://doi.org/10.1007/s00403-010-1046-3

Chang SL, Huang YH, Yang CH, Hu S, Hong HS (2008) Clinical manifestations and characteristics of patients with acute generalized exanthematous pustulosis in Asia. Acta Derm Venereol 88:363–365. https://doi.org/10.2340/00015555-0438

Charfi O, Kastalli S, Sahnoun R, Lakhoua G (2015) Hydroxychloroquine-induced acute generalized exanthematous pustulosis with positive patch-testing. Indian J Pharmacol 47(6):693–694. https://doi.org/10.4103/0253-7613.169589

Choi MJ, Kim HS, Park HJ, Park CJ, Lee JD, Lee JY, Kim HO, Park YM (2010) Clinicopathologic manifestations of 36 korean patients with acute generalized exanthematous pustulosis: a case series and review of the literature. Ann Dermatol 22:163–169. https://doi.org/10.5021/ad.2010.22.2.163

Chtioui M, Cousin-Testard F, Zimmermann U, Amar A, Saiag P, Mahe E (2008) Fluindione-induced acute generalised exanthematous pustulosis confirmed by patch testing. Ann Dermatol Venereol 135:295–298. https://doi.org/10.1016/j.annder.2007.07.004

Cohen AD, Cagnano E, Halevy S (2001) Acute generalized exanthematous pustulosis mimicking toxic epidermal necrolysis. Int J Dermatol 40:458–461

Davidovici B, Dodiuk-Gad R, Rozenman D, Halevy S (2008) Profile of acute generalized exanthematous pustulosis in Israel during 2002–2005: results of the RegiSCAR Study. Isr Med Assoc J 10:410–412

Davidovici BB, Pavel D, Cagnano E, Rozenman D, Halevy S (2006) Acute generalized exanthematous pustulosis following a spider bite: report of 3 cases. J Am Acad Dermatol 55:525–529. https://doi.org/10.1016/j.jaad.2006.05.010

De Cruz R, Ferguson J, Wee JS, Akhras V (2015) Acute localised exanthematous pustulosis (ALEP) induced by clindamycin in pregnancy. Australas J Dermatol 56:e55–e58. https://doi.org/10.1111/ajd.12135

Demitsu T, Kosuge A, Yamada T, Usui K, Katayama H, Yaoita H (1996) Acute generalized exanthematous pustulosis induced by dexamethasone injection. Dermatology 193:56–58

Di Lernia V, Ricci C (2015) Fluconazole-induced acute generalized exanthematous pustulosis. Indian J Dermatol 60(2):212. https://doi.org/10.4103/0019-5154.152572

Eeckhout I, Noens L, Ongenae K, al Sarraf Z, Schelfhout A, Naeyaert JM (1997) Acute generalized exanthematic pustulosis: a case with a lymphoma-like presentation. Dermatology 194:408–410

Ermertcan AT, Demirer O, Inanir I, Bilac C, Temiz P (2010) Acute generalized exanthematous pustulosis with lymphangitis triggered by a spider bite. Cutan Ocul Toxicol 29:67–69. https://doi.org/10.3109/15569520903455916

Feio AB, Apetato M, Costa MM, Sa J, Alcantara J (1997) Acute generalized exanthematous pustulosis due to Coxsackie B4 virus. Acta Medica Port 10:487–491

Gabay C, Towne JE (2015) Regulation and function of interleukin-36 cytokines in homeostasis and pathological conditions. J Leukoc Biol 97:645–652. https://doi.org/10.1189/jlb.3RI1014-495R

Gensch K, Hodzic-Avdagic N, Megahed M, Ruzicka T, Kuhn A (2007) Acute generalized exanthematous pustulosis with confirmed type IV allergy. Report of 3 cases. Hautarzt 58:250–252. https://doi.org/10.1007/s00105-006-1161-4, 254–255.

Girardi M, Duncan KO, Tigelaar RE, Imaeda S, Watsky KL, McNiff JM (2005) Cross-comparison of patch test and lymphocyte proliferation responses in patients with a history of acute generalized exanthematous pustulosis. Am J Dermatopathol 27:343–346

Goh TK, Pang SM, Thirumoorthy T, Goh SG (2008) Acute generalised exanthematous pustulosis and toxic epidermal necrolysis induced by carbamazepine. Singap Med J 49:507–510

Halevy S (2009) Acute generalized exanthematous pustulosis. Curr Opin Allergy Clin Immunol 9:322–328. https://doi.org/10.1097/ACI.0b013e32832cf64e

Halevy S, Cohen AD, Grossman N (2005) Clinical implications of in vitro drug-induced interferon gamma release from peripheral blood lymphocytes in cutaneous adverse drug reactions. J Am Acad Dermatol 52:254–261

Halevy S, Cohen AD, Livni E (2000) Acute generalized exanthematous pustulosis associated with polysensitivity to paracetamol and bromhexine. The diagnostic role of in vitro interferon-g release test. Clin Exp Dermatol 25:652–654

Halevy S, Kardaun SH, Davidovici B, Wechsler J, EuroSCAR and RegiSCAR study group (2010) The spectrum of histopathological features in acute generalized exanthematous pustulosis: a study of 102 cases. Br J Dermatol 163:1245–1252. https://doi.org/10.1111/j.1365-2133.2010.09967.x

Haro-Gabaldon V, Sanchez-Sanchez-Vizcaino J, Ruiz-Avila P, Gutierrez-Fernandez J, Linares J, Naranjo-Sintes R (1996) Acute generalized exanthematous pustulosis with cytomegalovirus infection. Int J Dermatol 35:735–737

Hausermann P, Scherer K, Weber M, Bircher AJ (2005) Ciprofloxacin-induced acute generalized exanthematous pustulosis mimicking bullous drug eruption confirmed by a positive patch test. Dermatology 211:277–280. https://doi.org/10.1159/000087024

Hogan CJ, Barbaro KC, Winkel K (2004) Loxoscelism: old obstacles, new directions. Ann Emerg Med 44(6):608–624. https://doi.org/10.1016/S0196064404013149

Hotz C, Valeyrie-Allanore L, Haddad C, Bouvresse S, Ortonne N, Duong TA, Ingen-Housz-Oro S, Roujeau JC, Wolkenstein P, Chosidow O (2013) Systemic involvement of acute generalized exanthematous pustulosis: a retrospective study on 58 patients. Br J Dermatol 169:1223–1232. https://doi.org/10.1111/bjd.12502

Kabashima R, Sugita K, Sawada Y, Hino R, Nakamura M, Tokura Y (2011) Increased circulating Th17 frequencies and serum IL-22 levels in patients with acute generalized exanthematous pustulosis. J Eur Acad Dermatol Venereol 25:485–488. https://doi.org/10.1111/j.1468-3083.2010.03771.x

Kanazawa N, Nakamura T, Mikita N, Furukawa F (2013) Novel IL36RN mutation in a Japanese case of early onset generalized pustular psoriasis. J Dermatol 40:749–751. https://doi.org/10.1111/1346-8138.12227

Kardaun SH, Kuiper H, Fidler V, Jonkman MF (2010) The histopathological spectrum of acute generalized exanthematous pustulosis (AGEP) and its differentiation from generalized pustular psoriasis. J Cutan Pathol 37:1220–1229. https://doi.org/10.1111/j.1600-0560.2010.01612.x

Kawaguchi M, Mitsuhashi Y, Kondo S (1999) Acute generalized exanthematous pustulosis induced by salazosulfapyridine in a patient with ulcerative colitis. J Dermatol 26(6):359–362

Klein N, Hartmann M, Helmbold P, Enk A (2009) Acute generalized exanthematous pustulosis associated with recurrent urinary tract infections. Hautarzt 60(3):226–228. https://doi.org/10.1007/s00105-008-1604-1

Lane L, McCoppin HH, Dyer J (2011) Acute generalized exanthematous pustulosis and coombs-positive hemolytic anemia in a child following Loxosceles reclusa envenomation. Pediatr Dermatol 28:685–688. https://doi.org/10.1111/j.1525-1470.2010.01302.x

Lateef A, Tan KB, Lau TC (2009) Acute generalized exanthematous pustulosis and toxic epidermal necrolysis induced by hydroxychloroquine. Clin Rheumatol 28:1449–1452. https://doi.org/10.1007/s10067-009-1262-4

Lazarov A, Livni E, Halevy S (1998) Generalized pustular drug eruptions: confirmation by in vitro tests. J Eur Acad Dermatol Venereol 10:36–41

Lee D, Kang JN, Hwang SH, Lee YS, Kim H, Seo JK, Sung HS (2014) Acute generalized exanthematous pustulosis induced by parvovirus b19 infection. Ann Dermatol 26:399–400. https://doi.org/10.5021/ad.2014.26.3.399

Lerch M, Bircher AJ (2004) Systemically induced allergic exanthem from mercury. Contact Dermatitis 50:349–353. https://doi.org/10.1111/j.0105-1873.2004.00366.xCOD366

Lim CS, Lim SL (2009) Acute generalized exanthematous pustulosis associated with asymptomatic Mycoplasma pneumoniae infection. Arch Dermatol 145:848–849. https://doi.org/10.1001/archdermatol.2009.127

Macmillan AL (1973) Generalised pustular drug rash. Dermatologica 146(5):285–291

Makela L, Lammintausta K (2008) Etoricoxib-induced acute generalized exanthematous pustulosis. Acta Derm Venereol 88:200–201. https://doi.org/10.2340/00015555-0381

Makris M, Spanoudaki N, Giannoula F, Chliva C, Antoniadou A, Kalogeromitros D (2009) Acute generalized exanthematous pustulosis (AGEP) triggered by a spider bite. Allergol Int 58:301–303. https://doi.org/10.2332/allergolint.08-CR-0035

Manzano S, Guggisberg D, Hammann C, Laubscher B (2006) Acute generalized exanthematous pustulosis: first case associated with a Chlamydia pneumoniae infection. Arch Pediatr 13:1230–1232. https://doi.org/10.1016/j.arcped.2006.06.004

Marrakchi S, Guigue P, Renshaw BR, Puel A, Pei XY, Fraitag S, Zribi J, Bal E, Cluzeau C, Chrabieh M, Towne JE, Douangpanya J, Pons C, Mansour S, Serre V, Makni H, Mahfoudh N, Fakhfakh F, Bodemer C, Feingold J, Hadj-Rabia S, Favre M, Genin E, Sahbatou M, Munnich A, Casanova JL, Sims JE, Turki H, Bachelez H, Smahi A (2011) Interleukin-36-receptor antagonist deficiency and generalized pustular psoriasis. N Engl J Med 365(7):620–628. https://doi.org/10.1056/NEJMoa1013068

Mashiah J, Brenner S (2003) A systemic reaction to patch testing for the evaluation of acute generalized exanthematous pustulosis. Arch Dermatol 139:1181–1183. https://doi.org/10.1001/archderm.139.9.1181139/9/1181 [pii]

Matsumoto Y, Okubo Y, Yamamoto T, Ito T, Tsuboi R (2008) Case of acute generalized exanthematous pustulosis caused by ampicillin/cloxacillin sodium in a pregnant woman. J Dermatol 35:362–364. https://doi.org/10.1111/j.1346-8138.2008.00484.x

Matsushita H, Ishiguro T, Kurabayashi T, Shibuya M (2012) Acute generalized exanthematous pustulosis during the puerperal period: a case report. Clin Exp Obstet Gynecol 39:414–416

Meiss F, Helmbold P, Meykadeh N, Gaber G, Marsch W, Fischer M (2007) Overlap of acute generalized exanthematous pustulosis and toxic epidermal necrolysis: response to antitumour necrosis factor-alpha antibody infliximab: report of three cases. J Eur Acad Dermatol Venereol 21:717–719. https://doi.org/10.1111/j.1468-3083.2006.02026.x

Milman Lde M, Muller GP, Souza PR, Grill AB, Rhoden DL, Mello-da-Silva CA, Vettorato G (2016) Acute generalized exanthematous pustulosis associated with spider bite. An Bras Dermatol 91:524–527. https://doi.org/10.1590/abd1806-4841.20164045

Nacaroglu HT, Celegen M, Ozek G, Umac O, Karkiner CS, Yildirim HT, Can D (2014) Acute generalized exanthematous pustulosis induced by ceftriaxone use. Postepy Dermatol Alergol 31:269–271. https://doi.org/10.5114/pdia.2014.40938

Nakai N, Sugiura K, Akiyama M, Katoh N (2015) Acute generalized exanthematous pustulosis caused by dihydrocodeine phosphate in a patient with psoriasis vulgaris and a heterozygous IL36RN mutation. JAMA Dermatol 151:311–315. https://doi.org/10.1001/jamadermatol.2014.3002

Nantes Castillejo O, Zozaya Urmeneta JM, Valcayo Penalba A, Martinez-Penuela Virseda JM (2008) Acute generalized exanthematous pustulosis induced by omeprazole. Gastroenterol Hepatol 31:295–298

Navarini AA, Valeyrie-Allanore L, Setta-Kaffetzi N, Barker JN, Capon F, Creamer D, Roujeau JC, Sekula P, Simpson MA, Trembath RC, Mockenhaupt M, Smith CH (2013) Rare variations in IL36RN in severe adverse drug reactions manifesting as acute generalized exanthematous pustulosis. J Invest Dermatol 133:1904–1907. https://doi.org/10.1038/jid.2013.44

Noce R, Paredes BE, Pichler WJ, Krahenbuhl S (2000) Acute generalized exanthematic pustulosis (AGEP) in a patient treated with furosemide. Am J Med Sci 320:331–333

Ofuji S, Yamamoto O (2007) Acute generalized exanthematous pustulosis associated with a human parvovirus B19 infection. J Dermatol 34:121–123. https://doi.org/10.1111/j.1346-8138.2006.00230.x

Onoufriadis A, Simpson MA, Pink AE, Di Meglio P, Smith CH, Pullabhatla V, Knight J, Spain SL, Nestle FO, Burden AD, Capon F, Trembath RC, Barker JN (2011) Mutations in IL36RN/IL1F5 are associated with the severe episodic inflammatory skin disease known as generalized pustular psoriasis. Am J Hum Genet 89:432–437. https://doi.org/10.1016/j.ajhg.2011.07.022

Padial MA, Alvarez-Ferreira J, Tapia B, Blanco R, Manas C, Blanca M, Bellon T (2004) Acute generalized exanthematous pustulosis associated with pseudoephedrine. Br J Dermatol 150:139–142

Paradisi A, Bugatti L, Sisto T, Filosa G, Amerio PL, Capizzi R (2008) Acute generalized exanthematous pustulosis induced by hydroxychloroquine: three cases and a review of the literature. Clin Ther 30:930–940. https://doi.org/10.1016/j.clinthera.2008.05.014

Park MY, Kang HY (2008) Acute generalized exanthematous pustulosis after ingestion of lacquer chicken. Ann Dermatol 20:209–211. https://doi.org/10.5021/ad.2008.20.4.209

Park JJ, Yun SJ, Lee JB, Kim SJ, Won YH, Lee SC (2010) A case of hydroxychloroquine induced acute generalized exanthematous pustulosis confirmed by accidental oral provocation. Ann Dermatol 22:102–105. https://doi.org/10.5021/ad.2010.22.1.102

Pennisi RS (2006) Acute generalised exanthematous pustulosis induced by the herbal remedy Ginkgo biloba. Med J Australia 184:583–584

Pinho A, Coutinho I, Gameiro A, Gouveia M, Goncalo M (2017) Patch testing – a valuable tool for investigating non-immediate cutaneous adverse drug reactions to antibiotics. J Eur Acad Dermatol Venereol 31:280–287. https://doi.org/10.1111/jdv.13796

Rastogi S, Modi M, Dhawan V (2009) Acute localized exanthematous pustulosis (ALEP) caused by Ibuprofen a case report. Br J Oral Maxillofac Surg 47(2):132–134. https://doi.org/10.1016/j.bjoms.2008.07.185

Roujeau JC (2005) Clinical heterogeneity of drug hypersensitivity. Toxicology 209:123–129. https://doi.org/10.1016/j.tox.2004.12.022

Roujeau JC, Bioulac-Sage P, Bourseau C, Guillaume JC, Bernard P, Lok C, Plantin P, Claudy A, Delavierre C, Vaillant L et al (1991) Acute generalized exanthematous pustulosis. Analysis of 63 cases. Arch Dermatol 127:1333–1338

Schaerli P, Britschgi M, Keller M, Steiner UC, Steinmann LS, Moser B, Pichler WJ (2004) Characterization of human T cells that regulate neutrophilic skin inflammation. J Immunol 173:2151–2158

Schlapbach C, Zawodniak A, Irla N, Adam J, Hunger RE, Yerly D, Pichler WJ, Yawalkar N (2011) NKp46+ cells express granulysin in multiple cutaneous adverse drug reactions. Allergy 66:1469–1476. https://doi.org/10.1111/j.1398-9995.2011.02677.x

Schmid S, Kuechler PC, Britschgi M, Steiner UC, Yawalkar N, Limat A, Baltensperger K, Braathen L, Pichler WJ (2002) Acute generalized exanthematous pustulosis: role of cytotoxic T cells in pustule formation. Am J Pathol 161(6):2079–2086

Schwarz M, Kreuzer KA, Baskaynak G, Dorken B, le Coutre P (2002) Imatinib-induced acute generalized exanthematous pustulosis (AGEP) in two patients with chronic myeloid leukemia. Eur J Haematol 69:254–256

Scott AD, Lee M, Kubba F, Chu A (2015) Acute generalized exanthematous pustulosis (AGEP) secondary to imatinib in a patient with chronic myeloid leukaemia. Clin Exp Dermatol 40:926–927. https://doi.org/10.1111/ced.12479

Serrao V, Caldas Lopes L, Campos Lopes JM, Lobo L, Ferreira A (2008) Acute generalized exanthematous pustulosis associated with diltiazem. Acta Medica Port 21:99–102

Shin HT, Park SW, Lee KT, Park HY, Park JH, Lee DY, Lee JH, Yang JM, Lee ES (2011) A case of celecoxib induced acute generalized exanthematous pustulosis. Ann Dermatol 23(Suppl 3):S380–S382. https://doi.org/10.5021/ad.2011.23.S3.S380

Sidoroff A, Dunant A, Viboud C, Halevy S, Bavinck JN, Naldi L, Mockenhaupt M, Fagot JP, Roujeau JC (2007) Risk factors for acute generalized exanthematous pustulosis (AGEP)-results of a multinational case-control study (EuroSCAR). Br J Dermatol 157:989–996. https://doi.org/10.1111/j.1365-2133.2007.08156.x

Sidoroff A, Halevy S, Bavinck JN, Vaillant L, Roujeau JC (2001) Acute generalized exanthematous pustulosis (AGEP)--a clinical reaction pattern. J Cutan Pathol 28:113–119

Smeets TJ, Jessurun N, Harmark L, Kardaun SH (2016) Clindamycin-induced acute generalised exanthematous pustulosis: five cases and a review of the literature. Neth J Med 74:421–428

Son CH, Lee CU, Roh MS, Lee SK, Kim KH, Yang DK (2008) Acute generalized exanthematous pustulosis as a manifestation of carbamazepine hypersensitivity syndrome. J Investig Allergol Clin Immunol 18:461–464

Song HS, Kim SJ, Park TI, Jang YH, Lee ES (2016) Immunohistochemical comparison of IL-36 and the IL-23/Th17 Axis of generalized pustular psoriasis and acute generalized exanthematous pustulosis. Ann Dermatol 28:451–456. https://doi.org/10.5021/ad.2016.28.4.451

Song HS, Yun SJ, Park S, Lee ES (2014) Gene mutation analysis in a Korean patient with early-onset and recalcitrant generalized pustular psoriasis. Ann Dermatol 26:424–425. https://doi.org/10.5021/ad.2014.26.3.424

Speck LM, Wilkerson MG, Perri AJ, Kelly BC (2008) Acute generalized exanthematous pustulosis caused by terazosin hydrochloride. J Drugs Dermatol 7:395–397

Spencer JM, Silvers DN, Grossman ME (1994) Pustular eruption after drug exposure: is it pustular psoriasis or a pustular drug eruption? Br J Dermatol 130:514–519

Staughton RC, Payne CM, Harper JI, McMichen H (1984) Toxic pustuloderma--a new entity? J Royal Soc Med 77(Suppl 4):6–8

Sugita K, Nishio D, Kabashima K, Tokura Y (2008) Acute generalized exanthematous pustulosis caused by sennoside in a patient with multiple myeloma. J Eur Acad Dermatol Venereol 22:517–319. https://doi.org/10.1111/j.1468-3083.2007.02378.x

Syrigou E, Grapsa D, Charpidou A, Syrigos K (2015) Acute generalized exanthematous pustulosis induced by amoxicillin/clavulanic acid: report of a case presenting with generalized lymphadenopathy. J Cutan Med Surg 19:592–594. https://doi.org/10.1177/1203475415588003

Taguchi K, Oka M, Bito T, Nishigori C (2016) Acute generalized exanthematous pustulosis induced by Mycoplasma pneumoniae infection. J Dermatol 43:113–114. https://doi.org/10.1111/1346-8138.13151

Tamir E, Wohl Y, Mashiah J, Brenner S (2006) Acute generalized exanthematous pustulosis: a retrospective analysis showing a clear predilection for women. Skinmed 5:186–188

Thomas E, Bellon T, Barranco P, Padial A, Tapia B, Morel E, Alves-Ferreira J, Martin-Esteban M (2008) Acute generalized exanthematous pustulosis due to tetrazepam. J Investig Allergol Clin Immunol 18:119–122

Wolkenstein P, Chosidow O, Flechet ML, Robbiola O, Paul M, Dume L, Revuz J, Roujeau JC (1996) Patch testing in severe cutaneous adverse drug reactions, including Stevens-Johnson syndrome and toxic epidermal necrolysis. Contact Dermatitis 35:234–236

Yamamoto T, Minatohara K (1997) Minocycline-induced acute generalized exanthematous pustulosis in a patient with generalized pustular psoriasis showing elevated level of sELAM-1. Acta Derm Venereol 77:168–169

Urticarial Reactions to Drugs

9

Daniel F. Carr

Abbreviations

AU	Acute urticaria
CU	Chronic urticaria
IgE	Immunoglobulin E
RAST	Radioallergosorbent test
SSLR	Serum sickness-like reaction

Key Points

1. Urticaria is the second most common form of drug-induced cutaneous adverse drug reactions and can often present with angioedema. Urticarial eruptions are typically self-limiting and in most cases recede following drug withdrawal.
2. There are three distinct forms of drug-induced urticaria: Acute, chronic and contact.
3. Acute drug-urticarial eruptions can occur via immunological (Type I, IgE-mediated or Type III, complement activation) and non-immunological (direct drug degranulation of mast cells) mechanisms.
4. Chronic drug-induced urticarial reactions are non-immune-mediated and are typically an exacerbation of underlying idiopathic chronic urticaria.
5. Aspirins and NSAIDs can elicit a non-immune-mediated urticarial eruption via COX1 inhibition and subsequent alteration of the arachidonic acid pathway.

D. F. Carr (✉)
Wolfson Centre for Personalised Medicine, MRC Centre for Drug Safety Science, Institute of Translational Medicine, University of Liverpool, Liverpool, England, UK
e-mail: D.Carr@liverpool.ac.uk

N. H. Shear, R. P. Dodiuk-Gad (eds.), *Advances in Diagnosis and Management of Cutaneous Adverse Drug Reactions*, https://doi.org/10.1007/978-981-13-1489-6_9

9.1 Clinical Features and Epidemiology

Urticaria, often referred to as hives, is a common cutaneous disorder which is thought to occur in 15–25% of individuals over the course of a lifetime (Amar and Dreskin 2008; Poonawalla and Kelly 2009). Urticarial eruptions are characterised by recurrent pruritic, pink to red edematous lesions with pale centres (wheals). Lesions can range from a few millimetres to several centimetres in size (Kanani et al. 2011) and are transient in nature, often appearing and disappearing within 48 h. Approximately 40% of patients with urticarial eruptions will also present with angioedema (deeper swellings of the subcutaneous or mucosal tissues) (Amar and Dreskin 2008) which in some cases can be very severe with swelling of the lips and tongue causing impairment of swallowing and ventilation.

Though most urticarial eruptions (50%) are idiopathic, it has shown that a drug aetiology accounts for a significant proportion of cases. Indeed, in an outpatient dermatology setting, drugs have been shown to account for the aetiology of 9.1% of all urticaria or angioedema (Kozel et al. 1998). Of all cutaneous drug eruptions, it is thought that urticaria is the second most common after exanthema (Hunziker et al. 1997) with overall incidence of drug-induced urticaria estimated at 0.16% and accounting for 5.9% of all rashes in an inpatient setting (Hunziker et al. 1997).

Urticarial eruption with drug aetiology is generally indistinguishable from reactions of alternative aetiology and most commonly attributable to penicillins and non-steroidal anti-inflammatory drugs though a wide spectrum of other drugs has also been observed to cause urticaria (Table 9.1).

Drug-induced urticarial reactions can be classified into three subtypes which will be discussed here in detail: acute, chronic and contact.

Acute urticaria (AU) is the most common of the three subtypes of drug-induced urticaria and is defined as a reaction persisting for less than 6 weeks. AU reactions are generally considered to occur through three distinct mechanisms which can be specific to the causal drug (Table 9.1) and differ significantly in their time course (Fig. 9.1).

(a) Type I hypersensitivity is an immune-mediated mechanism which requires an initial period of sensitisation at which time no allergic reaction usually occurs. During the sensitisation process, drug-specific immunoglobulin E (IgE) antibodies are synthesised. The Fc portion of IgE binds with high affinity to receptors (FcεRIs) on the surface of mast cells, the key mediator cells of urticarial reactions. The drug binds to the antigen binding site of drug-specific IgE molecules anchored to the mast cell membrane. This causes cross-linking of adjacent Fc receptors and activation of mast cells causing degranulation and release of mediators including histamine and vasodilators.

An immune-mediated reaction can occur upon first drug exposure but always within 3 weeks of treatment. After the uneventful sensitisation period, IgE-mediated urticarial reactions occur within 60 minutes of drug treatment and can be accompanied by more severe clinical manifestations, including angioedema and

Table 9.1 Drugs known to cause urticarial drug eruptions adapted from Mathelier-Fusade (2006)

Acute urticaria			Chronic urticaria		
Type I (IgE-mediated)	Type III (Serum sickness)	Non-immune	Non-immune	Pharmacological hypersensitivity	Contact urticaria
• Angiotensin-converting enzyme inhibitors • *Antifungal Agents* – Fluconazole – Ketoconazole • Dextran • Hydralazine • Hydantoins • NSAIDs/aspirin • *Muscle relaxants* – Curare • Opioids • Penicillins and cephalosporins • Progesterone • Protamine • Quinidine • Sorbitol complexes • Steroids • Vaccines • Vitamins	• Allopurinol • Aspirin • Barbiturates • Captopril • Penicillins and cephalosporins • Furazolidone • Gold salts • Griseofulvin • Halothane • Hydralazine • Iodides • Methyldopa • Penicillamine • Phenytoin • Piperazine • Procainamide • Quinidine • Streptokinase • Sulfonamides • Thiouracils	• Amphetamine • Atropine • Hydralazine • Muscle relaxants • Pentamidine • Quinidine • Opioids • Radio-contrast media	• NSAIDs/aspirin • Codeine • Morphine	• NSAIDs/aspirin	• *Topical antibiotics* – Penicillins and cephalosporins – Bacitracin – Chloramphenicol – Gentamycin – Neomycin – Streptomycin • *Topical anaesthetics* – Benzocaine – Lidocaine

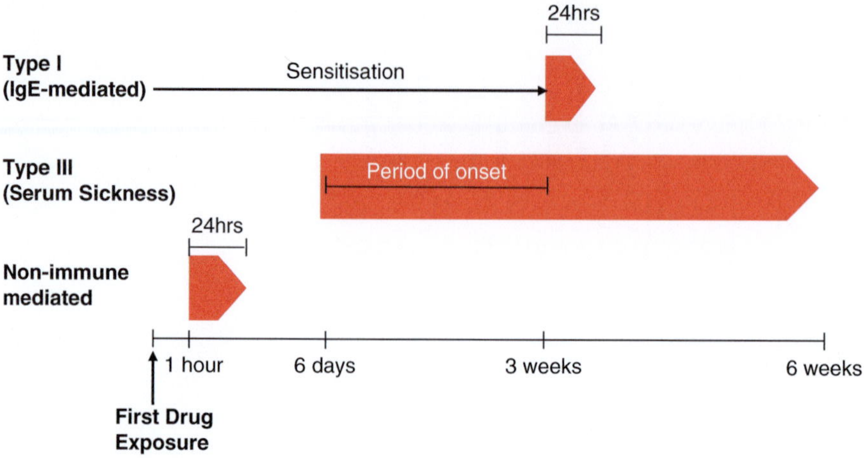

Fig. 9.1 Typical time course for the three types of drug-induced acute urticarial eruptions (indicated by red arrows)

anaphylaxis. IgE-mediated urticarial reactions typically subside within 24 hours of drug withdrawal.

(b) Acute urticaria can also occur immunologically via a type III hypersensitivity reaction. Such reactions occur when IgG or IgM antibodies combine with the drug antigen to form immune complexes. These complexes activate the classical complement cascade which produces anaphylatoxins which in turn act on mast cells to promote release of mediators. This pathophysiological mechanism is often referred to as "serum sickness" and is associated with systemic symptoms which can include fever, papular rash, arthritis, neuritis and nephritis.

In the case of type III reactions, the eruption usually appears from between 6 days and 3 weeks after initial drug exposure and subsides up to a few weeks after drug withdrawal.

In addition to true serum sickness, the possibility of serum sickness-like reaction (SSLR) should also be considered. Despite similar presentation, SSLR is a drug reaction typically occurring 7–21 days post-exposure and is believed to occur via a distinct mechanism to that of true serum sickness. The pathogenesis of SSLR is poorly understood but is not thought to be immune-mediated, with patients having no detectable immune complexes or hypocomplementaemia (Mathur and Mathes 2013) and no systemic involvement (e.g. nephritis, vasculitis). Cefaclor, a cephalosporin antibiotic, is the most commonly implicated drug in SSLR. Studies in patients with previous SSLR caused by cefaclor (Kearns et al. 1994) have suggested the aetiology may be due to inherited defects of metabolism of reactive metabolites leading to an as yet uncharacterised inflammatory response.

(c) Non-immune mechanisms can also elicit an acute urticarial eruption. This involves a drug acting directly to initiate degranulation of mast cells which subsequently release histamine and vasodilatory mediators. Since they act directly on mast cell mediator release, a period of sensitization is not needed.

Chronic urticaria (CU) differs from acute urticaria in its time course and is defined as having been continuous or intermittently present for at least 6 weeks (Mathelier-Fusade 2006). It is generally perceived that chronic urticaria is an idiopathic pre-existing condition which is exacerbated by the administration of a drug, of which there are a number thought to do so (Table 9.1). The mechanism of action is through the non-immune-mediated pathway whereby drugs directly cause release of mast cell mediators in the same way as for acute eruptions.

Another recognised mechanism of chronic urticaria is a specific pharmacological reaction related to use of non-steroidal anti-inflammatory drugs (NSAIDs) or aspirin and their interference with the arachidonic acid pathway. This is a pseudo-allergic reaction which is a consequence of the cyclooxygenase (COX) inhibition properties of aspirin and NSAIDs causing alteration of the arachidonic acid metabolism pathway. Inhibiting COX1 and COX2 increases leukotriene levels leading to vasodilation and edema and subsequent wheal-and-flare eruptions. Aspirin/NSAIDs and opioids (codeine) are most commonly known to exacerbate CU. Indeed, it is estimated that 12–30% of patients with CU will develop accelerated cutaneous symptoms within 1 min to 4 hours of receiving aspirin or NSAIDs (Sanchez-Borges et al. 2015; Szczeklik et al. 1977).

Contact urticaria. Most adverse drug reactions to topically applied medication tend to take the form of eczematous contact dermatitis. However, topical application of drugs can also result in urticarial eruptions (Table 9.1). Contact urticaria can occur as a result of either Type I (IgE-mediated) or non-immunological mechanisms. The immunological mechanism can result in generalised urticaria, but via non-immunological mechanisms, it tends to remain localised to the initial area of exposure/application. Typically, reactions occur from a few minutes to an hour with resolution occurring within 2 h of removal of the causal agent.

9.1.1 Diagnosis and Treatment

A comprehensive history is generally sufficient to confirm an accurate clinical diagnosis and ascertain causality of urticarial drug eruptions. However, it may be necessary to confirm diagnosis using a laboratory test. These typically take the form of a skin-prick test or a disease-specific IgE antibody assay, such as the radioallergosorbent test (RAST), though the latter is usually only available for a handful of drugs (e.g. penicillin, cephalosporin).

The first, and most important, step in management of drug-induced urticaria is the immediate withdrawal of the causal drug. This can be ascertained either by observation of the recent use of a drug known to elicit urticaria or by patient self-reported allergy. Since urticaria is self-limiting, withdrawal of the causal agent is usually sufficient. However, the main concern should be to rule out anaphylaxis via observation and relieve pruritic symptoms. Many symptoms of urticaria are mediated through the action of histamine on H1 receptors. As such, recent guidelines on the treatment and management of urticaria (Zuberbier et al. 2014) recommend first-line therapy which consists of second-generation H1 antihistamine administration. Second-line treatment is a dose escalation of H1 antihistamine up to fourfold. Finally, for individuals not responding to antihistamines, a third-line treatment consisting of anti-IgE therapy (omalizumab), a direct effector of mast cell mediator release (cyclosporine) or a leukotriene receptor antagonist (montelukast) can be used. For AU and acute exacerbations of CU, a short course of corticosteroid (prednisolone) can be used to limit disease duration/activity.

9.1.2 Summary

Urticarial eruptions (hives) are a prominent form of cutaneous adverse drug reactions which are (in acute cases) usually self-limiting and often resolve rapidly following drug withdrawal. They are typically divided into three distinct forms: (a) Acute urticarial eruptions can occur via immune (Type I (IgE-mediated) and Type II (Immune-complex)) and non-immune-mediated reactions and in many cases (40%) are associated with angioedema. Type I and Type II immune-mediated reactions occur immediately after drug administration but require a period of sensitisation of around 3 weeks. Non-immune reactions (direct mast cell activation) are typically immediate but usually as severe. (b) Drug-induced chronic urticaria (CU) is non-immune-mediated and is generally considered an exacerbation of underlying idiopathic CU. (c) Contact urticarial reactions occur due to topical exposure of casual agents and can occur by both immune and non-immune-mediated reactions. The former can result in generalised urticarial with latter usually localised to the area of exposure.

Since drug-induced urticarial eruptions can lead to angioedema, immediate causal agent withdrawal is vital upon diagnosis. First-line treatment should be concerned with management of pruritic symptoms and prevention of possible anaphylaxis.

References

Amar SM, Dreskin SC (2008) Urticaria. Prim Care 35(1):141–157., vii–viii. https://doi.org/10.1016/j.pop.2007.09.009

Hunziker T, Kunzi UP, Braunschweig S, Zehnder D, Hoigne R (1997) Comprehensive hospital drug monitoring (CHDM): adverse skin reactions, a 20-year survey. Allergy 52(4):388–393

Kanani A, Schellenberg R, Warrington R (2011) Urticaria and angioedema. Allergy Asthma Clin Immunol 7(Suppl 1):S9. https://doi.org/10.1186/1710-1492-7-S1-S9

Kearns GL, Wheeler JG, Childress SH, Letzig LG (1994) Serum sickness-like reactions to cefaclor: role of hepatic metabolism and individual susceptibility. J Pediatr 125(5 Pt 1):805–811

Kozel MM, Mekkes JR, Bossuyt PM, Bos JD (1998) The effectiveness of a history-based diagnostic approach in chronic urticaria and angioedema. Arch Dermatol 134(12):1575–1580

Mathelier-Fusade P (2006) Drug-induced urticarias. Clin Rev Allergy Immunol 30(1):19–23. https://doi.org/10.1385/CRIAI:30:1:019

Mathur AN, Mathes EF (2013) Urticaria mimickers in children. Dermatol Ther 26(6):467–475. https://doi.org/10.1111/dth.12103

Poonawalla T, Kelly B (2009) Urticaria: a review. Am J Clin Dermatol 10(1):9–21. https://doi.org/10.2165/0128071-200910010-00002

Sanchez-Borges M, Caballero-Fonseca F, Capriles-Hulett A, Gonzalez-Aveledo L (2015) Aspirin-exacerbated cutaneous disease (AECD) is a distinct subphenotype of chronic spontaneous urticaria. J Eur Acad Dermatol Venereol 29(4):698–701. https://doi.org/10.1111/jdv.12658

Szczeklik A, Gryglewski RJ, Czerniawska-Mysik G (1977) Clinical patterns of hypersensitivity to nonsteroidal anti-inflammatory drugs and their pathogenesis. J Allergy Clin Immunol 60(5):276–284

Zuberbier T, Aberer W, Asero R, Bindslev-Jensen C, Brzoza Z, Canonica GW, Church MK, Ensina LF, Gimenez-Arnau A, Godse K, Goncalo M, Grattan C, Hebert J, Hide M, Kaplan A, Kapp A, Abdul Latiff AH, Mathelier-Fusade P, Metz M, Nast A, Saini SS, Sanchez-Borges M, Schmid-Grendelmeier P, Simons FE, Staubach P, Sussman G, Toubi E, Vena GA, Wedi B, Zhu XJ, Maurer M, European Academy of A, Clinical I, Global A, Asthma European N, European Dermatology F, World Allergy O (2014) The EAACI/GA(2) LEN/EDF/WAO Guideline for the definition, classification, diagnosis, and management of urticaria: the 2013 revision and update. Allergy 69(7):868–887. https://doi.org/10.1111/all.12313

Dermatologic Adverse Events from Cancer Treatments

10

Jennifer Wu, Alina Markova, and Mario E. Lacouture

Abbreviations

ADL	Activities of daily living
ADRs	Adverse drug reactions
AGA	Androgenetic alopecia
AK	Actinic keratoses
CAR-T Cell	Chimeric antigen receptor-modified T lymphocytes
CIA	Chemotherapy-induced alopecia
CombiDT	Combination of dabrafenib with trametinib
CRS	Cytokine release syndrome
CTLA-4	Cytotoxic T lymphocyte antigen-4
DRESS	Drug reaction with eosinophilia and systemic symptoms
EGFR	Epidermal growth factor receptor

J. Wu
Dermatology Service, Department of Medicine, Memorial Sloan Kettering Cancer Center, New York, NY, USA

Department of Dermatology, Drug Hypersensitivity Clinical and Research Center, Chang Gung Memorial Hospital, Taipei, Taiwan

College of Medicine, Chang Gung University, Taoyuan, Taiwan

A. Markova · M. E. Lacouture (✉)
Dermatology Service, Department of Medicine, Memorial Sloan Kettering Cancer Center, New York, NY, USA
e-mail: markovaa@mskcc.org; lacoutum@mskcc.org

N. H. Shear, R. P. Dodiuk-Gad (eds.), *Advances in Diagnosis and Management of Cutaneous Adverse Drug Reactions*, https://doi.org/10.1007/978-981-13-1489-6_10

FAERS	Food and Drug Administration Adverse Event Reporting System
FEC	Fluorouracil/epirubicin/cyclophosphamide
GI	gastrointestinal
GVHD	Graft versus host disease
HFSR	Hand-foot skin reaction
HSCT	Hematopoietic stem cell transplantation
ICIs	Immune checkpoint inhibitors
IHSR	Immediate hypersensitivity reactions
irAEs	Immune-related adverse events
irBP	Immune-related bullous pemphigoid
JAKIs	Janus kinase inhibitors
KAs	Keratoacanthomas
MKIs	Multi-targeted kinase inhibitors
MMF	Mycophenolate mofetil
MPR	Maculopapular rash
MSSA	Methicillin-sensitive Staphylococcus aureus
nbUVB	Narrow band ultraviolet B
NSCLC	Non-small cell lung cancer
NV	Nasal vestibulitis
pCIA	persistent CIA
PLD	Pegylated liposomal doxorubicin
PPE	Papulopustular eruption
QoL	Quality of life
RD	Radiation dermatitis
SCARs	Severe cutaneous adverse reactions
SCCs	Squamous cell carcinomas
SCIs	Systemic calcineurin inhibitors
SJS/TEN	Stevens-Johnson syndrome/toxic epidermal necrolysis
SK	Seborrheic keratoses
TCIs	Topical calcineurin inhibitors
TCR	T cell receptor
WHO	World Health Organization

Key Points

- Dermatologic adverse events (dAEs) vary by anticancer treatment modalities, including cytotoxic chemotherapy, targeted therapy, immunotherapy, radiation therapy, and hematopoietic stem cell transplantation.
- Rashes, alopecia, hand-foot syndrome, and nail changes are well-described dAEs in patient treated with cytotoxic chemotherapies.
- Papulopustular eruption/maculopapular rash, pruritus, xerosis, and hair and nail changes are frequently encountered in patients receiving targeted therapies.
- Immune-related dAEs such as vitiligo, rash, and pruritus are among the earliest and most common AEs of immunotherapies.

- Life-threatening severe cutaneous adverse reactions such as Stevens-Johnson syndrome and toxic epidermal necrolysis associated with cancer treatments have also been reported.
- Dermatological AEs may lead to decreased quality of life (QoL) and dose reduction or discontinuation of cancer treatments and may compromise clinical outcome. Prevention, early diagnosis, and proper management are crucial for optimizing anticancer response and maintaining a good QoL for cancer patients.

10.1 Background: Cancer Incidence and Types of Systemic Anticancer Therapies

According to the 2016 report of the World Health Organization (WHO), 14 million new cancer cases were diagnosed in 2012, 8.2 million people died from cancer, and 32.6 million are surviving with cancer (Santoni et al. 2015). New cancer treatments are being rapidly developed, and each year many of them are approved by regulatory bodies. In parallel, the incidences of adverse drug reactions (ADRs) to cancer treatments have increased dramatically (Giavina-Bianchi et al. 2017). Dermatologic adverse events (dAEs) vary by cancer treatment modalities, including cytotoxic chemotherapy, targeted therapy, immunotherapy, radiation therapy, chimeric antigen receptor-modified T lymphocyte (CAR-T cell) therapy, and hematopoietic stem cell transplantation. These dAEs—which affect the skin, hair, nails, and mucous membranes—strongly impact patients' morbidity, mortality, as well as quality of life (QoL), self-esteem, and physical, psychosocial, and financial well-being. Serious dAEs often result in treatment interruption, dose reduction, and regimen changes, which can compromise clinical outcomes or even lead to life-threatening events (Lacouture 2015). Understanding the underlying biology of these dAEs, emphasizing early diagnosis, and timely and proper management are crucial for optimizing treatment response and maintaining a good QoL for cancer patients. Before initiation of any cancer treatment, it is of good practice getting patients educated regarding potential dAEs and strategies for prevention.

10.2 Adverse Drug Reactions to Anticancer Therapies (See Table 10.1 for a Summary)

10.2.1 Cytotoxic Chemotherapy

10.2.1.1 Hand-Foot Syndrome (HFS)

HFS, also known as palmar-plantar erythrodysesthesia, is a well-described dAE of certain chemotherapeutic agents (Bolognia et al. 2008; Parker et al. 2013), mainly capecitabine, 5-fluorouracil, cytarabine, docetaxel, doxorubicin, and pegylated liposomal doxorubicin (PLD) (Hackbarth et al. 2008; Saif et al. 2008; Chew and Chuen 2009; Balagula et al. 2011b; Lorusso et al. 2007). Dysesthesia, symmetrical painful erythema, and edema located on palms and soles are the most characteristic manifestations (Fig. 10.1a, b). Without proper interventions, the lesions may progress to

Table 10.1 Summary of dermatologic adverse events from cancer treatments

Types of systemic anticancer therapies	Dermatologic adverse events	Common culprits (incidence %)	Clinical manifestation (incidence %)	Histology/risk factors/proposed pathomechanism
Chemotherapy				
	Hand-foot syndrome (HFS) (palmar-plantar erythrodysesthesia)	Capecitabine (43–63%) (Sibaud et al. 2016), continuously infused 5-fluorouracil, cytarabine, docetaxel (5–10%) (Sibaud et al. 2016), doxorubicin, and pegylated liposomal doxorubicin (PLD) (45%) (Hackbarth et al. 2008; Saif et al. 2008; Chew and Chuen 2009; Balagula et al. 2011b; Lorusso et al. 2007; Lacouture et al. 2008a).	Onset: days to months after initiation of treatment Symptoms: dysesthesia, followed by symmetrical painful erythema and edema located on palms and soles; the lesions may progress to blisters, crusts, ulcerations, or even epidermal necrosis (Lorusso et al. 2007)	The pathophysiology is not fully understood. Studies suggested that capecitabine (Chen et al. 2017) and PLD (Chen et al. 2017), or accumulation of metabolites could significantly induce keratinocytes apoptosis, which may be enhanced through the transport by sweat (Lou et al. 2016). The involvement of an inflammatory process mediated by the overexpression of cyclooxygenase 2 (COX-2) was also reported (Zhang et al. 2012)
	Immediate hypersensitivity reactions (IHSR)	Taxanes (30% if without premedication) (Giavina-Bianchi et al. 2017; Sibaud et al. 2016; Aoyama et al. 2017); platinum-based regimens (12–24%) (Park et al. 2016)	Onset: during the first two cycles of treatment with a rapid onset within minutes (Sibaud et al. 2016). Symptoms: maculopapular rash, urticaria, flushing, angioedema, and pruritus, with or without systemic signs, e.g., hypotension, dyspnea, or chills (Sibaud et al. 2016; Syrigou et al. 2011); severe anaphylaxis (docetaxel) (Syrigou et al. 2011)	The underlying mechanism is poorly understood. A hypersensitivity reaction to the solvent for paclitaxel (Cremophor EL®, castor oil vehicle) may play a crucial role, while the solvent for docetaxel (Tween 80, polyoxyethylene-20-sorbitan monooleate) is less frequently addressed (Gelmon 1994)

	Extravasation reactions	Irritants: platinum-based alkylating agents, taxanes, and topoisomerase inhibitors Vesicants: anthracyclines, vinca alkaloids, and nitrogen mustards incidence: 0.1–6% (Sibaud et al. 2016; Langer 2010)	The severity of the reaction depends on the volume, concentration, and type of chemotherapeutic agents. Irritants usually cause milder inflammatory reaction with the presentation of erythema, edema, and pain. Vesicants can lead to blister formation, ulceration, and tissue necrosis (Kyllo and Anadkat 2014b).	The extravasation of chemotherapeutic drugs into soft tissues in the vicinity of an infusion site.
	Pigmentary changes	Busulfan, cyclophosphamide, ifosfamide, bleomycin, 5-FU, vinorelbine, fotemustine, docetaxel, etc.	Busulfan: Addison-like generalized skin hyperpigmentation Cyclophosphamide and ifosfamide: localized hyperpigmentation of the nails, palms, and soles (Teresi et al. 1993; Chittari et al. 2009). Bleomycin: flagellate hyperpigmentation(20%) (Abess et al. 2003; Vuerstaek et al. 2007) 5-FU, vinorelbine, fotemustine, or docetaxel: serpentine supravenous hyperpigmentation (Huang and Anadkat 2011; Suvirya et al. 2014)	

(continued)

Table 10.1 (continued)

Types of systemic anticancer therapies	Dermatologic adverse events	Common culprits (incidence %)	Clinical manifestation (incidence %)	Histology/risk factors/proposed pathomechanism
	Onychodystrophy	Beau's lines: bleomycin, cisplatin, docetaxel, doxorubicin, melphalan, and vincristine (Kyllo and Anadkat 2014a). Onycholysis: mitoxantrone, docetaxel, anthracyclines, and paclitaxel	Beau's lines, onycholysis, hyperpigmentation, discoloration, splinter hemorrhages, subungual hematomas, and nail loss (Capriotti et al. 2015); paronychia, granulation tissue formation, and secondary bacterial infection with abscess formation may occur with pain (Capriotti et al. 2015) Overall incidence of skin, nail, and hair side effects to chemotherapeutic agents, including taxanes ($n = 42$, 46%), PEG doxorubicin ($n = 17$, 7%), other anthracyclines (epirubicin and doxorubicin; $n = 6$, 19%), topotecan ($n = 13$, 14%), and other agents ($n = 13$, 14%), was 86.8% ($n = 76$), and 23.1% ($n = 23$) developed nail changes (Hackbarth et al. 2008)	
	Chemotherapy-induced alopecia (CIA)		Incidence: 65% (Trueb 2010)	
	Chemotherapy-induced acute reversible alopecia	Taxanes are one of the top CIA-inducing drugs (Trueb 2010; Tallon et al. 2010)	Chemotherapy-induced acute reversible alopecia is commonly induced by anagen effluvium and typically occurs after the first treatment cycle (Trueb 2007). Any hair-bearing areas (scalp hair, eyelashes, eyebrows, beard, axillae, pubis, and body) can be involved. The hair usually starts to regrow 3–6 months after the last cycle of chemotherapy and gradually returns to baseline with one third of patients undergoing texture and color change of the regrown hair (Lindner et al. 2012)	

	Persistent chemotherapy-induced alopecia (pCIA)	Busulfan, thiotepa, fluorouracil/epirubicin/cyclophosphamide (FEC), and taxanes	The incidence is not clear and suspected to be underestimated. Kluger et al. estimated the incidence is around 2% in breast cancer patients treated with docetaxel (Kluger et al. 2012). The hair loss presents as suboptimal or absence of regrowth of scalp and body hair, >6 months after the completion of chemotherapy (Tallon et al. 2010). CIPAL usually manifests as diffuse hair loss or hair thinning and tends to be accentuated in vertex areas prone to androgenetic alopecia (Lindner et al. 2012; Palamaras et al. 2011; Kluger et al. 2012; Miteva et al. 2011; Fonia et al. 2017; Asz-Sigall et al. 2016). Eyelashes, eyebrows, axillae, pubis, and body hair can also be affected (Kluger et al. 2012; Miteva et al. 2011; Prevezas et al. 2009)	The histological findings of CIPAL are similar to androgenetic alopecia (AGA) or female pattern hair loss (Lindner et al. 2012; Miteva et al. 2011; Fonia et al. 2017) The pathomechanism of CIPAL has not been fully understood, and a separation of the matrix cells from the dermal papilla, as well as a direct cytotoxic action of taxanes on hair matrix keratinocytes or hair bulge stem cells, has been postulated (Tallon et al. 2010; Kluger et al. 2012; Miteva et al. 2011)
	Radiation recall	Doxorubicin, taxanes, 5-FU, gemcitabine, and capecitabine were most commonly reported (Kyllo and Anadkat 2014b; Sanborn and Sauer 2008; Wyatt et al. 2006; Burris and Hurtig 2010; Korman et al. 2017)	Radiation recall is an acute inflammatory reaction confined to previously irradiated areas triggered by chemotherapy administered after radiotherapy. Incidence: drug dependent; varies from 1.8 to 11.5% (Kyllo and Anadkat 2014b; Sanborn and Sauer 2008; Wyatt et al. 2006) The latency period for the radiation recall ranges from several months to years (Sanborn and Sauer 2008; Wyatt et al. 2006)	The underlying pathogenesis remain unclear; however, some proposed that a cytotoxic chemotherapy-induced, memory-cell-mediated hypersensitivity reaction may be involved (Burris and Hurtig 2010; Korman et al. 2017)

(continued)

Table 10.1 (continued)

Types of systemic anticancer therapies	Dermatologic adverse events	Common culprits (incidence %)	Clinical manifestation (incidence %)	Histology/risk factors/proposed pathomechanism
Targeted anticancer therapy				
EGFR inhibitors (EGFRIs)	Papulopustular eruption (PPE)	EGFR inhibitors are used to treat advanced or metastatic non-small cell lung cancer (afatinib, erlotinib, gefitinib, necitumumab), pancreatic cancer (erlotinib), breast cancer (lapatinib, neratinib), colon cancer (cetuximab, panitumumab), and head and neck cancer (cetuximab) and in even more broad clinical settings based on individual mutations of the tumor (Tang and Ratner 2016; Kyllo and Anadkat 2014b; Tischer et al. 2017)	Early-onset: usually occurs during the first 2 weeks of treatment (Drilon et al. 2016) The incidence is higher with monoclonal antibodies such as cetuximab and panitumumab (90%) than with tyrosine kinase inhibitors such as gefitinib, erlotinib, lapatinib, and afatinib (44–75%) (Kyllo and Anadkat 2014b; Hofheinz et al. 2016) The severity in most patients are mild (grade 1) to moderate (grade 2), but severe skin reaction (grade 3) is seen in 18% of patients (Hofheinz et al. 2016)	The normal expression profile of EGFR includes epidermal keratinocytes, sebaceous glands, hair follicle epithelium, and periungual tissues. (Tischer et al. 2017; Drilon et al. 2016) These agents not only inhibit specific signaling pathways on tumor cells but also interfere signal transduction in normal tissues of various organ systems, including the skin, hair and nails, leading to the toxicity. (Lacouture et al. 2014; Kyllo and Anadkat 2014b; Tischer et al. 2017)
	Pigmentary changes		A systematic review showed the overall incidences of targeted cancer therapy-induced all-grade pigmentary changes in the skin and hair were 17.7 and 21.5%, respectively, and EGFRI and imatinib inhibitors were the most common culprits (Julia Dai et al. 2017)	

	Changes in hair texture, nonscarring and scarring alopecia, facial hypertrichosis, and eyelash trichomegaly (Lacouture et al. 2011; Kyllo and Anadkat 2014b; Drilon et al. 2016; Gandhi et al. 2014; Belum et al. 2015a)		Change in hair texture: increased brittleness and curliness (Belum et al. 2015a) Nonscarring alopecia: frontal, patchy, or diffuse pattern; typically develops 2–3 months after initiation of EGFRI therapy (5%) and resolves spontaneously after discontinuation of the drug (Lacouture et al. 2011) Scarring alopecia: consequent to PPE, results in permanent hair loss (Lacouture et al. 2011) Facial hypertrichosis and eyelash trichomegaly: develop after 1–2 months of EGFRI treatment (20%) (Lacouture et al. 2011). Eyelash trichomegaly can lead to corneal abrasions and further ocular complications (Lacouture et al. 2011)	
	Paronychia (Lacouture et al. 2011; Kyllo and Anadkat 2014b; Drilon et al. 2016; Gandhi et al. 2014; Belum et al. 2015a)		Periungual erythema, swelling, pain, and periungual pyogenic granuloma-like lesions can be observed (Gandhi et al. 2014): develop approximately 2–3 months after initiation of EGFRI therapy with the incidence varying with different EGFRIs from 12 to 58% (Lacouture et al. 2011). The lesion is initially sterile but can become superinfected. (Kyllo and Anadkat 2014b)	The hypothesized pathogenesis is periungual inflammation related to keratinocyte cytokine dysregulation, an effect which may be aggravated by ingrown nails and local trauma (Kyllo and Anadkat 2014b)

(continued)

Table 10.1 (continued)

Types of systemic anticancer therapies	Dermatologic adverse events	Common culprits (incidence %)	Clinical manifestation (incidence %)	Histology/risk factors/proposed pathomechanism
	Nasal vestibulitis (NV)		NV is an acute inflammation of the tissue around the nasal vestibule—a part of the anterior nasal cavity Local erythema, nasal tenderness, crusting, and/or epistaxis. (Ruiz et al. 2015) The frequently noted clinico-morphological features include xerosis, fissures, erythema, crusting, impetiginization, furunculosis, folliculitis, epistaxis, and edematous and painful nose. The occurrence of NV simultaneously with rash or xerosis in patients receiving EGFRIs was reported	Patients treated with targeted therapies frequently develop dAEs characterized by epidermal disruption of the skin and mucosa which makes them more susceptible to NV and secondary skin infections from spreading of pathogenic organisms from the nares (Ruiz et al. 2015) The most frequent organism identified was methicillin-sensitive *Staphylococcus aureus* (MSSA) (43%) with 18% of MSSA resistant to tetracycline (Ruiz et al. 2015) Methicillin-resistant *S. aureus* (MRSA) was also found
Multi-targeted kinase inhibitors (MKIs)	Hand-foot skin reaction (FHSR)	9–62% patients exposed to sorafenib, sunitinib, regorafenib, axitinib, and pazopanib (Belum et al. 2013d; Fischer et al. 2013; McLellan et al. 2015; Balagula et al. 2012)	HFSR most commonly develops within the first 6 weeks of treatment. Symptoms include localized paresthesia; tingling, burning, or painful sensations; and a decreased tolerance for touching hot objects, usually developing on pressure-bearing and friction-prone areas such as the palms and soles; symmetric acral erythematous and edematous lesions associated with desquamation and fissures; hyperkeratosis, presenting as yellowish painful plaques encompassed by an erythematous/edematous halo, usually develops after blister formation on pressure areas (54%) (Gomez and Lacouture 2011)	The proposed pathogenesis of HFSR involves direct pressure and friction to the hands and feet causing the blistering and capillary endothelial damage, disruption of endothelial healing by inhibition of VEGFR and PDGFR, and direct keratinocyte toxicity from the drug probably related to dysregulation of the Fas/FasL signaling pathway which contribute to the apoptosis of keratinocytes and following inflammatory response (Belum et al. 2013a; Lacouture et al. 2008b; Yeh et al. 2014)

BRAF inhibitors (BRAFIs)	Nonmalignant hyperkeratotic skin eruptions (Choi 2014; Belum et al. 2013b; Carlos et al. 2015)	Vemurafenib and dabrafenib	Squamoproliferative/keratinocytic lesions (60–85%), verrucal keratosis (most common, >60%; early onset, 1 week after the initiation of treatment); skin papillomas,; verruca vulgaris; seborrheic keratoses (SK); warty dyskeratomas; palmar/plantar hyperkeratosis over pressure or friction points (40%); inflamed actinic keratoses (AK); and keratoacanthomas (KAs) (Belum et al. 2013b)	BRAF is a serine-threonine protein kinase functioning in the RAS/RAF/MEK/MAPK signaling pathway triggered by activation of multiple receptor tyrosine kinases, including those of the EGFR/ErbB family. This pathway regulates cellular proliferation, differentiation, migration, survival, and apoptosis (Belum et al. 2013a, d; ; Choi 2014; Carlos et al. 2015) Paradoxical activation of wild-type BRAF cells which potentiates the activity of the MAPK pathway and subsequent keratinocyte hyperproliferation (Choi 2014; Belum et al. 2013b; Carlos et al. 2015) Paradoxical activation of the MAPK pathway in cells that harbor a RAS mutation or activation of CRAF in wild-type-BRAF cells by a BRAFI (Pugliese et al. 2015; Carlos et al. 2015)
	Cutaneous squamous cell carcinomas (SCCs) (Choi 2014; Belum et al. 2013b; Carlos et al. 2015)		Cutaneous SCCs, usually KA type, presenting as rapid growing, dome-shaped crateriform nodules, located on sun-exposed skin area (4–36%) (Choi 2014; Belum et al. 2013b; Carlos et al. 2015), appear early during the course of treatment (median time: 8 weeks) with vemurafenib but may occur from 1 to 9 months (Belum et al. 2013b)	

(continued)

Table 10.1 (continued)

Types of systemic anticancer therapies	Dermatologic adverse events	Common culprits (incidence %)	Clinical manifestation (incidence %)	Histology/risk factors/proposed pathomechanism
	Photosensitivity		More common in patients treated with vemurafenib (30–52%) Acute erythema, burning, and even painful blistering on sun-exposed skin (Belum et al. 2013b) Rapid onset: usually within 24 h of sun exposure	
	Maculopapular rash (MPR), PPE, or folliculocentric rashes with or without pruritus (Belum et al. 2013b); keratosis pilaris (KP)-like skin eruption on the proximal limbs, trunk, and face (5–9%); and HFSR. (Belum et al. 2013b; Pugliese et al. 2015; Chandrakumar and Yeung 2014)		Incidence: 8–20%, more commonly with vemurafenib than with dabrafenib Early onset: within 2 weeks after initiation of treatment	
MEK inhibitors (MEKIs)		Trametinib, cobimetinib	The dAEs of MEKI are similar to those of EGFRIs: PPE (52–93%, most common), xerosis, pruritus, alopecia (9–17%), paronychia, hyperpigmentation, trichomegaly of eyelashes, changes in hair texture, and hypertrichosis of the face (Choi 2014; Balagula et al. 2011a; Carlos et al. 2015; Dreno et al. 2017; Keating 2016); secondary bacterial infection to affected skin area	

BRAF inhibitors plus MEK inhibitors			Combination therapy seems to show an improved skin toxicity profile than a BRAFI alone: the combination of dabrafenib with trametinib (CombiDT study) showed a higher frequency of folliculitis (40 vs. 6.7%) and a significant decrease of cutaneous SCCs (0 vs. 26.1%), verrucal keratosis (0 vs. 66.4%), and Grover's disease (0 vs. 42.9%) (Choi 2014; Carlos et al. 2015; Dreno et al. 2017; Keating 2016)	
Hedgehog inhibitors	Alopecia, follicular dermatitis, hypersensitivity reaction, KAs, and cutaneous SCCs (Sekulic et al. 2012; LoRusso et al. 2011; US 2012; European Medicines Agency 2016; Aasi et al. 2013; Kwong et al. 2017; Sekulic et al. 2017; Lacouture et al. 2016)	Vismodegib, sonidegib	Common AEs include alopecia (58%), muscle spasms (71%), and dysgeusia (71%) (LoRusso et al. 2011; Kwong et al. 2017; Sekulic et al. 2017) Follicular dermatitis, hypersensitivity reaction, KAs, and cutaneous SCCs have been reported to occur after vismodegib treatment (Aasi et al. 2013; Kwong et al. 2017; Sekulic et al. 2017)	The hedgehog pathway plays an important role in normal hair follicle function, follicle-based toxicities such as alopecia and folliculitis are hypothesized to be a possible clinical indicator of treatment response (Kwong et al. 2017)

(continued)

Table 10.1 (continued)

Types of systemic anticancer therapies	Dermatologic adverse events	Common culprits (incidence %)	Clinical manifestation (incidence %)	Histology/risk factors/proposed pathomechanism
Immunotherapy				
Immune checkpoint inhibitors (ICIs)	Rash, pruritus, vitiligo	Anti-CTLA4, anti-PD1, anti-PD-L1	Incidence of all-grade rash: ipilimumab 24.3%, pembrolizumab 16.7%, nivolumab 14.3% Incidence of all-grade pruritus was ipilimumab 31%, pembrolizumab 20.2%, and nivolumab 13.2% (Belum et al. 2016) Incidence of all-grade vitiligo was ipilimumab 1.6–8.7%, nivolumab 7.5%, pembrolizumab 8.3–25% (Belum et al. 2016; Larsabal et al. 2017) The time to onset of vitiligo-like lesions ranged from 16 to 52 weeks. (Larsabal et al. 2017)	As ICIs restore antitumor immunity which leads to durable anticancer effect, by interrupting normal inhibitory and immune escape mechanisms induced by tumor cells; they may concurrently induce autoimmunity that results in organ dysfunction, referred to as immune-related adverse events (irAEs). (Michot et al. 2016; Wolchok et al. 2010)
	Autoimmune bullous dermatosis	Anti-PD1 and anti-PD-L1		
	Severe cutaneous adverse reactions (SCARs)	Anti-CTLA4, anti-PD1, and anti-PD-L1		
Chimeric antigen receptor-modified T lymphocytes (CAR-T cell) therapy	Cytokine release syndrome (CRS)	CAR-T cell therapy	CRS can be observed shortly after administration of CAR-T cells (Weber et al. 2015) The clinical manifestation resembles sepsis, presenting with fever, tachycardia, vascular leak, oliguria, hypotension, and even multiorgan failure in severe cases. When proteins of melanocytic origin were targeted with TCRs against MART-1 and gp100, cutaneous, ocular, and internal ear toxicities occurred (Weber et al. 2015)	Autoimmunity may occur when a T cell receptor (TCR) targeting a protein was expressed in normal tissue

Radiation therapy				
Radiation therapy	Radiation dermatitis (RD) (Lacouture et al. 2010a; Wong et al. 2013; Shaitelman et al. 2015)	Ionized radiation	RD often occurs approximately 2–3 weeks following the start of radiotherapy (Wong et al. 2013) Acute RD is self-limiting and usually resolves after 2–3 weeks: mild erythema, dry and moist desquamation, and ulceration Late toxicities (occurring >90 days of treatment) may persist and result in a persistent negative impact on patients' QOL (Lacouture et al. 2010a): telangiectasia, atrophy, fibrosis, edema, and ulceration	The risks of radiation injury are dose- and location-dependent (Wong et al. 2013)
Hematopoietic stem cell transplantation (HSCT)				
Hematopoietic stem cell transplantation (HSCT)	Cutaneous graft versus host disease (GVHD)	HSCT	Clinical manifestations include fever, rash, severe gastrointestinal (GI) manifestations, and impaired liver function Cutaneous GVHD is usually the earliest and most common manifestations of GVHD (Hymes et al. 2012a) Early cutaneous signs and symptoms include pruritus, dysesthesias, or macular erythema and edema, followed by a folliculocentric or morbilliform eruption, often first appearing on the trunk and then becoming confluent over time (Hymes et al. 2012a); bullae formation or epidermal detachment may occur (Hymes et al. 2012a); eyes and mucous membranes can also be involved (Hymes et al. 2012a)	The risk of GVHD increases with certain conditions such as unrelated donors, mismatched donors, older donors, multiparous female donors, older recipients, and different chemotherapy regimens (Wolchok et al. 2010). A biopsy can be performed to confirm the diagnosis, although the pathologic changes of GVHD are nonspecific (Villarreal et al. 2016)

(continued)

Table 10.1 (continued)

Types of systemic anticancer therapies	Dermatologic adverse events	Common culprits (incidence %)	Clinical manifestation (incidence %)	Histology/risk factors/proposed pathomechanism
Others				
Other cutaneous adverse reactions from cancer treatment	Skin infections associated with anticancer treatment (Gandhi et al. 2014)		29% of 221 patients on EGFRI in a case series developed secondary infection at affected skin area of PPE: 78% *S. aureus*, 6.3% MRSA. (Gandhi et al. 2014) The incidence of herpes simplex infection and herpes zoster while on EGFRI treatment was reported to be 13% (Gandhi et al. 2014) Other anticancer treatments such as bortezomib, rituximab, and temozolomide have also been linked to varicella zoster virus infection. (Gandhi et al. 2014)	Studies suggest that cancer patients with neutropenia and preexisting skin toxicity are susceptible to secondary infection
	Stevens-Johnson syndrome/toxic epidermal necrolysis (SJS/TEN)	SJS: bendamustine TEN: bendamustine, busulfan, chlorambucil, fludarabine, lomustine, and procarbazine (Food and Drug Administration Adverse Event Reporting System (FAERS)) (Rosen et al. 2014)	The incidences of life-threatening toxicities such as SJS/TEN are inconsistently reported: A systematic review showed there were 46 SJS and 37 TEN cases associated with 18 and 22 anticancer drugs in the literature (Rosen et al. 2014)	

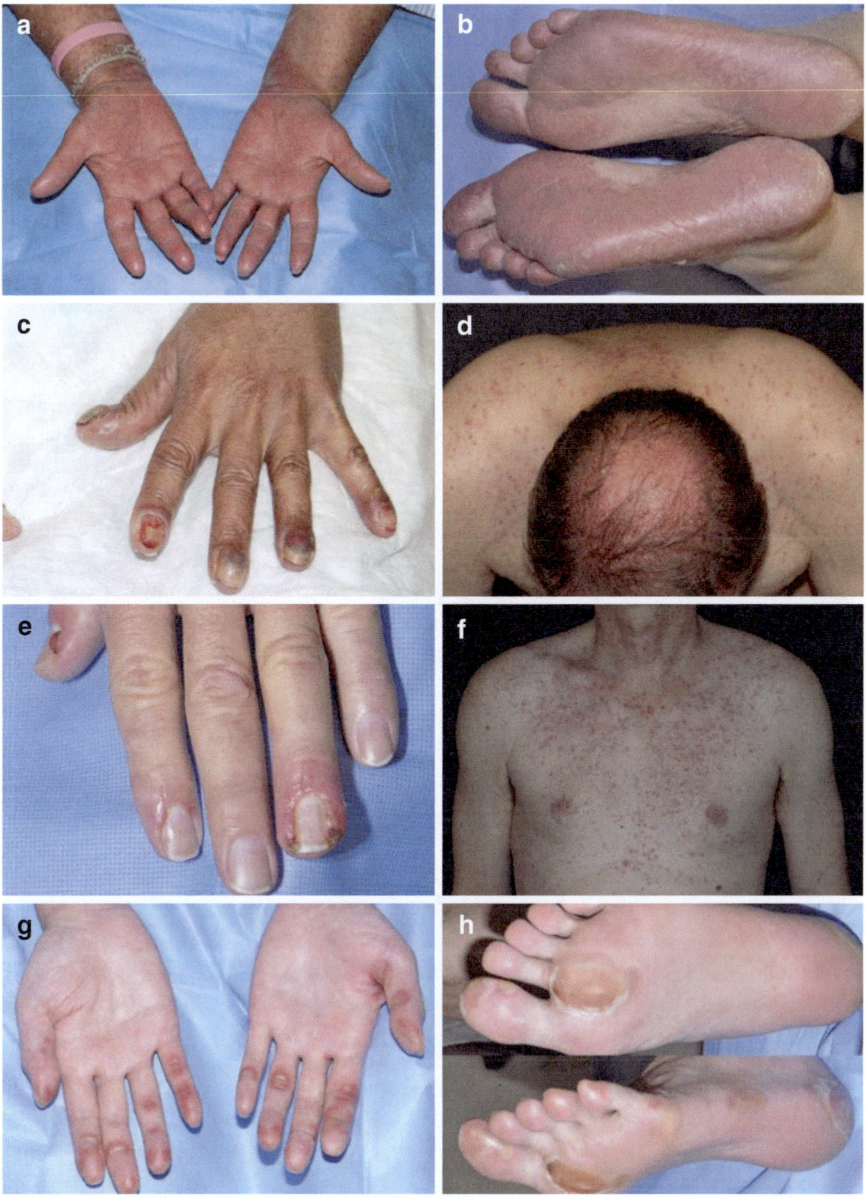

Fig. 10.1 Dermatologic adverse events from cancer treatments. (**a**) Hand-foot syndrome (HFS) induced by chemotherapy, palms; (**b**) HFS induced by chemotherapy, soles; (**c**) swelling of fingertips, subungual hemorrhage, onycholysis, and nail loss induced by chemotherapy; (**d**) papulopustular eruption (PPE) induced by EGFRIs on the scalp and upper trunk with secondary bacterial infection; (**e**) paronychia induced by EGFRIs; (**f**) PPE induced by MKIs; (**g**) hand-foot skin reaction (HFSR) induced by MKIs, palms; (**h**) HFSR induced by MKIs, soles

blisters, crusts, ulcerations, or even epidermal necrosis which can significantly affect patient's QoL and necessitate therapeutic modifications or even treatment discontinuation (Lorusso et al. 2007; von Moos et al. 2008; Nikolaou et al. 2016).

10.2.1.2 Pigmentary Changes

Alkylating agents are commonly associated with mucocutaneous hyperpigmentation which usually spontaneously resolves over time and may not warrant discontinuation of chemotherapy (Teresi et al. 1993; Chittari et al. 2009; Abess et al. 2003; Vuerstaek et al. 2007; Huang and Anadkat 2011; Suvirya et al. 2014; Jain et al. 2005).

10.2.1.3 Hair and Nail Changes

Nail Toxicities

Damage to the nail matrix induced by cytotoxic chemotherapeutic agents characteristically manifests as Beau's lines, which resolve after completion of chemotherapy (Kyllo and Anadkat 2014a). The nail bed is also commonly affected, resulting in onycholysis, which sometimes need intervention. Other nail changes include hyperpigmentation, discoloration, splinter hemorrhages, and subungual hematomas (Capriotti et al. 2015) (Fig. 10.1c). Paronychia, granulation tissue formation, and secondary bacterial infection with abscess formation may occur with pain that significantly interferes with patients' daily activities and QoL (Capriotti et al. 2015).

Chemotherapy-Induced Alopecia (CIA)

CIA is estimated to occur in 65% patients receiving chemotherapy and is considered the most traumatic aspect of chemotherapy by 47% of female patients (Trueb 2010). CIA is commonly presented as anagen effluvium and typically occurs after four cycles of chemotherapy (Trueb 2007). Taxanes and anthracyclines are the top CIA-inducing drugs (Trueb 2010; Tallon et al. 2010; Lindner et al. 2012; Nangia et al. 2017). There is increasing evidence that certain chemotherapy regimens, including busulfan, thiotepa, fluorouracil/epirubicin/cyclophosphamide (FEC), and taxanes, can cause persistent CIA (pCIA) (Tallon et al. 2010; Lindner et al. 2012; Palamaras et al. 2011; Kluger et al. 2012; Miteva et al. 2011; Prevezas et al. 2009; Fonia et al. 2017; Asz-Sigall et al. 2016).

10.2.2 Targeted Anticancer Therapy

In recent years, several therapeutic agents have been developed that inhibit the epidermal growth factor receptor (EGFR) and the intracellular RAS/RAF/MEK/MAPK signaling pathway, which play a central role in tumor growth of certain cancers (Belum et al. 2013a; Tang and Ratner 2016). Incidence and severity of dAEs vary with specific targeted therapies and different doses (Lacouture et al. 2011, 2014; Kyllo and Anadkat 2014b; Belum et al. 2013c; Tischer et al. 2017).

10.2.2.1 EGFR Inhibitors (EGFRIs)

EGFRIs are used to treat advanced/metastatic non-small cell lung cancer (NSCLC) (afatinib, erlotinib, gefitinib, necitumumab), pancreatic cancer (erlotinib), breast cancer (lapatinib, neratinib), colon cancer (cetuximab, panitumumab), and head and neck cancer (cetuximab) and in even broader clinical settings based on individual mutations of the tumor (Tang and Ratner 2016; Kyllo and Anadkat 2014b; Tischer et al. 2017). Skin reactions are the most common EGFRI-related AEs, which may be painful and debilitating and may have a negative impact on patients' daily activity, QoL, and treatment durability (Lacouture et al. 2010a, 2011, 2014; Kyllo and Anadkat 2014b).

Papulopustular Eruption (PPE)

The most common dAE of EGFRIs is PPE, affecting 75–90% of patients (Kyllo and Anadkat 2014b; Hofheinz et al. 2016). PPE consists of acneiform folliculocentric papules and sterile pustules with a predilection for seborrheic areas, often accompanied by xerosis, pruritus, or even pain (Fig. 10.1d) (Hsiao et al. 2011). PPE is a relatively early-onset AE which usually occurs during the first 2 weeks of treatment (Drilon et al. 2016). Skin reactions are transient, usually most prominent in the beginning, abating after the completion of treatment; however, postinflammatory erythema or hyperpigmentation may persist (Hofheinz et al. 2016; Clabbers et al. 2016). Interestingly, the development and severity of skin toxicity have been correlated to a more favorable prognosis (Liu et al. 2013; Lacouture et al. 2010b).
Hair and nail changes (Fig. 10.1e)

10.2.2.2 Multi-targeted Kinase Inhibitors (MKIs)

The MKIs such as sorafenib, sunitinib, regorafenib, axitinib, and pazopanib exert their antitumor effects by interfering with molecular signaling mechanisms important for cell growth and angiogenesis (Lacouture et al. 2008b). Dermatologic AEs are among the most commonly reported AEs in patients receiving MKIs which include skin rash (Fig. 10.1f), xerosis, and pruritus (Kyllo and Anadkat 2014b; Valentine et al. 2015; Ensslin et al. 2013).

Hand-Foot Skin Reaction (HFSR)

HFSR is one of the most common dAEs encountered by 9–62% patients exposed to MKIs, and incidence and severity appear to be dose dependent (Belum et al. 2013a, d; Lacouture et al. 2008a, b, 2013a; Gomez and Lacouture 2011; Yeh et al. 2014; Fischer et al. 2013; McLellan et al. 2015; Balagula et al. 2012). Localized paresthesia and tingling, burning, or painful sensations accompanied by symmetric acral erythema and edema with desquamation and fissures usually develop on pressure-bearing/friction-prone areas, which negatively affect walking in 35% of patients (Lacouture et al. 2008b, 2013a; Gomez and Lacouture 2011). Hyperkeratosis, presenting as yellowish painful plaques encompassed by an erythematous/edematous halo, develops after blister formation on pressure areas of the soles and is a defining feature of HFSR (Gomez and Lacouture 2011) (Fig. 10.1g, h).

10.2.2.3 BRAF Inhibitors (BRAFIs)

Dermatologic AEs are among the most significant and frequent AEs associated with the use of BRAFIs (vemurafenib and dabrafenib), occurring in 92–95% of patients, and can be generally categorized into inflammatory conditions, squamoproliferative/keratinocytic lesions, melanocytic proliferations, and hair and nail changes (Belum et al. 2013a, b, d; Choi 2014; Lacouture et al. 2013b).

Skin rashes

Photosensitivity

Photosensitivity is a well-known AE reported in 30–52% of patients treated with vemurafenib, presenting as acute erythema, with burning and even painful blistering on sun-exposed skin (Choi 2014; Belum et al. 2013b; Pugliese et al. 2015).

Nonmalignant hyperkeratotic skin eruptions

Cutaneous squamous cell carcinomas (SCCs)

10.2.2.4 MEK Inhibitors (MEKIs)

The dAEs of MEKIs are similar to those of EGFRIs (Balagula et al. 2011a).

10.2.2.5 Hedgehog Pathway Inhibitors (Vismodegib, Sonidegib) (Table 10.1)

10.2.3 Immune Checkpoint Inhibitors (ICIs)

The cytotoxic T lymphocyte antigen-4 (CTLA-4) signaling pathway and the programmed cell death receptor-1 (PD-1)/PD ligand-1/2 (PD-L1/PD-L2) signaling pathway have been increasingly recognized as the immune checkpoint of tumor-induced immune suppression (Weber et al. 2015). As immune checkpoint inhibitors (ICIs) restore antitumor immunity which leads to durable anticancer effect, by unbalancing the immune system, they may induce autoimmunity that results in organ dysfunction, referred to as immune-related adverse events (irAEs) (Michot et al. 2016; Wolchok et al. 2010).

10.2.3.1 Rash, Pruritus, and Vitiligo

Rash, pruritus, and vitiligo (Fig. 10.2a, b) are among the earliest and most common AEs of ICIs (Wolchok et al. 2010; Belum et al. 2016; Robert et al. 2015; Larsabal et al. 2017). Autoimmune bullous dermatoses (Naidoo et al. 2016), lichenoid reactions (Sibaud et al. 2017), psoriasis, alopecia areata/universalis (Damsky and King 2017; Shreberk-Hassidim et al. 2017), Stevens-Johnson syndrome (SJS), and toxic epidermal necrosis (TEN)-like eruptions have been anecdotally reported (Michot et al. 2016; Robert et al. 2015; Weber et al. 2013; Curry et al. 2017). Increasing evidence supports that vitiligo and/or cutaneous reactions emerging during ICI

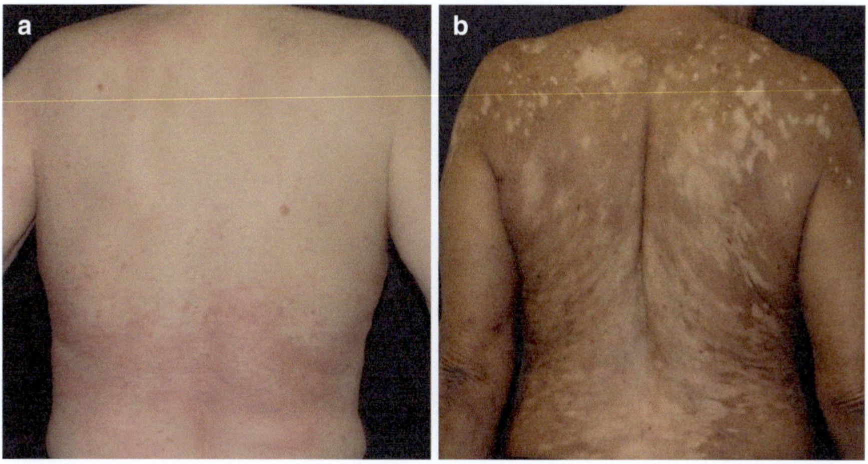

Fig. 10.2 Common dermatologic adverse events associated with immune checkpoint inhibitors. (**a**) Maculopapular rash, (**b**) vitiligo-like lesions

treatments are associated with favorable prognosis (Weber et al. 2012, 2013, 2015; Freeman-Keller et al. 2016; Goldinger et al. 2016).

10.2.3.2 Autoimmune Bullous Dermatosis

Patients receiving an anti-PD-1/PD-L1 treatment may induce immune-related bullous pemphigoid (irBP), which may be mediated by both T-cell and B-cell responses (Naidoo et al. 2016; Jour et al. 2016). BP associated with ICIs may occur months later, accompanied or preceded by pruritus, and persist after cessation of treatment (Naidoo et al. 2016).

10.2.3.3 Severe Cutaneous Adverse Reactions (SCARs)

Grade 3/4 reactions are rare, but TEN-like reaction associated with nivolumab in a patient with ipilimumab refractory metastatic melanoma (Nayar et al. 2016) and drug reaction with eosinophilia and systemic symptoms (DRESS) syndrome with anti-CTLA4 and anti-PD-1 agents (Johnson et al. 2013; Voskens et al. 2013) were reported in the literature.

10.2.4 Chimeric Antigen Receptor-Modified T Lymphocytes (CAR-T Cell) Therapy

Cytokine release syndrome (CRS) can be observed shortly after administration of CAR-T cells (Weber et al. 2015). Autoimmunity may be induced when a T cell receptor (TCR) targets a protein expressed in normal tissue. Cutaneous, ocular, and internal ear toxicities were reported (Weber et al. 2015).

10.2.5 Radiation Therapy

10.2.5.1 Radiation Dermatitis (Table 10.1)

10.2.6 Hematopoietic Stem Cell Transplantation (HSCT)

10.2.6.1 Cutaneous Graft Versus Host Disease (GVHD)

GVHD is a major cause of morbidity and mortality, affecting 40–60% of allogeneic HSCT (allo-HSCT) recipients and accounting for 15% of deaths (Hymes et al. 2012a; Villarreal et al. 2016). Cutaneous GVHD is the most common complication after transplantation, reported in 60–80% of patients, with initial skin involvement in 75–90% of cases followed by the oral mucosa, liver, and eye, often resulting in long-term complications (Hymes et al. 2012a; Villarreal et al. 2016). Characteristic skin manifestations of cutaneous GVHD include poikiloderma; lichen planus (LP)-, lichen sclerosus-, or morphea-like lesions; and deep sclerosis/fasciitis (Hymes et al. 2012a). LP-like lesions of the oral and genital areas, hyperkeratotic plaques/leukoplakia, esophageal strictures, and joint stiffness are additional diagnostic features (Hymes et al. 2012a).

10.2.7 Other Cutaneous Adverse Reactions from Cancer Treatments

10.2.7.1 Skin Infections (Table 10.1) (Gandhi et al. 2014)

10.2.7.2 Stevens-Johnson Syndrome (SJS)/Toxic Epidermal Necrolysis (TEN) (Table 10.1) (Rosen et al. 2014; Bastuji-Garin et al. 2000; Wu et al. 2015)

10.3 Treatment of Adverse Drug Reactions to Cancer Therapies

10.3.1 Cytotoxic Chemotherapy

10.3.1.1 Hand-Foot Syndrome, Mucositis, and Anagen Effluvium

Prevention: Regional cooling (supportive cryotherapy) significantly reduces severity of HFS, onychodystrophy/onycholysis, mucositis, and anagen effluvium, respectively, via cold-mediated vasoconstriction and subsequent decreased concentration of toxic metabolites delivered to the cooled skin (Nikolaou et al. 2016; Gomez and Lacouture 2011; Scotte et al. 2005; Mangili et al. 2008; Gilbar et al. 2009). Regional cooling devices should be used as tolerated from 15 min before, during, and through 15 min after the infusion (Scotte et al. 2005, 2008; Riley et al. 2015). *Initial skin-directed therapies for grade 1/2 HFS*: High-potency topical corticosteroids for erythema/edema and lidocaine 5% patches for associated pain (Sibaud et al. 2016).

Therapies for severe HFS: Addition of systemic corticosteroids may be necessary (von Moos et al. 2008; Brown et al. 1991). Celecoxib 200 mg orally twice daily is a safe and effective management to prevent moderate-severe capecitabine-related HFS (Macedo et al. 2014).

10.3.1.2 Pigmentary Changes

Skin-directed therapy with keratolytics (ammonium lactate, salicylic acid 6%, urea, retinoids), bleaching agents (hydroquinone), azelaic acid, chemical peels, and sun protection may facilitate cosmetic improvement; full coverage concealers may be used to camouflage in interim (Lacouture 2014).

10.3.1.3 Hair and Nail Changes

Chemotherapy-Induced Alopecia (CIA)

Scalp cooling 30 min prior to, during, and 90 min after each infusion leads to a 50% reduction in hair loss in 50–75% of patients with breast cancers receiving taxane or anthracycline (Nangia et al. 2017; Rugo et al. 2017; Betticher et al. 2013; Komen et al. 2013; van den Hurk et al. 2012). Topical minoxidil (2–5%) 1–2 times daily application initiated at the start of chemotherapy may accelerate hair regrowth rate in CIA (Tallon et al. 2010; Palamaras et al. 2011; Kluger et al. 2012; Prevezas et al. 2009; Glaser et al. 2015).

Onychodystrophy and nailfold lesions (Table 10.2) (Lacouture 2014)

10.3.2 Targeted Anticancer Therapy

10.3.2.1 EGFR Inhibitors (EGFRIs)

Papulopustular Eruption

Gentle cleansing, moisturizing creams, and sun protection followed by prophylactic rather than reactive management of EGFRI skin toxicities with oral tetracyclines significantly reduce (>50%) the severity (Kyllo and Anadkat 2014b; Hofheinz et al. 2016; Lacouture et al. 2010b; Gandhi et al. 2014). Addition of topical antibiotics and topical corticosteroids may be necessary for mild-moderate reactions already on tetracyclines (Belum et al. 2017).

Hair and nail changes (Table 10.2) (Lacouture et al. 2011; Belum et al. 2015b)

10.3.2.2 Multi-targeted Kinase Inhibitors (MKIs)

Hand-Foot Skin Reaction (HFSR) of Antiangiogenic (Anti-VEGF) MKIs

Grade 1/2 HFSR is managed with topical keratolytics and avoidance of friction. Topical analgesics and oral NSAIDs may be used for pain. High-grade HFSR results in a significant impact on a patient's daily activity and QoL which necessitates dose modification (Lacouture et al. 2008b; Gomez and Lacouture 2011). HFSR usually resolves spontaneously 3–4 weeks after cessation of MKIs without long-term sequelae (Kyllo and Anadkat 2014b). No systemic therapies (pyridoxine, systemic steroids) have demonstrated benefit for HFSR.

Table 10.2 Summary of grading and treatment algorithms of dermatologic adverse events from cancer treatments

Grading and treatment algorithms for dAEs from cancer treatments						
Adverse events		Grading				
		1	2	3	4	5
Severity		Mild	Moderate	Severe or medically significant but not immediately life-threatening	Life-threatening consequences	Death
Description		Asymptomatic or mild symptoms; clinical or diagnostic observations only; intervention not indicated	Minimal, local, or noninvasive intervention indicated; limiting age-appropriate instrumental ADL[a]	Hospitalization or prolongation of hospitalization indicated; disabling; limiting self-care ADL[b]	Urgent intervention indicated	Death related to AE
General approach	Moisturizer, sunscreen, gentle skin care instructions	Continue anticancer treatment at current dose, and monitor for change in severity	Continue anticancer treatment at current dose, and monitor for change in severity; continue treatment of skin reaction	Interrupt anticancer treatment until severity decreases to grade 1/2 and dose modify per label, and monitor for change in severity; continue treatment of skin reaction; reassess after 2 weeks, if reactions worsen, dose reduction or discontinuation may be necessary		
		Reassess after 2 weeks (either by healthcare professional or patient self-report); if reactions worsen or do not improve proceed to next grade therapy				

Hand-foot syndrome (HFS) A disorder characterized by redness, marked discomfort, swelling, and tingling in the palms of the hands or the soles of the feet	Minimal skin changes or dermatitis (e.g., erythema, edema, or hyperkeratosis) without pain	Skin changes (e.g., peeling, blisters, bleeding, edema, or hyperkeratosis) with pain; limiting instrumental ADL	Severe skin changes (e.g., peeling, blisters, bleeding, edema, or hyperkeratosis) with pain; limiting self-care ADL		
Management	High-potency topical steroids for erythema/edema; and lidocaine 5% patches for associated pain amifostine, topical antiperspirant, dexamethasone with H2 blockers, oral cod liver oil, oral pyridoxine, topical antioxidant/silymarin, and topical urea have demonstrated limited efficacy in preventing or reducing HFS (Mangili et al. 2008; Macedo et al. 2014; Elyasi et al. 2017).	Additional systemic steroids may be necessary; celecoxib 200 mg BID to prevent moderate-severe capecitabine-related HFS			

(continued)

Table 10.2 (continued)

Grading and treatment algorithms for dAEs from cancer treatments						
Adverse events		Grading				
		1	2	3	4	5
Rash acneiform (PPE) A disorder characterized by an eruption of papules and pustules, typically appearing in the face, scalp, upper chest, and back		Papules and/or pustules covering <10% BSA, which may or may not be associated with symptoms of pruritus or tenderness	Papules and/or pustules covering 10–30% BSA, which may or may not be associated with symptoms of pruritus or tenderness; associated with psychosocial impact; limiting instrumental ADL	Papules and/or pustules covering >30% BSA, which may or may not be associated with symptoms of pruritus or tenderness; limiting self-care ADL; associated with local superinfection with oral antibiotics indicated	Papules and/or pustules covering any % BSA, which may or may not be associated with symptoms of pruritus or tenderness and are associated with extensive superinfection with IV antibiotics indicated; life-threatening consequences	Death
Management	Preventive treatment for the first 6–8 weeks	Hydrocortisone 2.5% cream Clindamycin 1% gel or dapsone 5% gel (Belum et al. 2017) Doxycycline 100 mg BID or minocycline 100 mg QD				

	Reactive treatment	Hydrocortisone 2.5% cream Clindamycin 1% gel or dapsone 5% gel (Belum et al. 2017)	Hydrocortisone 2.5% cream/alclometasone 0.05% cream/fluocinonide 0.05% cream BID Doxycycline 100 mg BID or minocycline 100 mg QD	Hydrocortisone 2.5% cream/alclometasone 0.05% cream/ fluocinonide 0.05% cream BID Doxycycline 100 mg BID or minocycline 100 mg QD Oral prednisone (0.5 mg/kg/day) for 5 days		
Rash maculopapular (MPR) A disorder characterized by the presence of macules (flat) and papules (elevated). Also known as morbilliform rash, it is one of the most common cutaneous adverse events, frequently affecting the upper trunk, spreading centripetally and associated with pruritus		Macules/papules covering <10% BSA with or without symptoms (e.g., pruritus, burning, tightness)	Macules/papules covering 10–30% BSA with or without symptoms (e.g., pruritus, burning, tightness); limiting instrumental ADL	Macules/papules covering >30% BSA with or without associated symptoms; limiting self-care ADL		
Management		Hydrocortisone 2.5% cream to the face Ttriamcinolone 0.1% cream to the body and extremities BID	Hydrocortisone 2.5% cream to the face Fluocinonide 0.1% cream to the body and extremities BID	Hydrocortisone 2.5% cream to the face Fluocinonide 0.1% cream to the body and extremities Prednisone 0.5 mg/kg for 10 days		

(continued)

Table 10.2 (continued)

Grading and treatment algorithms for dAEs from cancer treatments

Adverse events		Grading				
		1	2	3	4	5
Pruritus A disorder characterized by an intense itching sensation		Mild or localized; topical intervention indicated	Intense or widespread; intermittent; skin changes from scratching (e.g., edema, papulation, excoriations, lichenification, oozing/crusts); oral intervention indicated; limiting instrumental ADL	Intense or widespread; constant; limiting self-care ADL or sleep; oral corticosteroid or immunosuppressive therapy indicated		
Management		Topical treatments: doxepin Medium- to high-potency steroids (triamcinolone acetonide 0.025%; desonide 0.05%; fluticasone propionate 0.05%; alclometasone 0.05%)	Topical treatments Oral antihistamines	Topical treatments Oral antihistamines Gabapentin/pregabalin/doxepin Prednisone		
Dry skin A disorder characterized by flaky and dull skin; the pores are generally fine; the texture is a papery thin texture		Covering <10% BSA and no associated erythema or pruritus	Covering 10–30% BSA and associated with erythema or pruritus; limiting instrumental ADL	Covering >30% BSA and associated with pruritus; limiting self-care ADL		
Management	Preventive treatment	Bathing techniques using bath oils or mild moisturizing soaps and bathing in tepid water; Regular moisturizing creams; Avoid extreme temperatures and direct sunlight				

	Reactive treatment	OTC moisturizing cream or ointment to the face bid Ammonium lactate 12% cream to the body	OTC moisturizing cream or ointment to the face bid Ammonium lactate 12% cream or salicylic acid 6% or lactic acid cream 12% or urea creams 10–40% to the body bid	OTC moisturizing cream or ointment to face bid Ammonium lactate 12% cream or salicylic acid 6% or lactic acid cream 12% or urea creams 10–40% to the body bid Medium- to high-potency steroid creams (triamcinolone acetonide 0.025%; desonide 0.05%; fluticasone propionate 0.05%; alclometasone 0.05%)		
Photosensitivity A disorder characterized by an increase in sensitivity of the skin to light		Painless erythema and erythema covering <10% BSA	Tender erythema covering 10–30% BSA	Erythema covering >30% BSA and erythema with blistering; photosensitivity; oral corticosteroid therapy indicated; pain control indicated (e.g., narcotics or NSAIDs)	Life-threatening consequences; urgent intervention indicated	Death
Management		Sun protection Photosensitivity is commonly reported with use of EGFR inhibitors (Belum et al. 2015a). Patients should be counseled regarding sun protection including the use of broad-spectrum sunscreen, sun-protective clothing, broad-brimmed hats, and avoidance of sun exposure during peak UV hours, especially when concurrent photosensitizing antibiotics such as doxycycline or sulfamethoxazole/trimethoprim are prescribed (Pugliese et al. 2015). Follow MPR algorithm; add oral antihistamine (grade 2 /3) if necessary				

(continued)

Table 10.2 (continued)

Grading and treatment algorithms for dAEs from cancer treatments						
Adverse events		Grading				
		1	2	3	4	5
Alopecia A disorder characterized by a decrease in density of hair compared to normal for a given individual at a given age and body location		Hair loss of <50% of normal for that individual that is not obvious from a distance but only on close inspection; a different hair style may be required to cover the hair loss but it does not require a wig or hair piece to camouflage	Hair loss of ≥50% normal for that individual that is readily apparent to others; a wig or hair piece is necessary if the patient desires to completely camouflage the hair loss; associated with psychosocial impact			
Management	Preventive treatment	Scarring alopecia from targeted therapy: follow PPE algorithm, high-potency topical steroids, antibacterial wash Chemotherapy-induced alopecia (CIA): scalp cooling (Nangia et al. 2017; Rugo et al. 2017; Betticher et al. 2013; Komen et al. 2013; van den Hurk et al. 2012)				

	Reactive treatment	Refer to a dermatologist for evaluation and treatment Hair camouflage includes partial/full wigs, concealing powders and sprays Chemotherapy-induced alopecia (CIA): topical minoxidil (2–5%) BID (Tallon et al. 2010; Palamaras et al. 2011; Kluger et al. 2012; Prevezas et al. 2009) Chemotherapy-induced hypotrichosis of eyelash, brow, and scalp: topical bimatoprost (Glaser et al. 2015) Scarring alopecia from targeted therapy: high-potency topical steroids, antibacterial wash				
Hair and nail changes related to targeted therapy						
Management	Preventive treatment	Prophylactic treatment with doxycycline with addition of topical steroids for anti-inflammatory effect may minimize the risk of scarring alopecia (Lacouture et al. 2011; Belum et al. 2015b)				
	Reactive treatment	Facial hypertrichosis and eyelash trichomegaly develop after 1–2 months of EGFRI treatment in approximately 20% of patients (Lacouture et al. 2011). Eyelashes may need trimming to reduce risk of corneal abrasions; facial hypertrichosis may be treated with depilatory/bleaching creams, eflornithine cream, or laser hair removal				
Hand-foot skin reaction (HFSR) A disorder characterized by redness, marked discomfort, swelling, and tingling in the palms of the hands or the soles of the feet		Minimal skin changes or dermatitis (e.g., erythema, edema, or hyperkeratosis) without pain	Skin changes (e.g., peeling, blisters, bleeding, edema, or hyperkeratosis) with pain; limiting instrumental ADL	Severe skin changes (e.g., peeling, blisters, bleeding, edema, or hyperkeratosis) with pain; limiting self-care ADL	–	–

(continued)

Table 10.2 (continued)

Grading and treatment algorithms for dAEs from cancer treatments					
Adverse events	Grading				
	1	2	3	4	5
Management	Topicals (e.g., keratolytics: salicylic acid 6 %, urea 10–20%, ammonium lactate 12%; clobetasol 0.05%) (Belum et al. 2013c)	Topicals (e.g., keratolytics: urea 20%, salicylic acid 6%, ammonium lactate 12%; clobetasol 0.05%) Topical analgesia (topical creams ad libitum, e.g., lidocaine 3% or lidocaine patches, EMLA, diclofenac gel)	Topical high-potency corticosteroid creams BID (e.g., clobetasol 0.05%) Topical analgesia (topical creams ad libitum e.g., lidocaine 3% or lidocaine patches, EMLA, diclofenac gel) Oral medications: NSAIDs, GABA agonists, opioids (Belum et al. 2013c)		
Radiation dermatitis	Faint erythema or dry desquamation (Lacouture et al. 2010a)	Moderate to brisk erythema; patchy moist desquamation, mostly confined to skin folds and creases; moderate edema (Lacouture et al. 2010a)	Moist desquamation other than skin folds and creases; bleeding induced by minor trauma or abrasion (Lacouture et al. 2010a)	Skin necrosis or ulceration of full thickness dermis; spontaneous bleeding from involved site (Lacouture et al. 2010a)	

Management	Preventive treatment	Maintain hygiene and gently clean and dry the skin in the radiation field, shortly before radiation treatment Topical mometasone cream after radiation treatment		
	Reactive treatment	Topical mometasone cream or mid-to-high potency topical steroids for anti-inflammation; Silver sulfadiazine cream may be considered to reduce the severity; Pentoxifylline and vitamin E can be used to improve the fibrosis (for breast cancer patients, combination therapy with pentoxifylline and vitamin E may prevent severe contracture and implant loss, allowing for immediate reconstruction with implant or tissue expander even if radiation is planned after mastectomy. (Cook et al. 2016))		
Chemotherapy-associated extravasation reactions				
Management		Immediate cessation of the infusion, aspiration of the drug from the catheter, ice packing (or warm packing for Vinca alkaloids), and use of salvage medications, e.g., intravenous dexrazoxane for anthracyclines, subcutaneous injection of sodium thiosulfate for nitrogen mustards, or hyaluronidase for Vinca alkaloids and taxanes, may be applied (Kyllo and Anadkat 2014b). Close clinical monitoring, wound care, and a prompt surgical intervention should be performed if indicated		
Nasal vestibulitis (NV)				
Management		Mild/moderate NV (with intranasal symptoms including erythema, crusting, impetigo, furunculosis, epistaxis, etc.) responded to intranasal antibiotics (mupirocin), while severe cases (with edematous and painful nose) required oral antibiotics. (Ruiz et al. 2015)		

(continued)

Table 10.2 (continued)

Grading and treatment algorithms for dAEs from cancer treatments					
Adverse events	Grading				
	1	2	3	4	5
Onychodystrophy/nail fold lesions					
Management	Nail fragility may improve with oral biotin and topical nail polish/hardeners (Lacouture 2014); trimming or debridement of nail plate, followed by antiseptic soaks with dilute acetic acid or sodium hypochlorite; podiatry evaluation of symptomatic onychocryptosis/ingrown toenail Presence of erythema and drainage should raise concern for superinfection, wound cultures performed, and empiric treatment with topical mupirocin, or oral antibiotics (e.g., doxycycline or cephalexin) should be initiated. Periungual abscesses should be incised and drained Periungual pyogenic granulomas may be treated with topical or intralesional corticosteroids, chemical- (silver nitrate) or electrocautery, curettage with topical phenol application, and pulsed dye or carbon dioxide (CO_2) laser. Persistent lesions may benefit from oral doxycycline 100 mg twice daily For severe nail changes, dose reduction, cessation, or discontinuation of the offending agent may be necessary				

Adapted from CTCAE grading scale. https://evs.nci.nih.gov/ftp1/CTCAE/CTCAE_4.03_2010-06 14_QuickReference_5x7.pdf. Accessed on 27 July 2017

Note: A single dash (–) indicates a grade is not available. Not all grades are appropriate for all AEs. Therefore, some AEs are listed with fewer than five options for grade selection. Grade 5 (death) is not appropriate for some AEs and therefore is not an option

Activities of Daily Living (ADL): [a]Instrumental ADL refer to preparing meals, shopping for groceries or clothes, using the telephone, managing money, etc. [b]Self-care ADL refer to bathing, dressing and undressing, feeding self, using the toilet, and taking medications, not bedridden

10.3.2.3 BRAF Inhibitors (BRAFIs)

Nonmalignant Hyperkeratotic Skin Eruptions

Topical keratolytics used prior to and after the initiation of treatment, avoidance of trauma and friction, and treatment of reactive inflammation with high-potency topical corticosteroids may be recommended (Choi 2014; Pugliese et al. 2015).

Cutaneous Squamous Cell Carcinomas (SCCs)

Local management with cryotherapy, saucerization, conservative excision, or electrodessication and curettage is often adequate, and dose modification or discontinuation of BRAFIs is usually not necessary (Choi 2014; Pugliese et al. 2015). Photodynamic therapy, topical fluorouracil, nicotinamide, oral retinoids, and CO_2 laser can be considered for eruptive or multiple concurrent lesions (Choi 2014). Combination regimen of MEKIs and BRAFIs leads to significantly decreased development of SCCs (Long et al. 2014).

10.3.2.4 MEK Inhibitors (MEKIs)

Treatment strategies used for EGFRI-induced dAEs can be applied (Balagula et al. 2011a).

10.3.3 Immune Checkpoint Inhibitors (ICIs)

10.3.3.1 Rash

Associated morbilliform rashes may be managed with topical and systemic corticosteroids and narrow band ultraviolet B (nbUVB) phototherapy (Belum et al. 2016). New onset or exacerbations of psoriasis/psoriasiform dermatitis may be managed with topical steroids, vitamin D analogs, and nbUVB phototherapy; systemic treatment may rarely be required. Topical steroids, topical calcineurin inhibitors (TCIs), and systemic retinoids may be beneficial in cutaneous lichenoid dermatoses; mucosal lichenoid reactions may benefit from TCIs (tacrolimus ointment, cyclosporine rinse), topical corticosteroids (e.g., clobetasol cream, dexamethasone mouthwash), or low-level laser therapy (Spanemberg et al. 2016).

10.3.3.2 Pruritus

Skin-directed therapies with topical corticosteroids/menthol/doxepin, ice packs, and nbUVB phototherapy may be suggested for low-grade pruritus. Moderate- and high-grade pruritus may require systemic therapies including sedating antihistamines, tricyclic antidepressants (amitriptyline, doxepin), anticonvulsants (gabapentin, pregabalin), mirtazapine, aprepitant, systemic corticosteroids, or phototherapy (Vincenzi et al. 2010; Stander et al. 2010; Ito et al. 2017).

10.3.3.3 Vitiligo and Vitiligo-Like Lesions

Topical/intralesional(IL)/oral steroids, TCIs, topical Janus kinase inhibitors (JAKIs), nbUVB phototherapy, and camouflage (full-coverage concealers, sunless tanners) are available for cosmesis (Damsky and King 2017; Shreberk-Hassidim et al. 2017).

10.3.3.4 Alopecia Areata/Universalis

Topical/IL/oral steroids, TCIs, topical JAKIs, and hair camouflage may be used for these autoimmune sequelae (Damsky and King 2017; Shreberk-Hassidim et al. 2017).

10.3.3.5 Autoimmune Bullous Dermatosis

Discontinuation of ICIs may be required for extensive disease (Naidoo et al. 2016). Topical steroids, oral tetracyclines with nicotinamide, mycophenolate mofetil (MMF), dapsone, systemic steroids, omalizumab, IVIg, and rituximab may be used (Sowerby et al. 2017).

10.3.3.6 Severe Cutaneous Adverse Reactions (SCARs)

Drug withdrawal and systemic steroids are used for immunotherapy-associated grade 3/4 SCARs; cyclosporine, IVIg, rituximab, and MMF may be required in severe cases (Nayar et al. 2016; Tanaka et al. 2017).

10.3.4 Chimeric Antigen Receptor-Modified T Lymphocytes (CAR-T Cell) Therapy

Treatments typically include topical and systemic immunomodulators, while new targeted therapy, e.g., tocilizumab, an anti-IL-6 receptor mAb, has been used in clinical practice (Weber et al. 2015).

10.3.5 Radiation Therapy

10.3.5.1 Radiation Dermatitis

Use of topical prophylactic corticosteroids (mometasone) is recommended (Cook et al. 2016; Wong et al. 2013).

10.3.6 Hematopoietic Stem Cell Transplantation

10.3.6.1 Cutaneous GVHD

Acute cutaneous GVHD (aGVHD) therapy includes topical corticosteroids and/or TCIs for stage 1 (<10% BSA) disease and nbUVB or systemic corticosteroids with systemic calcineurin inhibitors (SCIs) for stage 2+. For steroid-dependent or steroid-refractory aGVHD, extracorporeal photophoresis, IVIg, mesenchymal stem cell therapy, systemic ruxolitinib, and antithymocyte globulin may be beneficial.

Lichenoid/sclerodermatous chronic GVHD (cGVHD) is managed with topical and systemic steroids, TCIs and SCIs, systemic ruxolitinib, systemic ibrutinib, nbUVB phototherapy, and extracorporeal photophoresis (Wolff et al. 2013; Capuano et al. 2015). Sclerodermatous cGVHD is additionally managed with systemic rapamycin inhibitors, imatinib, and systemic retinoids (Villarreal et al. 2016; Wolff et al. 2013; Hymes et al. 2012b).

Acknowledgment We would like to thank Ms. Bernadette Murphy for clinical photography.

References

Aasi S, Silkiss R, Tang JY et al (2013) New onset of keratoacanthomas after vismodegib treatment for locally advanced basal cell carcinomas: a report of 2 cases. JAMA Dermatol 149(2):242–243

Abess A, Keel DM, Graham BS (2003) Flagellate hyperpigmentation following intralesional bleomycin treatment of verruca plantaris. Arch Dermatol 139(3):337–339

Aoyama T, Takano M, Miyamoto M et al (2017) Is there any predictor for hypersensitivity reactions in gynecologic cancer patients treated with paclitaxel-based therapy? Cancer Chemother Pharmacol 80:65

Asz-Sigall D, Gonzalez-de-Cossio-Hernandez AC, Rodriguez-Lobato E, Ortega-Springall MF, Vega-Memije ME, Arenas Guzman R (2016) Differential diagnosis of female-pattern hair loss. Skin Appendage Disord 2(1–2):18–21

Balagula Y, Barth Huston K, Busam KJ, Lacouture ME, Chapman PB, Myskowski PL (2011a) Dermatologic side effects associated with the MEK 1/2 inhibitor selumetinib (AZD6244, ARRY-142886). Investig New Drugs 29(5):1114–1121

Balagula Y, Rosen ST, Lacouture ME (2011b) The emergence of supportive oncodermatology: the study of dermatologic adverse events to cancer therapies. J Am Acad Dermatol 65(3):624–635

Balagula Y, Wu S, Su X, Feldman DR, Lacouture ME (2012) The risk of hand foot skin reaction to pazopanib, a novel multikinase inhibitor: a systematic review of literature and meta-analysis. Investig New Drugs 30(4):1773–1781

Bastuji-Garin S, Fouchard N, Bertocchi M, Roujeau JC, Revuz J, Wolkenstein P (2000) SCORTEN: a severity-of-illness score for toxic epidermal necrolysis. J Invest Dermatol 115(2):149–153

Belum VR, Benhuri B, Postow MA et al (2016) Characterisation and management of dermatologic adverse events to agents targeting the PD-1 receptor. Eur J Cancer 60:12–25

Belum VR, Cercek A, Sanz-Motilva V, Lacouture ME (2013c) Dermatologic adverse events to targeted therapies in lower GI cancers: clinical presentation and management. Curr Treat Options in Oncol 14(3):389–404

Belum VR, Fischer A, Choi JN, Lacouture ME (2013b) Dermatological adverse events from BRAF inhibitors: a growing problem. Curr Oncol Rep 15(3):249–259

Belum VR, Fontanilla Patel H, Lacouture ME, Rodeck U (2013a) Skin toxicity of targeted cancer agents: mechanisms and intervention. Future Oncol 9(8):1161–1170

Belum VR, Marchetti MA, Dusza SW, Cercek A, Kemeny NE, Lacouture ME (2017) A prospective, randomized, double-blinded, split-face/chest study of prophylactic topical dapsone 5% gel versus moisturizer for the prevention of cetuximab-induced acneiform rash. J Am Acad Dermatol 77(3):577–579

Belum VR, Marulanda K, Ensslin C et al (2015b) Alopecia in patients treated with molecularly targeted anticancer therapies. Ann Oncol 26(12):2496–2502

Belum VR, Washington C, Pratilas CA, Sibaud V, Boralevi F, Lacouture ME (2015a) Dermatologic adverse events in pediatric patients receiving targeted anticancer therapies: a pooled analysis. Pediatr Blood Cancer 62(5):798–806

Belum VR, Wu S, Lacouture ME (2013d) Risk of hand-foot skin reaction with the novel multikinase inhibitor regorafenib: a meta-analysis. Investig New Drugs 31(4):1078–1086

Betticher DC, Delmore G, Breitenstein U et al (2013) Efficacy and tolerability of two scalp cooling systems for the prevention of alopecia associated with docetaxel treatment. Support Care Cancer 21(9):2565–2573

Bolognia JL, Cooper DL, Glusac EJ (2008) Toxic erythema of chemotherapy: a useful clinical term. J Am Acad Dermatol 59(3):524–529

Brown J, Burck K, Black D, Collins C (1991) Treatment of cytarabine acral erythema with corticosteroids. J Am Acad Dermatol 24(6 Pt 1):1023–1025

Burris HA 3rd, Hurtig J (2010) Radiation recall with anticancer agents. Oncologist 15(11):1227–1237

Capriotti K, Capriotti JA, Lessin S et al (2015) The risk of nail changes with taxane chemotherapy: a systematic review of the literature and meta-analysis. Br J Dermatol 173(3):842–845

Capuano M, Sommese L, Pignalosa O et al (2015) Current clinical applications of extracorporeal photochemotherapy. Ther Apher Dial 19(2):103–110

Carlos G, Anforth R, Clements A et al (2015) Cutaneous toxic effects of BRAF inhibitors alone and in combination with MEK inhibitors for metastatic melanoma. JAMA Dermatol 151(10):1103–1109

Chandrakumar SF, Yeung J (2014) Cutaneous adverse events during vemurafenib therapy. J Cutan Med Surg 18(4):223–228

Chen M, Chen J, Peng X et al (2017) The contribution of keratinocytes in capecitabine-stimulated hand-foot-syndrome. Environ Toxicol Pharmacol 49:81–88

Chew L, Chuen VS (2009) Cutaneous reaction associated with weekly docetaxel administration. J Oncol Pharm Pract 15(1):29–34

Chittari K, Tagboto S, Tan BB (2009) Cyclophosphamide-induced nail discoloration and skin hyperpigmentation: a rare presentation. Clin Exp Dermatol 34(3):405–406

Choi JN (2014) Dermatologic adverse events to chemotherapeutic agents, part 2: BRAF inhibitors, MEK inhibitors, and ipilimumab. Semin Cutan Med Surg 33(1):40–48

Clabbers JMK, Boers-Doets CB, Gelderblom H et al (2016) Xerosis and pruritus as major EGFRI-associated adverse events. Support Care Cancer 24(2):513–521

Cook M, Johnson N, Zegzula HD, Schray M, Glissmeyer M, Sorenson L (2016) Prophylactic use of pentoxifylline (Trental) and vitamin E to prevent capsular contracture after implant reconstruction in patients requiring adjuvant radiation. Am J Surg 211(5):854–859

Curry JL, Tetzlaff MT, Nagarajan P et al (2017) Diverse types of dermatologic toxicities from immune checkpoint blockade therapy. J Cutan Pathol 44(2):158–176

Damsky W, King BA (2017) JAK inhibitors in dermatology: the promise of a new drug class. J Am Acad Dermatol 76(4):736–744

Dreno B, Ribas A, Larkin J et al (2017) Incidence, course, and management of toxicities associated with cobimetinib in combination with vemurafenib in the coBRIM study. Ann Oncol 28(5):1137–1144

Drilon A, Eaton AA, Schindler K et al (2016) Beyond the dose-limiting toxicity period: dermatologic adverse events of patients on phase 1 trials of the cancer therapeutics evaluation program. Cancer 122(8):1228–1237

Elyasi S, Shojaee FSR, Allahyari A, Karimi G (2017) Topical Silymarin Administration for Prevention of Capecitabine-induced hand-foot syndrome: a randomized, double-blinded, placebo-controlled clinical trial. Phytother Res 31:1323

Ensslin CJ, Rosen AC, Wu S, Lacouture ME (2013) Pruritus in patients treated with targeted cancer therapies: systematic review and meta-analysis. J Am Acad Dermatol 69(5):708–720

European Medicines Agency (2016) European Public Assessment Report: Erivdege. http://www.ema.europa.eu/docs/en_GB/document_library/EPAR_-_Summary_for_the_public/human/002602/WC500146821.pdf

Fischer A, Wu S, Ho AL, Lacouture ME (2013) The risk of hand-foot skin reaction to axitinib, a novel VEGF inhibitor: a systematic review of literature and meta-analysis. Investig New Drugs 31(3):787–797

Fonia A, Cota C, Setterfield JF, Goldberg LJ, Fenton DA, Stefanato CM (2017) Permanent alopecia in patients with breast cancer after taxane chemotherapy and adjuvant hormonal therapy: Clinicopathologic findings in a cohort of 10 patients. J Am Acad Dermatol 76:948

Freeman-Keller M, Kim Y, Cronin H, Richards A, Gibney G, Weber JS (2016) Nivolumab in resected and unresectable metastatic melanoma: characteristics of immune-related adverse events and association with outcomes. Clin Cancer Res 22(4):886–894

Gandhi M, Brieva JC, Lacouture ME (2014) Dermatologic infections in cancer patients. Cancer Treat Res 161:299–317
Gelmon K (1994) The taxoids: paclitaxel and docetaxel. Lancet 344(8932):1267–1272
Giavina-Bianchi P, Patil SU, Banerji A (2017) Immediate hypersensitivity reaction to chemotherapeutic agents. J Allergy Clin Immunol Pract 5(3):593–599
Gilbar P, Hain A, Peereboom VM (2009) Nail toxicity induced by cancer chemotherapy. J Oncol Pharm Pract 15(3):143–155
Glaser DA, Hossain P, Perkins W et al (2015) Long-term safety and efficacy of bimatoprost solution 0.03% application to the eyelid margin for the treatment of idiopathic and chemotherapy-induced eyelash hypotrichosis: a randomized controlled trial. Br J Dermatol 172(5): 1384–1394
Goldinger SM, Stieger P, Meier B et al (2016) Cytotoxic cutaneous adverse drug reactions during anti-PD-1 therapy. Clin Cancer Res 22(16):4023–4029
Gomez P, Lacouture ME (2011) Clinical presentation and management of hand-foot skin reaction associated with sorafenib in combination with cytotoxic chemotherapy: experience in breast cancer. Oncologist 16(11):1508–1519
Hackbarth M, Haas N, Fotopoulou C, Lichtenegger W, Sehouli J (2008) Chemotherapy-induced dermatological toxicity: frequencies and impact on quality of life in women's cancers. Results of a prospective study. Support Care Cancer 16(3):267–273
Hofheinz RD, Deplanque G, Komatsu Y et al (2016) Recommendations for the prophylactic Management of Skin Reactions Induced by epidermal growth factor receptor inhibitors in patients with solid tumors. Oncologist 21(12):1483–1491
Hsiao YW, Lin YC, Hui RC, Yang CH (2011) Fulminant acneiform eruptions after administration of dovitinib in a patient with renal cell carcinoma. J Clin Oncol 29(12):e340–e341
Huang V, Anadkat M (2011) Dermatologic manifestations of cytotoxic therapy. Dermatol Ther 24(4):401–410
Hymes SR, Alousi AM, Cowen EW (2012a) Graft-versus-host disease: part I Pathogenesis and clinical manifestations of graft-versus-host disease. J Am Acad Dermatol 66(4):515 e1–18; quiz 33–4
Hymes SR, Alousi AM, Cowen EW (2012b) Graft-versus-host disease: part II Management of cutaneous graft-versus-host disease. J Am Acad Dermatol 66(4):535.e1–535.16 quiz 51–2
Ito J, Fujimoto D, Nakamura A et al (2017) Aprepitant for refractory nivolumab-induced pruritus. Lung Cancer 109:58–61
Jain V, Bhandary S, Prasad GN, Shenoi SD (2005) Serpentine supravenous streaks induced by 5-fluorouracil. J Am Acad Dermatol 53(3):529–530
Johnson DB, Wallender EK, Cohen DN et al (2013) Severe cutaneous and neurologic toxicity in melanoma patients during vemurafenib administration following anti-PD-1 therapy. Cancer Immunol Res 1(6):373–377
Jour G, Glitza IC, Ellis RM et al (2016) Autoimmune dermatologic toxicities from immune checkpoint blockade with anti-PD-1 antibody therapy: a report on bullous skin eruptions. J Cutan Pathol 43(8):688–696
Julia Dai VRB, Shenhong W, Sibaud V, Lacouture ME (2017) Pigmentary changes in patients treated with targeted anticancer agents: a systematic review and meta-analysis. J Am Acad Dermatol 77(5):902–910.e2. https://doi.org/10.1016/j.jaad.2017.06.044
Keating GM (2016) Cobimetinib plus Vemurafenib: a review in BRAF (V600) mutation-positive unresectable or metastatic melanoma. Drugs 76(5):605–615
Kluger N, Jacot W, Frouin E et al (2012) Permanent scalp alopecia related to breast cancer chemotherapy by sequential fluorouracil/epirubicin/cyclophosphamide (FEC) and docetaxel: a prospective study of 20 patients. Ann Oncol 23(11):2879–2884
Komen MM, Smorenburg CH, van den Hurk CJ, Nortier JW (2013) Factors influencing the effectiveness of scalp cooling in the prevention of chemotherapy-induced alopecia. Oncologist 18(7):885–891
Korman AM, Tyler KH, Kaffenberger BH (2017) Radiation recall dermatitis associated with nivolumab for metastatic malignant melanoma. Int J Dermatol 56(4):e75–ee7

Kwong B, Danial C, Liu A, Chun KA, Chang AL (2017) Reversible cutaneous side effects of vismodegib treatment. Cutis 99(3):E19–e20

Kyllo RL, Anadkat MJ (2014a) Dermatologic adverse events to chemotherapeutic agents, part 1: cytotoxics, epidermal growth factor receptors, multikinase inhibitors, and proteasome inhibitors. Semin Cutan Med Surg 33(1):28–39

Kyllo R, Anadkat M (2014b) Dermatologic adverse events to chemotherapeutic agents, part 1: cytotoxic agents, epidermal growth factor inhibitors, multikinase inhibitors, and proteasome inhibitors. Semin Cutan Med Surg 33(1):28–39

Lacouture ME (2014) Dermatologic principles and practice in oncology: conditions of the skin, hair, and nails in cancer patients. John Wiley & Sons, Hoboken, NJ

Lacouture ME (2015) Management of dermatologic toxicities. J Natl Compr Canc Netw 13(5 Suppl):686–689

Lacouture ME, Anadkat MJ, Bensadoun RJ et al (2011) Clinical practice guidelines for the prevention and treatment of EGFR inhibitor-associated dermatologic toxicities. Support Care Cancer 19(8):1079–1095

Lacouture ME, Ciccolini K, Kloos RT, Agulnik M (2014) Overview and management of dermatologic events associated with targeted therapies for medullary thyroid cancer. Thyroid 24(9):1329–1340

Lacouture ME, Dreno B, Ascierto PA et al (2016) Characterization and management of hedgehog pathway inhibitor-related adverse events in patients with advanced basal cell carcinoma. Oncologist 21(10):1218–1229

Lacouture ME, Duvic M, Hauschild A et al (2013b) Analysis of dermatologic events in vemurafenib-treated patients with melanoma. Oncologist 18(3):314–322

Lacouture ME, Maitland ML, Segaert S et al (2010a) A proposed EGFR inhibitor dermatologic adverse event-specific grading scale from the MASCC skin toxicity study group. Support Care Cancer 18(4):509–522

Lacouture ME, Mitchell EP, Piperdi B et al (2010b) Skin toxicity evaluation protocol with panitumumab (STEPP), a phase II, open-label, randomized trial evaluating the impact of a pre-Emptive skin treatment regimen on skin toxicities and quality of life in patients with metastatic colorectal cancer. J Clin Oncol 28(8):1351–1357

Lacouture ME, Reilly LM, Gerami P, Guitart J (2008a) Hand foot skin reaction in cancer patients treated with the multikinase inhibitors sorafenib and sunitinib. Ann Oncol 19(11):1955–1961

Lacouture ME, Schadendorf D, Chu CY et al (2013a) Dermatologic adverse events associated with afatinib: an oral ErbB family blocker. Expert Rev Anticancer Ther 13(6):721–728

Lacouture ME, Wu S, Robert C et al (2008b) Evolving strategies for the management of hand-foot skin reaction associated with the multitargeted kinase inhibitors sorafenib and sunitinib. Oncologist 13(9):1001–1011

Langer SW (2010) Extravasation of chemotherapy. Curr Oncol Rep 12(4):242–246

Larsabal M, Marti A, Jacquemin C et al (2017) Vitiligo-like lesions occurring in patients receiving anti-programmed cell death-1 therapies are clinically and biologically distinct from vitiligo. J Am Acad Dermatol 76:863

Lindner J, Hillmann K, Blume-Peytavi U et al (2012) Hair shaft abnormalities after chemotherapy and tamoxifen therapy in patients with breast cancer evaluated by optical coherence tomography. Br J Dermatol 167(6):1272–1278

Liu HB, Wu Y, Lv TF et al (2013) Skin rash could predict the response to EGFR tyrosine kinase inhibitor and the prognosis for patients with non-small cell lung cancer: a systematic review and meta-analysis. PLoS One 8(1):e55128

Long GV, Stroyakovskiy D, Gogas H et al (2014) Combined BRAF and MEK inhibition versus BRAF inhibition alone in melanoma. N Engl J Med 371(20):1877–1888

Lorusso D, Di Stefano A, Carone V, Fagotti A, Pisconti S, Scambia G (2007) Pegylated liposomal doxorubicin-related palmar-plantar erythrodysesthesia ('hand-foot' syndrome). Ann Oncol 18(7):1159–1164

LoRusso PM, Rudin CM, Reddy JC et al (2011) Phase I trial of hedgehog pathway inhibitor vismodegib (GDC-0449) in patients with refractory, locally advanced or metastatic solid tumors. Clin Cancer Res 17(8):2502–2511

Lou Y, Wang Q, Zheng J et al (2016) Possible pathways of Capecitabine-induced hand-foot syndrome. Chem Res Toxicol 29(10):1591–1601

Macedo LT, Lima JP, dos Santos LV, Sasse AD (2014) Prevention strategies for chemotherapy-induced hand-foot syndrome: a systematic review and meta-analysis of prospective randomised trials. Support Care Cancer 22(6):1585–1593

Mangili G, Petrone M, Gentile C, De Marzi P, Vigano R, Rabaiotti E (2008) Prevention strategies in palmar-plantar erythrodysesthesia onset: the role of regional cooling. Gynecol Oncol 108(2):332–335

McLellan B, Ciardiello F, Lacouture ME, Segaert S, Van Cutsem E (2015) Regorafenib-associated hand-foot skin reaction: practical advice on diagnosis, prevention, and management. Ann Oncol 26(10):2017–2026

Michot JM, Bigenwald C, Champiat S et al (2016) Immune-related adverse events with immune checkpoint blockade: a comprehensive review. Eur J Cancer 54:139–148

Miteva M, Misciali C, Fanti PA, Vincenzi C, Romanelli P, Tosti A (2011) Permanent alopecia after systemic chemotherapy: a clinicopathological study of 10 cases. Am J Dermatopathol 33(4):345–350

Naidoo J, Schindler K, Querfeld C et al (2016) Autoimmune bullous skin disorders with immune checkpoint inhibitors targeting PD-1 and PD-L1. Cancer Immunol Res 4(5):383–389

Nangia J, Wang T, Osborne C et al (2017) Effect of a scalp cooling device on alopecia in women undergoing chemotherapy for breast cancer: the SCALP randomized clinical trial. JAMA 317(6):596–605

Nayar N, Briscoe K, Fernandez Penas P (2016) Toxic epidermal necrolysis-like reaction with severe satellite cell necrosis associated with Nivolumab in a patient with Ipilimumab refractory metastatic melanoma. J Immunother 39(3):149–152

Nikolaou V, Syrigos K, Saif MW (2016) Incidence and implications of chemotherapy related hand-foot syndrome. Expert Opin Drug Saf 15(12):1625–1633

Palamaras I, Misciali C, Vincenzi C, Robles WS, Tosti A (2011) Permanent chemotherapy-induced alopecia: a review. J Am Acad Dermatol 64(3):604–606

Park HJ, Lee JH, Kim SR et al (2016) A new practical desensitization protocol for Oxaliplatin-induced immediate hypersensitivity reactions: a necessary and useful approach. J Investig Allergol Clin Immunol 26(3):168–176

Parker TL, Cooper DL, Seropian SE, Bolognia JL (2013) Toxic erythema of chemotherapy following i.v. BU plus fludarabine for allogeneic PBSC transplant. Bone Marrow Transplant 48(5):646–650

Prevezas C, Matard B, Pinquier L, Reygagne P (2009) Irreversible and severe alopecia following docetaxel or paclitaxel cytotoxic therapy for breast cancer. Br J Dermatol 160(4):883–885

Pugliese SB, Neal JW, Kwong BY (2015) Management of Dermatologic Complications of lung Cancer therapies. Curr Treat Options in Oncol 16(10):50

Riley P, Glenny AM, Worthington HV, Littlewood A, Clarkson JE, McCabe MG (2015) Interventions for preventing oral mucositis in patients with cancer receiving treatment: oral cryotherapy. Cochrane Database Syst Rev 12:CD011552

Robert C, Schachter J, Long GV et al (2015) Pembrolizumab versus Ipilimumab in Advanced Melanoma. N Engl J Med 372(26):2521–2532

Rosen AC, Balagula Y, Raisch DW et al (2014) Life-threatening dermatologic adverse events in oncology. Anti-Cancer Drugs 25(2):225–234

Rugo HS, Melin SA, Voigt J (2017) Scalp cooling with adjuvant/neoadjuvant chemotherapy for breast cancer and the risk of scalp metastases: systematic review and meta-analysis. Breast Cancer Res Treat 163(2):199–205

Ruiz JN, Belum VR, Boers-Doets CB et al (2015) Nasal vestibulitis due to targeted therapies in cancer patients. Support Care Cancer 23(8):2391–2398

Saif MW, Katirtzoglou NA, Syrigos KN (2008) Capecitabine: an overview of the side effects and their management. Anti-Cancer Drugs 19(5):447–464

Sanborn RE, Sauer DA (2008) Cutaneous reactions to chemotherapy: commonly seen, less described, little understood. Dermatol Clin 26(1):103–119 ix

Santoni M, Conti A, Andrikou K et al (2015) Risk of pruritus in cancer patients treated with biological therapies: a systematic review and meta-analysis of clinical trials. Crit Rev Oncol Hematol 96(2):206–219

Scotte F, Banu E, Medioni J et al (2008) Matched case-control phase 2 study to evaluate the use of a frozen sock to prevent docetaxel-induced onycholysis and cutaneous toxicity of the foot. Cancer 112(7):1625–1631

Scotte F, Tourani JM, Banu E et al (2005) Multicenter study of a frozen glove to prevent docetaxel-induced onycholysis and cutaneous toxicity of the hand. J Clin Oncol 23(19):4424–4429

Sekulic A, Migden MR, Basset-Seguin N et al (2017) Long-term safety and efficacy of vismodegib in patients with advanced basal cell carcinoma: final update of the pivotal ERIVANCE BCC study. BMC Cancer 17(1):332

Sekulic A, Migden MR, Oro AE et al (2012) Efficacy and safety of vismodegib in advanced basal-cell carcinoma. N Engl J Med 366(23):2171–2179

Shaitelman SF, Schlembach PJ, Arzu I et al (2015) Acute and short-term toxic effects of conventionally fractionated vs hypofractionated whole-breast irradiation: a randomized clinical trial. JAMA Oncol 1(7):931–941

Shreberk-Hassidim R, Ramot Y, Zlotogorski A (2017) Janus kinase inhibitors in dermatology: a systematic review. J Am Acad Dermatol 76(4):745–753 e19

Sibaud V, Eid C, Belum VR et al (2017) Oral lichenoid reactions associated with anti-PD-1/PD-L1 therapies: clinicopathological findings. J Eur Acad Dermatol Venereol 31:e464

Sibaud V, Leboeuf NR, Roche H et al (2016) Dermatological adverse events with taxane chemotherapy. Eur J Dermatol 26(5):427–443

Sowerby L, Dewan AK, Granter S, Gandhi L, LeBoeuf NR (2017) Rituximab treatment of Nivolumab-induced bullous pemphigoid. JAMA Dermatol 153(6):603–605

Spanemberg JC, Figueiredo MA, Cherubini K, Salum FG (2016) Low-level laser therapy: a review of its applications in the management of oral mucosal disorders. Altern Ther Health Med 22(6):24–31

Stander S, Siepmann D, Herrgott I, Sunderkotter C, Luger TA (2010) Targeting the neurokinin receptor 1 with aprepitant: a novel antipruritic strategy. PLoS One 5(6):e10968

Suvirya S, Agrawal A, Parihar A (2014) 5-Fluorouracil-induced bilateral persistent serpentine supravenous hyperpigmented eruption, bilateral mottling of palms and diffuse hyperpigmentation of soles. BMJ Case Rep 2014:bcr2014206793

Syrigou E, Dannos I, Kotteas E et al (2011) Hypersensitivity reactions to docetaxel: retrospective evaluation and development of a desensitization protocol. Int Arch Allergy Immunol 156(3):320–324

Tallon B, Blanchard E, Goldberg LJ (2010) Permanent chemotherapy-induced alopecia: case report and review of the literature. J Am Acad Dermatol 63(2):333–336

Tanaka R, Fujisawa Y, Sae I et al (2017) Severe hepatitis arising from ipilimumab administration, following melanoma treatment with nivolumab. Jpn J Clin Oncol 47(2):175–178

Tang N, Ratner D (2016) Managing cutaneous side effects from targeted molecular inhibitors for melanoma and nonmelanoma skin cancer. Dermatol Surg 42(Suppl 1):S40–S48

Teresi ME, Murry DJ, Cornelius AS (1993) Ifosfamide-induced hyperpigmentation. Cancer 71(9):2873–2875

Tischer B, Huber R, Kraemer M, Lacouture ME (2017) Dermatologic events from EGFR inhibitors: the issue of the missing patient voice. Support Care Cancer 25(2):651–660

Trueb RM (2007) Chemotherapy-induced anagen effluvium: diffuse or patterned? Dermatology (Basel, Switzerland) 215(1):1–2

Trueb RM (2010) Chemotherapy-induced hair loss. Skin Therapy Lett 15(7):5–7

US (2012) Food and Drug Administration Web site. Vismodegib. https://www.accessdata.fda.gov/drugsatfda_docs/label/2012/203388lbl.pdf. Accessed 26 June 2017

Valentine J, Belum VR, Duran J et al (2015) Incidence and risk of xerosis with targeted anticancer therapies. J Am Acad Dermatol 72(4):656–667

van den Hurk CJ, Breed WP, Nortier JW (2012) Short post-infusion scalp cooling time in the prevention of docetaxel-induced alopecia. Support Care Cancer 20(12):3255–3260

Villarreal CD, Alanis JC, Perez JC, Candiani JO (2016) Cutaneous graft-versus-host disease after hematopoietic stem cell transplant – a review. An Bras Dermatol 91(3):336–343

Vincenzi B, Tonini G, Santini D (2010) Aprepitant for erlotinib-induced pruritus. N Engl J Med 363(4):397–398

von Moos R, Thuerlimann BJ, Aapro M et al (2008) Pegylated liposomal doxorubicin-associated hand-foot syndrome: recommendations of an international panel of experts. Eur J Cancer 44(6):781–790

Voskens CJ, Goldinger SM, Loquai C et al (2013) The price of tumor control: an analysis of rare side effects of anti-CTLA-4 therapy in metastatic melanoma from the ipilimumab network. PLoS One 8(1):e53745

Vuerstaek JD, Frank J, Poblete-Gutierrez P (2007) Bleomycin-induced flagellate dermatitis. Int J Dermatol 46(Suppl 3):3–5

Weber JS, Dummer R, de Pril V, Lebbe C, Hodi FS, Investigators MDX (2013) Patterns of onset and resolution of immune-related adverse events of special interest with ipilimumab: detailed safety analysis from a phase 3 trial in patients with advanced melanoma. Cancer 119(9):1675–1682

Weber JS, Kahler KC, Hauschild A (2012) Management of immune-related adverse events and kinetics of response with ipilimumab. J Clin Oncol 30(21):2691–2697

Weber JS, Yang JC, Atkins MB, Disis ML (2015) Toxicities of immunotherapy for the practitioner. J Clin Oncol 33(18):2092–2099

Wolchok JD, Neyns B, Linette G et al (2010) Ipilimumab monotherapy in patients with pretreated advanced melanoma: a randomised, double-blind, multicentre, phase 2, dose-ranging study. Lancet Oncol 11(2):155–164

Wolff D, Ayuk F, Elmaagacli A et al (2013) Current practice in diagnosis and treatment of acute graft-versus-host disease: results from a survey among German-Austrian-Swiss hematopoietic stem cell transplant centers. Biol Blood Marrow Transplant 19(5):767–776

Wong RK, Bensadoun RJ, Boers-Doets CB et al (2013) Clinical practice guidelines for the prevention and treatment of acute and late radiation reactions from the MASCC skin toxicity study group. Support Care Cancer 21(10):2933–2948

Wu J, Lee YY, Su SC et al (2015) Stevens-Johnson syndrome and toxic epidermal necrolysis in patients with malignancies. Br J Dermatol 173(5):1224–1231

Wyatt AJ, Leonard GD, Sachs DL (2006) Cutaneous reactions to chemotherapy and their management. Am J Clin Dermatol 7(1):45–63

Yeh CN, Chung WH, Su SC et al (2014) Fas/Fas ligand mediates keratinocyte death in sunitinib-induced hand-foot skin reaction. J Invest Dermatol 134(11):2768–2775

Zhang RX, Wu XJ, Wan DS et al (2012) Celecoxib can prevent capecitabine-related hand-foot syndrome in stage II and III colorectal cancer patients: result of a single-center, prospective randomized phase III trial. Ann Oncol 23(5):1348–1353

11 Cutaneous Adverse Drug Reactions in Pediatric Population

Ilan Fridental and Yaron Finkelstein

Abbreviations

ADR	Adverse drug reactions
AGEP	Acute generalized exanthematous pustulosis
cADR	Cutaneous adverse drug reactions
CPNDS	Canadian pharmacogenomics network for drug safety
DIHS	Drug-induced hypersensitivity syndrome
DRESS	Drug reaction with eosinophilia and systemic symptoms
EM	Erythema multiforme
GI	Gastrointestinal
JIA	Juvenile idiopathic arthritis
MIRM	Mycoplasma-induced rash and mucositis
NICUs	Neonatal intensive care units
NSAIDs	Nonsteroidal anti-inflammatory drugs
SJS/TEN	Stevens–Johnson syndrome/toxic epidermal necrolysis
SSLR	Serum sickness-like reactions

I. Fridental
Paediatric Dermatology, The Hospital of Sick Children, Toronto, ON, Canada

Y. Finkelstein (✉)
Emergency Medicine, Clinical Pharmacology and Toxicology, The Hospital of Sick Children, Toronto, ON, Canada
e-mail: yaron.finkelstein@sickkids.ca

N. H. Shear, R. P. Dodiuk-Gad (eds.), *Advances in Diagnosis and Management of Cutaneous Adverse Drug Reactions*, https://doi.org/10.1007/978-981-13-1489-6_11

Key Points

- Concurrent illness should always be in the differential diagnosis of a possible CADR.
- Considering the high prevalence of exanthems in children, a full and comprehensive work-up should be performed before labeling a child as allergic to a drug.
- Different age groups have specific risk factors, as well as characteristic pharmacokinetics.
- The most common culprit drugs in the pediatric population are antibiotics, antipyretics, and antiepileptics.
- Overall, the prognosis of children with severe CADR is more favorable than in the adult population.

Cutaneous adverse drug reactions (CADRs) are the most common type of adverse drug reactions (ADRs) and comprise about 35% of all ADRs in children compared to 23% in adults (Star et al. 2011). Data collected by the Canadian Pharmacogenomics Network for Drug Safety (CPNDS) between 2005 and 2008 has shown that in admitted children, 66% of all CADRs were classified as severe (Castro-Pastrana et al. 2011). Anti-infectives are common offenders in children, and are 2–3 folds more prevalent as a trigger than in adults (Star et al. 2011; Dilek et al. 2014).

11.1 Unique Features of CADRs in Children

There are several distinct features of CADRs in children, which contribute to the complexity of managing CADRs in this population.

11.1.1 Diversity

The pediatric population is traditionally subdivided into age groups: neonates, infants, toddlers, school age, and adolescents. Each has unique characteristics, which can influence their reaction to medications. The neonatal and infancy periods bare several challenges. In Canada, for example, ~26% of neonates are still exclusively breastfed at 6 months of age (Statistics Canada 2013). FDA reported that 24% of the adverse events under 2 years of age occur in infancy due to maternal exposure during pregnancy or after delivery (Moore et al. 2002). Therefore, when encountering a skin eruption in a breastfed baby, one should always gather information about mother's medication usage. Furthermore, in infants, there is common usage of medications that are off-label or unlicensed (Conroy et al. 2000), and in neonatal intensive care units (NICUs), many patients receive at least one unlicensed or off-label medication (t Jong et al. 2000). Thus, there is scarce data on safety or efficacy of medications in this age group as most clinical trials exclude infants (Food and Drug Administration 2001). Adolescents also have unique challenges. One in three adolescents misuses medications, either prescription or over-the-counter medications (Lewis et al. 2013). This behavior may lead to more frequent ADRs and may not be disclosed by the adolescent, for medicolegal and other reasons.

11.1.2 Concurrent Illness

Exanthems are significantly more frequent in children. There are seven classic exanthems in childhood (measles, scarlet fever, rubella, staphylococcal scalded skin syndrome [SSSS], erythema infectiosum, roseola infantum, and chickenpox) and many more atypical exanthems which differ in morphologies and etiologies. The main etiology for exanthems in children is infectious, either viral or less commonly bacterial (Drago et al. 2012). Thus, when encountering a child with an acute illness who received supportive or anti-infective drugs and now presents with a rash, it may be challenging to differentiate between an infection-induced exanthem and an ADR. Therefore, clinicians should avoid a hasty labeling of an "antibiotic allergy," which could accompany the child throughout life and be a cause for prescribing less effective and more costly antibiotics and other medications in the future. True drug allergy is found in only ~5% of suspected patients when proper investigative measures are taken (Rebelo Gomes et al. 2008). Another diagnostic challenge in children is distinguishing between severe CADRs and milder infectious rashes, e.g., Stevens–Johnson syndrome/toxic epidermal necrolysis (SJS/TEN) versus Mycoplasma-induced-rash and mucositis (MIRM), which is several-fold more common in children. MIRM is considered a distinct entity, with a characteristic clinical course and a favorable prognosis, and yet most cases are designated as SJS/TEN or erythema multiforme (Canavan et al. 2015).

11.1.3 Pharmacokinetics

Several pharmacokinetic aspects are age-dependent and evolve throughout childhood (i.e., ontogeny). These changes play a role in probability, occurrence, and severity of CADRs in children. Neonates and infants' gastrointestinal (GI) absorption undergoes maturation in terms of emptying, metabolism, enzymatic activity, and GI flora. In other forms of administration such as transdermal or inhalation, there is an increased absorption compared to adults, which might lead to greater systemic exposure and effect (Lugo and Ward 2004).The volume of distribution is also changing during childhood and is influenced by increased total body water-to-body fat ratio, decreased plasma-binding protein levels, and differences in tissue binding of medications. Renal function reaches full maturation at around the age of 3 years; thus, slower drug elimination via the kidneys can lead to unintended toxicity. In addition, biotransformation of drugs in the liver occurs mainly via the CYP450 pathway and the uridine diphosphate-glucuronosyltransferase pathways. These enzyme pathways are age-dependent. For example, CYP-dependent metabolism is low at birth, ~50–70% of adult levels; however, by 2–3 years, enzymatic activity exceeds adult values. Also, the different CYP450 isomers mature at different ages. For example, the higher risk of idiosyncratic lamotrigine rash in young children is frequently attributed to their higher metabolism rate (Anderson 2002).

11.2 Approach to a Child with Suspected CADR

The approach suggested in this chapter is based on articles by Heelan K and Shear NH (2013) and Noguera-Morel L et al. (2014). Diagnosis of a CADR is based on recognizing the morphology, determining a probability, followed by laboratory investigations when appropriate and further definitive diagnostic tests.

11.2.1 Probability of Causality

When examining a child with suspected drug eruption, as in adults, we aim to establish the probability that cutaneous eruption is related to the administered drug. Naranjo, in a paper published in 1981, suggested an algorithm, which includes ten questions relating to the drug exposure and ADR, is still widely used to assess the probability of an ADR, and has been repeatedly validated in adults. The Naranjo ADR Probability Scale algorithm has been used in pediatric research as well but has not been validated (Avner et al. 2007). More recently, Du et al. suggested a revised algorithm, which is more suitable for the complex population of neonates and preterm babies in the NICU (Du et al. 2013). The main differences were more relevant time relationship between drug exposure and appearance of the eruption, published reports specifically in children, evidence of an alternative cause that could explain the reaction (reduced probability), improvement without discontinuation (reduced probability), and evidence of toxic levels of the drug in bodily fluids. Both algorithms classify ADRs into definite, probable, possible, and doubtful. In children, alternative etiologies (such as viral exanthems) are more common and should be considered as part of the diagnostic process. The timing factor is also crucial in causality assessment.

11.2.2 Morphology and Severity

The clinical assessment is based on four main rash morphologies which are further divided into simple and complex/severe. Systemic signs and symptoms and laboratory tests help in differentiating simple from complex/severe reactions.

11.2.2.1 Maculopapular Exanthems

Simple maculopapular exanthems, also referred to as morbilliform, are the most common CADRs in children. These exanthems are considered to be T-cell-mediated hypersensitivity reactions, type IVc. Common drugs associated with these rashes are penicillins, sulfonamides, cephalosporins, and antiepileptics (Ott 2011). These eruptions may appear 7–14 days after the first drug exposure (even after discontinuation of the drug) and in as early as 2 h in previously sensitized patients. These eruptions can mimic an infection-induced exanthem or worsen in the presence of a viral infection (Thompson and Ramos 2017). Systemic involvement is absent, and the eruption is self-limited. Resolution occurs within 1–2 weeks. Maculopapular rashes are mild and do not lead to serious outcomes. Therefore, if the offending drug is a clinical necessity for the management of the patient's condition, and a sufficient substitute is not available, drug administration can be continued under strict monitoring. Management of the eruption itself is symptomatic.

Complex maculopapular eruptions—Drug reaction with eosinophilia and systemic symptoms (DRESS) and drug-induced hypersensitivity syndrome (DIHS) are rare and severe cutaneous drug reactions. Both are considered type IVb hypersensitivity reactions, although other mechanisms have been proposed, such as reactivation of a viral infection (especially Herpes virus 6) (Ferrero et al. 2013). Predisposition was found in patients with certain HLA haplotypes, who were exposed to specific medications (Pavlos et al. 2012). The most commonly associated drugs are antiepileptics, allopurinol, sulfonamides, dapsone, and other antibiotics (Kardaun et al. 2013). Clinically, in DRESS/DIHS symptoms appear 1–6 weeks after exposure. Fever and malaise usually precede the rash. There may be lymph node enlargement, hematologic abnormalities such as eosinophilia or atypical lymphocytes, and multiple internal organ dysfunction (Husain et al. 2013). In children, the most commonly involved internal organ is the liver (Sasidharanpillai et al. 2016; Dibek Misirlioglu et al. 2017). The eruption could persist for several weeks after withdrawal of the offending drug. The mortality rate in adults is ~10%. Data on outcomes in children is scarce, and mortality rate is unknown, although likely much lower than in adults. Management of DRESS requires systemic medical treatment in most cases, mainly with corticosteroids. Surely, prompt withdrawal of the offending drug is essential (Pichler et al. 2011).

11.2.2.2 Urticarial Eruptions

Simple urticarial eruptions—Urticaria is a common skin reaction in children, and is caused mainly by infection. Medications account for approximately 30% of urticaria cases (Tsakok et al. 2014). As previously mentioned, this figure should be considered carefully since a large proportion of children are treated with antibiotics during a viral illness and develop urticaria. Pathogenesis is usually either a type I, IgE-mediated hypersensitivity in which the main drugs involved are beta-lactam antibiotics and nonsteroidal anti-inflammatory drugs (NSAIDs) or direct degranulation of mast cells in which the main offending drugs are NSAIDs and contrast media. Angioedema is more common in children. It usually involves the lips, eyes, and mucous membranes. The angioedema could occur with or without urticaria. Upon evaluating a child with urticarial ADR, one should actively seek systemic features of anaphylaxis, such as bronchospasm, hypotension, hoarseness, vomiting/abdominal cramps, and swollen lips/tongue.

Complex urticarial eruptions—Serum sickness-like reactions (SSLR) do not exhibit immune complexes. The mechanism of action is not well understood. This reaction consists of a triad of fever, arthritis, and a rash that could present as simple urticaria or polycyclic wheals. Some authors suggest that joint involvement may be due to fluid in the skin around the joints rather than the arthritis. The skin is the most frequent finding in SSLR, including erythema that progresses to urticarial lesions (pruritic and migratory), urticarial wheals with dusty to purple centers ("purple urticaria") that morphologically resemble erythema multiforme (EM) (Emer et al. 2013). The rash usually appears between 1 to 3 weeks after drug exposure. Originally, this reaction was described in association with cefaclor (Murray et al. 1980). Later on, the reaction was described in relation to numerous other drugs, including antibiotics, biological agents, antimycotics, and more. Management is symptomatic. The rash usually self-resolves within a few days to 2 weeks but sometimes requires oral corticosteroids.

11.2.2.3 Bullous Eruptions

Simple bullous eruptions—Pseudoporphyria is an erythematous, blistering eruption that occurs in sun-exposed areas. It was described as common (10–12%) in children with juvenile idiopathic arthritis (JIA) treated with naproxen and other NSAIDs (De Silva et al. 2000). Treatment entails discontinuation of suspected agents and sun protection.

Complex bullous eruptions—Stevens–Johnson syndrome (SJS) and toxic epidermal necrolysis (TEN) are severe bullous adverse drug reactions on the same spectrum, which differ by the extent of skin involvement. The incidence per million children for this bullous ADR is 4.3 to 5.8 for SJS, 0.6 to 1.4 for SJS-TEN, and 0 to 0.7 for TEN (Hsu et al. 2017). The overall mortality rate of SJS and TEN reported in KID database of children in the US was 1.5% in 2009 and 0.3% in 2012 (Okubo et al. 2017). Data from the NIS database reported mortality rates of 0% for SJS, 4% for SJS/TEN, and 16% for TEN (Hsu et al. 2017) and are much lower than in adults (1–5% in SJS and up to 30% in TEN). Common culprit drugs associated with this ADR are sulfa antibiotics, phenobarbital, lamotrigine, carbamazepine, and NSAIDs (Alerhand et al. 2016). The reaction usually starts 1–3 weeks after the initiation of the drug. The initial presentation is a nonspecific prodrome—fever, malaise, myalgia and arthralgia, eye stinging, and dysphagia. The skin and mucous membranes involvement will start 1–3 days later. Management includes prompt withdrawal of the suspected causative drug and referral for admission in a pediatric intensive care unit or a burn center. Treatment should include supportive measures such as hydration, wound care, and nutritional support. The patient should be managed by a multidisciplinary team which includes an intensive care physician, ophthalmologist, plastic surgeon, and a dermatologist. There is no consensus regarding systemic treatment. Long-term complications of SJS/TEN in children are primarily (1) dermatologic (scarring and hypopigmentation) (Finkelstein et al. 2011), (2) ocular (symblepharon, corneal opacification, limbal stem cell failure, and corneal vascularization) (Catt et al. 2016), and (3) urogenital (phimosis and labial adhesions) (Van Batavia et al. 2017). Recurrence of SJS/TEN has been reported in children. In a retrospective analysis from two pediatric tertiary care hospitals in North America, the rate of recurrence was 1 out of 5, although most were infection-related (mycoplasma and herpes), and few had negative serologies and developed after exposure to structurally dissimilar drugs (Finkelstein et al. 2011). An important entity in the differential diagnosis of SJS/TEN is *Mycoplasma*-induced rash and mucositis (MIRM), which has been described primarily in children. In this entity, in contrast to SJS/TEN, there is a predominance of mucosal involvement and excellent prognosis of the majority of patients (Canavan et al. 2015).

11.2.2.4 Acneiform Eruptions

Simple acneiform eruptions—drug-induced acneiform eruptions were originally described after systemic corticosteroid use. A recent review reported that 10.8% of the total ADRs in children treated with corticosteroids were acneiform eruptions (Aljebab et al. 2017). Other drugs associated with acneiform eruptions are testosterone, B12 supplements, and, more recently, targeted cancer therapies (Kazandjieva and Tsankov 2017; Macdonald et al. 2015).

Complex acneiform eruptions—Drug-induced acute generalized exanthematous pustulosis (AGEP) is extremely rare in children. Available data is based mainly on case reports, and the knowledge about the course, treatment, and prognosis is extrapolated from adults. The main offending drugs in pediatric AGEP are aminopenicillins, cephalosporins, acetaminophen, methylphenidate, oral ketoconazole, paroxetine, bufexamac, lindane, carbamazepine, and contrast agents (Posso-De Los Rios and Pope 2014; Nacaroglu et al. 2014). The rash erupts at day 1–6 of treatment and resolves shortly after discontinuation of the offending drug with excellent prognosis (Lansang et al. 2011).

11.2.2.5 Other Eruptions

Some eruptions do not fit into one of the main morphologies discussed above, such as fixed-drug eruption (Morelli et al. 1999; Nussinovitch et al. 2002) and psoriasiform eruption (Gul Mert et al. 2013; Smith et al. 2013; Sherlock et al. 2013; Romiti et al. 2016).

11.3 Conclusions

Cutaneous adverse drug reactions are the most common ADRs in children. The diversity of this population, along with developmental changes, concurrent illnesses, and the paucity of evidence-based data, constitutes a unique diagnostic challenge in this population. Keeping these complexities in mind while establishing probability via an organized algorithm with the aid of proper recognition of morphology and severity is advised in assessing ADRs in a pediatric population. Moreover, these aforementioned relatively simple techniques will also prevent false allergy labeling. Hopefully, in the near future, available genetic tests will aid in achieving personalized treatments, decreasing the burden of CADRs in children.

References

Alerhand S, Cassella C, Koyfman A (2016) Stevens-Johnson syndrome and toxic epidermal necrolysis in the pediatric population: a review. Pediatr Emerg Care 32(7):472–476

Aljebab F, Choonara I, Conroy S (2017) Systematic review of the toxicity of long-course oral corticosteroids in children. PLoS One 12(1):e0170259. https://doi.org/10.1371/journal.pone.0170259 eCollection 2017

Anderson GD (2002) Children versus adults: pharmacokinetic and adverse-effect differences. Epilepsia 43(Suppl 3):53–59

Avner M, Finkelstein Y, Hackam D, Koren G (2007) Establishing causality in pediatric adverse drug reactions. Pediatr Drugs 9(4):267–270
Canavan TN, Mathes EF, Frieden I, Shinkai K (2015) Mycoplasma pneumoniae-induced rash and mucositis as a syndrome distinct from Stevens-Johnson syndrome and erythema multiforme: a systematic review. J Am Acad Dermatol 72(2):239–245. https://doi.org/10.1016/j.jaad.2014.06.026
Castro-Pastrana LI, Ghannadan R, Rieder MJ, Dahlke E, Hayden M, Carleton B (2011) Cutaneous adverse drug reactions in children: an analysis of reports from the Canadian pharmacogenomics network for drug safety (CPNDS). J Popul Ther Clin Pharmacol 18:e106–e120
Catt CJ, Hamilton GM, Fish J, Mireskandari K, Ali A (2016) Ocular manifestations of Stevens-Johnson syndrome and toxic epidermal necrolysis in children. Am J Ophthalmol 166:68–75. https://doi.org/10.1016/j.ajo.2016.03.020
Conroy S, Choonara I, Impicciatore P et al (2000) Survey of unlicensed and off label drug use in paediatric wards in European countries. European network for drug investigation in children. BMJ 320:79–82
De Silva B, Banney L, Uttley W, Luqmani R, Schofield O (2000) Pseudoporphyria and nonsteroidal antiinflammatory agents in children with juvenile idiopathic arthritis. Pediatr Dermatol 17(6):480–483
Dibek Misirlioglu E, Guvenir H, Bahceci S, Haktanir Abul M, Can D, Usta Guc BE, Erkocoğlu M, Toyran M, Nacaroglu HT, Civelek E, Buyuktiryaki B, Ginis T, Orhan F, Kocabas CN (2017) Severe cutaneous adverse drug reactions in pediatric patients: a multicenter study. J Allergy Clin Immunol Pract 5:757. https://doi.org/10.1016/j.jaip.2017.02.013
Dilek N, Özkol HU, Akbaş A, Kılınç F, Dilek AR, Saral Y, Metin A, Çalka Ö (2014) Cutaneous drug reactions in children: a multicentric study. Postep Derm Alergol XXXI(6):368–371
Drago F, Paolino S, Rebora A, Broccolo F, Drago F, Cardo P, Parodi A (2012) The challenge of diagnosing atypical exanthems: a clinico-laboratory study original research article. J Am Acad Dermatol 67(6):1282–1288
Du W, Lehr VT, Lieh-Lai M, Koo W, Ward RM, Rieder MJ, Van Den Anker JN, Reeves JH, Mathew M, Lulic-Botica M, Aranda JV (2013) An algorithm to detect adverse drug reactions in the neonatal intensive care unit. J Clin Pharmacol 53(1):87–95. https://doi.org/10.1177/0091270011433327
Emer JJ, Bernardo SG, Kovalerchik O, Ahmad M (2013) Urticaria multiforme. J Clin Aesthet Dermatol 6(3):34–39
Ferrero NA, Pearson KC, Zedek DC et al (2013) Case report of drug rash with eosinophilia and systemic symptoms demonstrating human herpesvirus-6 reactivaion. Pediatr Dermatol 30(5):608–613
Finkelstein Y, Soon GS, Acuna P, George M, Pope E, Ito S, Shear NH, Koren G, Shannon MW, Garcia-Bournissen F (2011) Recurrence and outcomes of Stevens-Johnson syndrome and toxic epidermal necrolysis in children. Pediatrics 128(4):723–728
Food and Drug Administration (2001) The pediatric exclusivity provision: January 2001 status report to congress. Food and Drug Administration, Rockville, MD
Gul Mert G, Incecik F, Gunasti S, Herguner O, Altunbasak S (2013) Psoriasiform drug eruption associated with sodium valproate. Case Rep Pediatr 2013:823469
Heelan K, Shear NH (2013) Cutaneous drug reactions in children: an update. Pediatr Drugs 15:493–503
Hsu DY, Brieva J, Silverberg NB, Paller AS, Silverberg JI (2017) Pediatric Stevens-Johnson syndrome and toxic epidermal necrolysis in the United States. J Am Acad Dermatol 76(5):811–817.e4. https://doi.org/10.1016/j.jaad.2016.12.024
Husain Z, Reddy BY, Schwartz RA (2013) DRESS syndrome: Part I Clinical perspectives. J Am Acad Dermatol 68(5):693.e1–693.14. https://doi.org/10.1016/j.jaad.2013.01.033; quiz 706–8.
Kardaun SH, Sekula P, Valeyrie-Allanore L et al (2013) Drug reaction with eosinophilia and systemic symptoms (DRESS): an original multisystem adverse drug reaction. Results from the prospective RegiSCAR study. Br J Dermatol 169(5):1071–1080
Kazandjieva J, Tsankov N (2017) Drug-induced acne. Clin Dermatol 35(2):156–162

Lansang P, Weinstein M, Shear N (2011) Drug reactions. In: Schachner LA, Hansen RC (eds) Pediatric dermatology, 4th edn. Mosby Elsevier, London, pp 1698–1711

Lewis AL, M. Klintworth E, O. Hinton J, M. Gray K (2013) Adolescent medication misuse: results from the MUSC inventory of medication experiences (MIME). Adolesc Psychiatry (Hilversum) 3(2):184–189

Lugo R, Ward R (2004) Basic pharmacokinetic principles. In: Polin R, Fox W, Abman S (eds) Fetal and neonatal physiology, 3rd edn. Harcourt Health Sciences, Philadelphia, pp 190–197

Macdonald JB, Macdonald B, Golitz LE, Lorusso P, Sekulic A (2015) Cutaneous adverse effects of targeted therapies. J Am Acad Dermatol 72(2):203–218, 221–236.

Moore TJ, Weiss SR, Kaplan S, Blaisdell CJ (2002) Reported adverse drug events in infants and children under 2 years of age. Pediatrics 110(5):e53

Morelli JG, Tay YK, Rogers M, Halbert A, Krafchik B, Weston WL (1999) Fixed drug eruptions in children. J Pediatr 134(3):365–367

Murray DL, Singer DA, Singer AB, Veldman JP (1980) Cefaclor--a cluster of adverse reactions. N Engl J Med 303(17):1003

Nacaroglu HT, Celegen M, Ozek G, Umac O, Karkıner CS, Yıldırım HT, Can D (2014) Acute generalized exanthematous pustulosis induced by ceftriaxone use. Postepy Dermatol Alergol 31(4):269–271

Noguera-Morel L, Hernández-Martín A, Torrelo A (2014) Cutaneous drug reactions in the pediatric population. Pediatr Clin N Am 61:403–426

Nussinovitch M, Prais D, Ben-Amitai D, Amir J, Volovitz B (2002) Fixed drug eruption in the genital area in 15 boys. Pediatr Dermatol 19(3):216–219

Okubo Y, Nochioka K, Testa MA (2017) Nationwide survey of Stevens-Johnson syndrome and toxic epidermal necrolysis in children in the United States. Pediatr Dermatol 34(2):206–208. https://doi.org/10.1111/pde.13050

Ott H (2011) Chapter 183. Hypersensitivity reactions to drugs. In: Harper's textbook of pediatric dermatology. Wiley Blackwell, Oxford

Pavlos R, Mallal S, Phillips E (2012) HLA and pharmacogenetics of drug hypersensitivity. Pharmacogenomics 13(11):1285–1306

Pichler WJ, Daubner B, Kawabata T (2011) Drug hypersensitivity: flare-up reactions, cross-reactivity and multiple drug hypersensitivity. J Dermatol 38(3):216–221. https://doi.org/10.1111/j.1346-8138.2010.01142.x

Posso-De Los Rios CJ, Pope E (2014) New insights into pustular dermatoses in pediatric patients. J Am Acad Dermatol 70(4):767–773

Rebelo Gomes E, Fonseca J, Araujo L, Demoly P (2008) Drug allergy claims in children: from self-reporting to confirmed diagnosis. Clin Exp Allergy 38(1):191–198

Romiti R, Araujo KM, Steinwurz F, Denadai R (2016) Anti-tumor necrosis factor α-related psoriatic lesions in children with inflammatory bowel disease: case report and systematic literature review. Pediatr Dermatol 33(2):e174–e178

Sasidharanpillai S, Sabitha S, Riyaz N, Binitha MP, Muhammed K, Riyaz A, Jayakrishnan MP, Reyila VP (2016) Drug reaction with eosinophilia and systemic symptoms in children: a prospective study. Pediatr Dermatol 33(2):e162–e165. https://doi.org/10.1111/pde.12803

Sherlock ME, Walters T, Tabbers MM, Frost K, Zachos M, Muise A, Pope E, Griffiths AM (2013) Infliximab-induced psoriasis and psoriasiform skin lesions in pediatric Crohn disease and a potential association with IL-23 receptor polymorphisms. J Pediatr Gastroenterol Nutr 56(5):512–518

Smith WA, Siegel D, Lyon VB, Holland KE (2013) Psoriasiform eruption and oral ulcerations as adverse effects of topical 5% imiquimod treatment in children: a report of four cases. Pediatr Dermatol 30(6):e157–e160

Star K, Noren GN, Nordin K, Edwards IR (2011) Suspected adverse drug reactions reported for children worldwide: an exploratory study using VigiBase. Drug Saf 34(5):415–428

Statistics Canada 2013 http://www.statcan.gc.ca/pub/82-624-x/2013001/article/11879-eng.htm. Accessed 10 July 2017

t Jong GW, Vulto AG, de Hoog M et al (2000) Unapproved and off-label use of drugs in a children's hospital. N Engl J Med 343:1125

Thompson DF, Ramos CL (2017) Antibiotic-induced rash in patients with infectious mononucleosis. Ann Pharmacother 51(2):154–162. https://doi.org/10.1177/1060028016669525

Tsakok T, Du Toit G, Flohr C (2014) Pediatric urticaria. Immunol Allergy Clin N Am 34(1):117–139. https://doi.org/10.1016/j.iac.2013.09.008

Van Batavia JP, Chu DI, Long CJ, Jen M, Canning DA, Weiss DA (2017) Genitourinary involvement and management in children with Stevens-Johnson syndrome and toxic epidermal necrolysis. J Pediatr Urol 13:490.e1. https://doi.org/10.1016/j.jpurol.2017.01.018

Cutaneous Drug Reactions in the Elderly 12

James W. S. Young

Abbreviations

AGEP	Acute generalized exanthematous pustulosis
AMD	Age-related macular degeneration
cADR	Cutaneous adverse drug reaction
DRESS	Drug reaction with eosinophilia and systemic symptoms
GBFDE	Generalized bullous fixed drug eruption
HCTZ	Hydrochlorothiazide
ICU	Intensive care unit
PIR	Proportional impairment ratio
SJS/TEN	Stevens-Johnson syndrome/toxic epidermal necrolysis

Key Points

1. Elderly patients are at increased risk of CADRs due to comorbidity and polypharmacy.
2. Older individuals have reduced reserve to cope with medical stressors including CADRs due to frailty, comorbidity, and the presence of geriatric syndromes.
3. Older individuals may have a seemingly disproportionate change in health status from a CADR.
4. The effects of a CADR may be persistent after the initial event.

J. W. S. Young (✉)
Department of Medicine, University of Toronto, Toronto, ON, Canada

Brampton Civic Hospital, Brampton, ON, Canada
e-mail: james.young@williamoslerhs.ca

N. H. Shear, R. P. Dodiuk-Gad (eds.), *Advances in Diagnosis and Management of Cutaneous Adverse Drug Reactions*, https://doi.org/10.1007/978-981-13-1489-6_12

5. Geriatricians have expertise applying a comprehensive approach to multifactorial problems which may be helpful in the management of CADRs, especially when severe.

Understanding the importance of cutaneous adverse drug reactions (CADRs) in the elderly requires understanding some general principles of geriatric medicine. This chapter discusses relevant principles as they apply to the diagnosis and management of CADRs in the elderly. Extensive detail on specific drug reactions will be found in other chapters.

The most important points are that CADRs often have far-reaching implications for the aged patient, and a broad perspective is necessary to appreciate their scope and provide optimal care. During an acute illness or medical stress, older patients often have seemingly disproportionate changes in their health status. It is essential to consider this when thinking about the effects of a CADR, as well as the selection of treatments, and follow-up care. The reasons for this are related to polypharmacy, multimorbidity, frailty, and the presence of geriatric syndromes.

Multimorbidity, the presence of multiple chronic diseases, is common in the elderly and generally increases with age. Perhaps not surprisingly, the presence of multimorbidity correlates with polypharmacy and frailty (Woo and Leung 2014; Aarts et al. 2015; Rolland and Morley 2016). Frailty is a separate but related concept which entails aspects of physical aging which are not due to diseases per se but contribute to declining physiologic reserve, such as sarcopenia or reduced gait speed (Rockwood 2005; Clegg et al. 2013). Polypharmacy results from the accumulation of prescribed medications to manage underlying multimorbidity (Maher et al. 2014).

The presence of polypharmacy should prompt the clinician to consider several related issues. First and most obvious, the medications on a patient's list may be the cause of a CADR. Second, drug interactions may have contributed to the CADR (Guthrie et al. 2015). Third, other drug interactions may occur when initiating treatment for a CADR. Finally, the anticholinergic burden should be considered. Many medications which are not typically viewed as anticholinergic actually have a measurable degree anticholinergic activity (Rudolph et al. 2008; Chew et al. 2008). While the importance of this is usually limited for any single drug, as the list of prescribed medications lengthens, the cumulative effects of this anticholinergic load may become significant (Salahudeen et al. 2015). Geriatricians worry about the cumulative effects of anticholinergic load because of the increased risk of delirium, cognitive decline/dementia, falls, and perhaps even mortality (Han et al. 2001; Ancelin 2006; Gray et al. 2015; Ruxton et al. 2015; Gutiérrez-Valencia et al. 2017).

Geriatric syndromes, often called the "geriatric giants," refer to problems which are common in old age. Whereas a typical medical disease is defined by a constellation of symptoms, geriatric syndromes are better thought of as "symptoms" resulting from a constellation of diseases. The geriatric giants are generally considered to be cognitive decline, mobility decline, incontinence, and frailty (Crome and Lally 2011). The defining characteristic of these syndromes is that they are "multifactorial." For example, an older person who develops a pruritus from a drug reaction may take an antihistamine for symptomatic relief but become excessively sedated

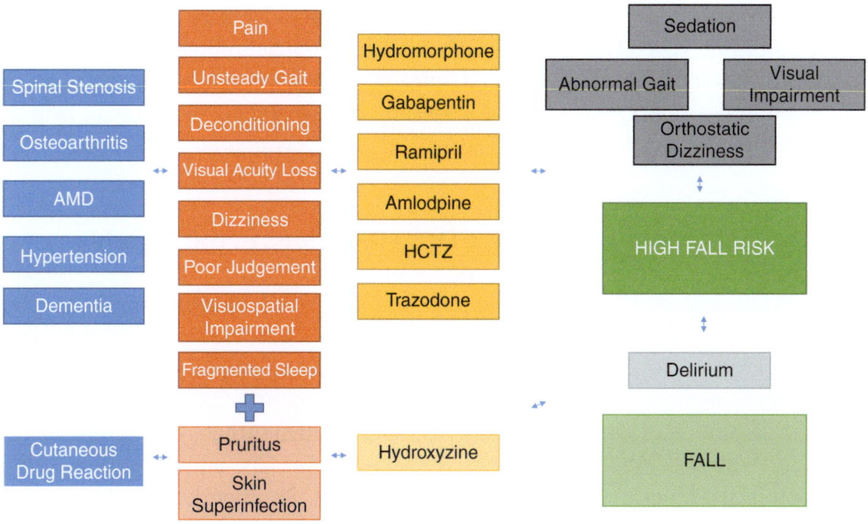

Fig. 12.1 CADRs in the elderly do not occur in isolation. Instead, these reactions occur in the context of a complex web of interrelated medical problems. The context is important to understand as it has major implications for the impact of the reaction, the tolerability of potential treatments, and the final outcomes. A representative example is shown above, where a CADR, its complications, and treatment result in a fall (which may not initially seem like an obvious complication to expect from this reaction). Several of the drugs listed above could have caused the CADR in this example. *AMD* age-related macular degeneration, *HCTZ* hydrochlorothiazide

leading to a fall and hip fracture. Whereas a younger person tolerates the same dose of antihistamine without incident, the older person may have mild cognitive impairment, reduced renal clearance of the drug, concomitant use of other sedating medications, arthritis of the knees, sarcopenia, visual impairment, and osteoporosis which together lead to a serious adverse outcome. Multimorbidity and frailty are independently associated with worse health outcomes for older individuals including falls, functional decline, hospitalization, discharge from hospital to an institutional setting, and mortality (Woo and Leung 2014; Clegg et al. 2013; Evans et al. 2014; Kahlon et al. 2015; Hubbard et al. 2017). Thus, the significance of a CADR must be considered in the context of the whole patient (Fig. 12.1).

12.1 Introduction

The clinical approach to diagnosing CADRs in the elderly is generally similar to other age groups. CADRS can be classified by their immune mechanism, although this is not very helpful in assessing the undifferentiated rash. The initial clinical approach should assess the morphology of the rash and look for any clues to internal organ involvement. Rash morphology informs the differential diagnosis. Seven morphologic groups encompass the spectrum of CADRs: exanthematous, dermatitic, urticarial, erythrodermic, blistering, pustular, and purpuric (Young and Shear

2017). The medication list should be reviewed carefully including medications used in the preceding year since some CADRs can have latencies of many months (drug-induced pemphigus and drug-induced subacute cutaneous lupus are notorious in this regard). Scoring systems exist for specific drug reactions, which may help to more firmly establish causality for a suspected drug (Sassolas et al. 2010).

12.1.1 Mild Cutaneous Adverse Drug Reactions in the Elderly

Mild CADRs are usually benign and therefore should be managed conservatively. The necessity of symptomatic treatments should be considered carefully to avoid using medications where the risk of adverse effects potentially outweighs their benefits. Simple exanthems are probably one of the commonest CADRs. Topical therapy with emollients or low-potency corticosteroids is often sufficient for symptomatic relief in these self-limited conditions. Pruritus, dermatitis, and eczema are also common in the elderly. Cholesterol and other lipids are important in skin barrier functions, and the use of statins can disturb this function causing dry skin and eczema (Proksch 1995). Diuretics may reduce skin water content. Anticholinergic drugs contribute to skin dryness by reducing perspiration. Dry skin may be asymptomatic but can lead to pruritus, asteatotic dermatitis, or eczema. Opioids can cause intense pruritus as a result of the direct release of histamine. Antihistamines may be useful to treat this side effect, though both opioids and antihistamines have the potential to provoke confusion or delirium (Clegg and Young 2011). Urticarial lesions are mechanistically heterogeneous. Acetylsalicylic acid, nonsteroidal anti-inflammatories, and angiotensin-converting enzyme inhibitors are the common causes (Zingale et al. 2006; Miller et al. 2008; Kowalski et al. 2011). While often a nuisance, urticaria may be a presentation of severe reactions including angioedema and anaphylaxis which can be life-threatening. Many new targeted agents for the treatment of cancer have been brought to market in recent years. The various kinase inhibitors cause a multitude of cutaneous reactions, including dermatitis, xerosis, hair and nail changes, pigmentary changes, and hand-foot syndrome (Alley et al. 2002; Robert et al. 2005; Lee et al. 2009). Immune checkpoint inhibitors appear to be the next wave in oncology and cause their own unique set of CADRs (Naidoo et al. 2015).

12.2 Severe Cutaneous Adverse Drug Reactions in the Elderly

Most severe CADRs are rare. Their seriousness is in large part due to their direct effects on the skin. These include Stevens-Johnson syndrome (SJS)/toxic epidermal necrolysis (TEN), drug reaction with eosinophilia and systemic symptoms (DRESS), acute generalized exanthematous pustulosis (AGEP), generalized bullous fixed drug eruption (GBFDE), drug-induced pemphigus, and drug-induced bullous pemphigoid. Any reaction which involves significant loss of skin across large amounts of body surface area may lead to significant fluid losses, superinfections, pain, and reduced mobility. Every superimposed medical stress in the context of a severe skin reaction increases the risk for slower recovery and long-term complications. SJS/TEN often have mucocutaneous involvement in the mouth and eyes. Oral lesions may lead to nutritional deficiency with associated muscle loss and slower wound healing. At least mild ocular involvement is common in SJS/TEN, with incidence in the 70–80% range, but some lesions may result in permanent visual impairment (Gueudry et al. 2009; Morales et al. 2010). DRESS may significantly involve internal organs, with the commonest cause of death from DRESS being hepatic failure (Cacoub et al. 2011; Chen et al. 2013). DRESS and AGEP may lead to a state of erythroderma and associated high-output heart failure (Loukas 2010). Across the spectrum of severe drug reactions (or their non-drug-induced analogues), older age and pre-existing comorbidity usually correlate with hard outcomes such as mortality (Ahmed and Moy 1982; Roujeau et al. 1998; Rzany et al. 2002; Lipowicz et al. 2013; Hsu et al. 2016). The downstream effects of a severe CADR may persist for months or even years. For example, in a large European cohort of older patients with SJS/TEN, 6-week mortality rates were 23% (in-hospital mortality) but mortality rates at 1 year were 34%, indicative of ongoing mortality risk well beyond 6 weeks (Sekula et al. 2013). This included many patients who were discharged from hospital. Mortality rates at 3 months tended to level off for younger patients or those with fewer comorbidities, whereas 25% of older/higher comorbidity patients died between 3 months and 1 year, and this was unrelated to the severity of the initial reaction.

12.3 Special Clinical Considerations in Treating Cutaneous Adverse Drug Reactions in the Elderly

Pharmacological treatment of CADRs may entail additional risks to the older patient (Table 12.1). While these treatments are often essential and therefore unavoidable, changes to dose, duration of treatment, or route of application may have help reduce these risks. For example, topical corticosteroids in bullous pemphigoid may have comparable efficacy and reduced risks versus systemic corticosteroids (Joly et al. 2002, 2005).

The treatment environment has important effects. Severe drug reactions are often managed in the intensive care unit (ICU). The incidence of delirium in the ICU setting is high (Agarwal et al. 2010). Cognitive impairment after critical illness is common; in some cases, previously healthy patients are left with the functional equivalent of mild dementia (Pandharipande et al. 2013). Prolonged immobility leads to loss of muscle and bone mass which is slow to recover. In the interim, patients with tenuous mobility, along with other issues such as bone loss, cognitive impairment, visual loss, and other lingering sequelae (Olteanu et al. 2017), will be a high risk for falls and fractures, increasing the risk of further complications or delays in recovery. Survivors of SJS/TEN (Dodiuk-Gad et al. 2016), critical illness, and delirium (Jones et al. 2001; Jackson et al. 2014) may have lasting post-traumatic

Table 12.1 Possible treatments for cutaneous drug reactions

Drug class	Drugs	Mechanism of side effects	Possible side effects	Anticholinergic risk score (if applicable) (Salahudeen et al. 2015)	Potential for sedation (FIR) (if applicable) (McDonald et al. 2008)
First-generation H1 antagonists	a. Chlorpheniramine b. Diphenhydramine c. Hydroxyzine d. Dimenhydrinate	Anti-histaminergic, anticholinergic, off-target effects (α- adrenergic antagonism, serotonergic effects)	Delirium, cognitive adverse effects, urinary retention, constipation	a. +++ b. +++ c. +++ d. +++	a. 1.956 b. 1.616 c. 2.104 d. 1.369
Second-generation H1 antagonists	a. Loratadine b. Desloratidine c. Cetirizine d. Levocetirizine e. Fexofenadine	Anti-histaminergic, anticholinergic	Delirium, cognitive adverse effects	a. +/++ b. + c. +/++ d. + e. ++	a. 0.357 b. 0.140 c. 0.193 d. 0.00 e. 0.021
Other H1 antagonists	a. Doxepin (tricyclic antidepressant sometimes used for its antihistamine effects)	Anti-histaminergic, anticholinergic, α-adrenergic antagonism	Delirium, cognitive adverse effects, urinary retention, constipation, postural hypotension	a. +++	
H2 antagonists	a. Ranitidine b. Cimetidine c. Nizatidine	Antihistamine, Anticholinergic	Delirium, cognitive adverse effects	a. +/++ b. +/++ c. +	
Systemic corticosteroids	a. Hydrocortisone b. Prednisone c. Methylprednisolone d. Triamcinolone	Glucocorticoid, Anticholinergic	Delirium, psychosis, accelerated bone loss, proximal myopathy, gastric ulceration, insomnia, diabetes, fluid retention/congestive heart failure, opportunistic infections, skin atrophy, secondary adrenal insufficiency	a. + b. + c. + d. +	

Drug class	Drugs	Mechanism of side effects	Possible side effects	Anticholinergic risk score (if applicable) (Salahudeen et al. 2015)	Potential for sedation (PIR) (if applicable) (McDonald et al. 2008)
Topical corticosteroids	Numerous	Glucocorticoid	Skin atrophy, systemic effects		

Many of these agents have risks which are especially significant in the elderly
Anticholinergic activity increases the risk for confusion, sedation, and other anticholinergic adverse events (+ low, ++ intermediate, +++ high)
PIR overall proportional impairment ratio; a composite score of subjective and objective measures of sedation; higher numbers are indicative of greater potential for sedation

anxiety and depression. These changes may all contribute to a state of increasing frailty and perhaps invite the use of other drugs.

The proactive involvement of a geriatrician should be considered in select cases, especially those of hospitalized elderly patients who have had a severe drug reaction. This may be beneficial in the identification of previously unidentified geriatric issues and minimization of treatment-related adverse outcomes. Identification of cognitive impairment may be important for safe medication use in the future. Qualitative identification of frailty can be easily performed using Rockwood's Clinical Frailty Scale, which has prognostic significance (Rockwood 2005; Evans et al. 2014). Because many geriatric problems are multifactorial, the solutions also tend to be multicomponent (Inouye et al. 1999; Gillespie et al. 2012). Management plans are usually developed and implemented with a multidisciplinary team of allied health professionals including physiotherapists, occupational therapists, dietitians, and others. Frail older people who receive inpatient comprehensive geriatric assessment are more likely to return home, less likely to experience cognitive or functional decline, and have lower in-hospital mortality (Ellis et al. 2011). The proactive approach of geriatrics has been shown to reduce delirium and medical complications in other inpatient settings (Marcantonio et al. 2001; Harari et al. 2007; Partridge et al. 2014). Given that recovery may be prolonged, and downstream risks linger for months after a CADR, periodic reassessment and optimization may be also facilitated by a geriatrician.

References

Aarts S, Patel KV, Garcia ME, Van den Akker M, Verhey FRJ, Metsemakers JFM, Van Boxtel MPJ, Gudnason V, Jonsdottir MK, Siggeirsdottir K, Jonsson PV, Harris TB, Launer LJ (2015) Co-presence of multimorbidity and disability with frailty: an examination of heterogeneity in the frail older population. J Frailty Aging 4:131–138. https://doi.org/10.14283/jfa.2015.45

Agarwal V, O'Neill PJ, Cotton BA, Pun BT, Haney S, Thompson J, Kassebaum N, Shintani A, Guy J, Ely EW, Pandharipande P (2010) Prevalence and risk factors for development of delirium in BURN intensive care unit patients. J Burn Care Res 31:706–715. https://doi.org/10.1097/BCR.0b013e3181eebee9

Ahmed AR, Moy R (1982) Death in pemphigus. J Am Acad Dermatol 7:221–228

Alley E, Green R, Schuchter L (2002) Cutaneous toxicities of cancer therapy. Curr Opin Oncol 14:212–216

Ancelin ML (2006) Non-degenerative mild cognitive impairment in elderly people and use of anticholinergic drugs: longitudinal cohort study. BMJ 332:455–459. https://doi.org/10.1136/bmj.38740.439664.DE

Cacoub P, Musette P, Descamps V, Meyer O, Speirs C, Finzi L, Roujeau JC (2011) The DRESS syndrome: a literature review. Am J Med 124:588–597. https://doi.org/10.1016/j.amjmed.2011.01.017

Chen Y-C, Chang C-Y, Cho Y-T, Chiu H-C, Chu C-Y (2013) Long-term sequelae of drug reaction with eosinophilia and systemic symptoms: a retrospective cohort study from Taiwan. J Am Acad Dermatol 68:459–465. https://doi.org/10.1016/j.jaad.2012.08.009

Chew ML, Mulsant BH, Pollock BG, Lehman ME, Greenspan A, Mahmoud RA, Kirshner MA, Sorisio DA, Bies RR, Gharabawi G (2008) Anticholinergic activity of 107 medications commonly used by older adults: anticholinergic activity of medication. J Am Geriatr Soc 56:1333–1341. https://doi.org/10.1111/j.1532-5415.2008.01737.x

Clegg A, Young JB (2011) Which medications to avoid in people at risk of delirium: a systematic review. Age Ageing 40:23–29. https://doi.org/10.1093/ageing/afq140

Clegg A, Young J, Iliffe S, Rikkert MO, Rockwood K (2013) Frailty in elderly people. Lancet 381:752–762. https://doi.org/10.1016/S0140-6736(12)62167-9

Crome P, Lally F (2011) Frailty: joining the giants. CMAJ Can Med Assoc J 183:889–890. https://doi.org/10.1503/cmaj.110626

Dodiuk-Gad RP, Olteanu C, Feinstein A, Hashimoto R, Alhusayen R, Whyte-Croasdaile S, Finkelstein Y, Burnett M, Sade S, Cartotto R, Jeschke M, Shear NH (2016) Major psychological complications and decreased health-related quality of life among survivors of Stevens-Johnson syndrome and toxic epidermal necrolysis. Br J Dermatol 175:422–424. https://doi.org/10.1111/bjd.14799

Ellis G, Whitehead MA, Robinson D, O'Neill D, Langhorne P (2011) Comprehensive geriatric assessment for older adults admitted to hospital: meta-analysis of randomised controlled trials. BMJ 343:d6553–d6553. https://doi.org/10.1136/bmj.d6553

Evans SJ, Sayers M, Mitnitski A, Rockwood K (2014) The risk of adverse outcomes in hospitalized older patients in relation to a frailty index based on a comprehensive geriatric assessment. Age Ageing 43:127–132. https://doi.org/10.1093/ageing/aft156

Gillespie LD, Robertson MC, Gillespie WJ, Sherrington C, Gates S, Clemson LM, Lamb SE (2012) Interventions for preventing falls in older people living in the community. In: The Cochrane Collaboration (ed) Cochrane database of systematic reviews. John Wiley & Sons, Ltd, Chichester

Gray SL, Anderson ML, Dublin S, Hanlon JT, Hubbard R, Walker R, Yu O, Crane PK, Larson EB (2015) Cumulative use of strong anticholinergics and incident dementia: a prospective cohort study. JAMA Intern Med 175:401. https://doi.org/10.1001/jamainternmed.2014.7663

Gueudry J, Roujeau J-C, Binaghi M, Soubrane G, Muraine M (2009) Risk factors for the development of ocular complications of Stevens-Johnson syndrome and toxic epidermal necrolysis. Arch Dermatol 145:157. https://doi.org/10.1001/archdermatol.2009.540

Guthrie B, Makubate B, Hernandez-Santiago V, Dreischulte T (2015) The rising tide of polypharmacy and drug-drug interactions: population database analysis 1995–2010. BMC Med 13(74):74. https://doi.org/10.1186/s12916-015-0322-7

Gutiérrez-Valencia M, Martínez-Velilla N, Vetrano DL, Corsonello A, Lattanzio F, Ladrón-Arana S, Onder G (2017) Anticholinergic burden and health outcomes among older adults discharged from hospital: results from the CRIME study. Eur J Clin Pharmacol 73:1467. https://doi.org/10.1007/s00228-017-2312-5

Han L, McCusker J, Cole M, Abrahamowicz M, Primeau F, Elie M (2001) Use of medications with anticholinergic effect predicts clinical severity of delirium symptoms in older medical inpatients. Arch Intern Med 161:1099–1105

Harari D, Hopper A, Dhesi J, Babic-Illman G, Lockwood L, Martin F (2007) Proactive care of older people undergoing surgery ('POPS'): designing, embedding, evaluating and funding a comprehensive geriatric assessment service for older elective surgical patients. Age Ageing 36:190–196. https://doi.org/10.1093/ageing/afl163

Hsu DY, Brieva J, Sinha AA, Langan SM, Silverberg JI (2016) Comorbidities and inpatient mortality for pemphigus in the U.S.A. Br J Dermatol 174:1290–1298. https://doi.org/10.1111/bjd.14463

Hubbard RE, Peel NM, Samanta M, Gray LC, Mitnitski A, Rockwood K (2017) Frailty status at admission to hospital predicts multiple adverse outcomes. Age Ageing 46:801–806. https://doi.org/10.1093/ageing/afx081

Inouye SK, Bogardus ST, Charpentier PA, Leo-Summers L, Acampora D, Holford TR, Cooney LM (1999) A multicomponent intervention to prevent delirium in hospitalized older patients. N Engl J Med 340:669–676. https://doi.org/10.1056/NEJM199903043400901

Jackson JC, Pandharipande PP, Girard TD, Brummel NE, Thompson JL, Hughes CG, Pun BT, Vasilevskis EE, Morandi A, Shintani AK, Hopkins RO, Bernard GR, Dittus RS, Ely EW (2014) Depression, posttraumatic stress disorder, and functional disability in survivors of critical illness: results from the BRAIN ICU (bringing to light the risk factors and incidence of neuropsychological dysfunction in ICU survivors) investigation: a longitudinal cohort study. Lancet Respir Med 2:369–379. https://doi.org/10.1016/S2213-2600(14)70051-7

Joly P, Fontaine J, Roujeau J-C (2005) The role of topical corticosteroids in bullous pemphigoid in the elderly. Drugs Aging 22:571–576

Joly P, Roujeau J-C, Benichou J, Picard C, Dreno B, Delaporte E, Vaillant L, Incan MD, Plantin P, Bedane C, Young P, Bernard P, Bullous Diseases French Study Group (2002) A comparison of oral and topical corticosteroids in patients with bullous pemphigoid. N Engl J Med 346:321–327. https://doi.org/10.1056/NEJMoa011592

Jones C, Griffiths RD, Humphris G, Skirrow PM (2001) Memory, delusions, and the development of acute posttraumatic stress disorder-related symptoms after intensive care. Crit Care Med 29:573–580

Kahlon S, Pederson J, Majumdar SR, Belga S, Lau D, Fradette M, Boyko D, Bakal JA, Johnston C, Padwal RS, McAlister FA (2015) Association between frailty and 30-day outcomes after discharge from hospital. Can Med Assoc J 187:799–804. https://doi.org/10.1503/cmaj.150100

Kowalski ML, Makowska JS, Blanca M, Bavbek S, Bochenek G, Bousquet J, Bousquet P, Celik G, Demoly P, Gomes ER, Niżankowska-Mogilnicka E, Romano A, Sanchez-Borges M, Sanz M, Torres MJ, De Weck A, Szczeklik A, Brockow K (2011) Hypersensitivity to nonsteroidal anti-inflammatory drugs (NSAIDs) – classification, diagnosis and management: review of the EAACI/ENDA# and GA2LEN/HANNA*: hypersensitivity to nonsteroidal anti-inflammatory drugs. Allergy 66:818–829. https://doi.org/10.1111/j.1398-9995.2011.02557.x

Lee WJ, Lee JL, Chang SE, Lee MW, Kang YK, Choi JH, Moon KC, Koh JK (2009) Cutaneous adverse effects in patients treated with the multitargeted kinase inhibitors sorafenib and sunitinib. Br J Dermatol 161:1045–1051. https://doi.org/10.1111/j.1365-2133.2009.09290.x

Lipowicz S, Sekula P, Ingen-Housz-Oro S, Liss Y, Sassolas B, Dunant A, Roujeau J-C, Mockenhaupt M (2013) Prognosis of generalized bullous fixed drug eruption: comparison with Stevens-Johnson syndrome and toxic epidermal necrolysis. Br J Dermatol 168:726–732. https://doi.org/10.1111/bjd.12133

Loukas E (2010) High-output heart failure in a patient with exfoliative Erythrodermic psoriasis. J Hosp Med 5:162–163

Maher RL, Hanlon J, Hajjar ER (2014) Clinical consequences of polypharmacy in elderly. Expert Opin Drug Saf 13:57–65. https://doi.org/10.1517/14740338.2013.827660

Marcantonio ER, Flacker JM, Wright RJ, Resnick NM (2001) Reducing delirium after hip fracture: a randomized trial. J Am Geriatr Soc 49:516–522

McDonald K, Trick L, Boyle J (2008) Sedation and antihistamines: an update. Review of inter-drug differences using proportional impairment ratios. Hum Psychopharmacol Clin Exp 23:555–570. https://doi.org/10.1002/hup.962

Miller DR, Oliveria SA, Berlowitz DR, Fincke BG, Stang P, Lillienfeld DE (2008) Angioedema incidence in US veterans initiating angiotensin-converting enzyme inhibitors. Hypertension 51:1624–1630. https://doi.org/10.1161/HYPERTENSIONAHA.108.110270

Morales ME, Purdue GF, Verity SM, Arnoldo BD, Blomquist PH (2010) Ophthalmic manifestations of Stevens-Johnson syndrome and toxic epidermal necrolysis and relation to SCORTEN. Am J Ophthalmol 150:505–510.e1. https://doi.org/10.1016/j.ajo.2010.04.026

Naidoo J, Page DB, Li BT, Connell LC, Schindler K, Lacouture ME, Postow MA, Wolchok JD (2015) Toxicities of the anti-PD-1 and anti-PD-L1 immune checkpoint antibodies. Ann Oncol 26:2375–2391. https://doi.org/10.1093/annonc/mdv383

Olteanu C, Shear NH, Chew HF, Hashimoto R, Alhusayen R, Whyte-Croasdaile S, Finkelstein Y, Burnett M, Ziv M, Sade S, Jeschke MG, Dodiuk-Gad RP (2017) Severe physical complications among survivors of Stevens–Johnson syndrome and toxic epidermal necrolysis. Drug Saf 41:277. https://doi.org/10.1007/s40264-017-0608-0

Pandharipande PP, Girard TD, Jackson JC, Morandi A, Thompson JL, Pun BT, Brummel NE, Hughes CG, Vasilevskis EE, Shintani AK, Moons KG, Geevarghese SK, Canonico A, Hopkins RO, Bernard GR, Dittus RS, Ely EW (2013) Long-term cognitive impairment after critical illness. N Engl J Med 369:1306–1316. https://doi.org/10.1056/NEJMoa1301372

Partridge JSL, Harari D, Martin FC, Dhesi JK (2014) The impact of pre-operative comprehensive geriatric assessment on postoperative outcomes in older patients undergoing scheduled surgery: a systematic review. Anaesthesia 69(Suppl 1):8–16. https://doi.org/10.1111/anae.12494

Proksch E (1995) Antilipemic drug-induced skin manifestations. Hautarzt Z Für Dermatol Venerol Verwandte Geb 46:76–80

Robert C, Soria J-C, Spatz A, Le Cesne A, Malka D, Pautier P, Wechsler J, Lhomme C, Escudier B, Boige V, Armand J-P, Le Chevalier T (2005) Cutaneous side-effects of kinase inhibitors and blocking antibodies. Lancet Oncol 6:491–500. https://doi.org/10.1016/S1470-2045(05)70243-6

Rockwood K (2005) A global clinical measure of fitness and frailty in elderly people. Can Med Assoc J 173:489–495. https://doi.org/10.1503/cmaj.050051

Rolland Y, Morley JE (2016) Frailty and polypharmacy. J Nutr Health Aging 20:645–646. https://doi.org/10.1007/s12603-015-0510-3

Roujeau J-C, Lok C, Bastuji-Garin S, Mhalla S, Enginger V, Bernard P (1998) High risk of death in elderly patients with extensive bullous pemphigoid. Arch Dermatol 134:465. https://doi.org/10.1001/archderm.134.4.465

Rudolph JL, Salow MJ, Angelini MC, McGlinchey RE (2008) The anticholinergic risk scale and anticholinergic adverse effects in older persons. Arch Intern Med 168:508–513. https://doi.org/10.1001/archinternmed.2007.106

Ruxton K, Woodman RJ, Mangoni AA (2015) Drugs with anticholinergic effects and cognitive impairment, falls and all-cause mortality in older adults: a systematic review and meta-analysis: anticholinergics and adverse outcomes in older adults. Br J Clin Pharmacol 80:209–220. https://doi.org/10.1111/bcp.12617

Rzany B, Partscht K, Jung M, Kippes W, Mecking D, Baima B, Prudlo C, Pawelczyk B, Messmer EM, Schuhmann M, Sinkgraven R, Büchner L, Büdinger L, Pfeiffer C, Sticherling M, Hertl M, Kaiser H-W, Meurer M, Zillikens D, Messer G (2002) Risk factors for lethal outcome in patients with bullous pemphigoid: low serum albumin level, high dosage of glucocorticosteroids, and old age. Arch Dermatol 138:903–908

Salahudeen MS, Duffull SB, Nishtala PS (2015) Anticholinergic burden quantified by anticholinergic risk scales and adverse outcomes in older people: a systematic review. BMC Geriatr 15:31. https://doi.org/10.1186/s12877-015-0029-9

Sassolas B, Haddad C, Mockenhaupt M, Dunant A, Liss Y, Bork K, Haustein UF, Vieluf D, Roujeau JC, Le Louet H (2010) ALDEN, an algorithm for assessment of drug causality in Stevens–Johnson syndrome and toxic epidermal necrolysis: comparison with case–control analysis. Clin Pharmacol Ther 88:60–68. https://doi.org/10.1038/clpt.2009.252

Sekula P, Dunant A, Mockenhaupt M, Naldi L, Bouwes Bavinck JN, Halevy S, Kardaun S, Sidoroff A, Liss Y, Schumacher M, Roujeau J-C, RegiSCAR Study Group (2013) Comprehensive survival analysis of a cohort of patients with Stevens-Johnson syndrome and toxic epidermal necrolysis. J Invest Dermatol 133:1197–1204. https://doi.org/10.1038/jid.2012.510

Woo J, Leung J (2014) Multi-morbidity, dependency, and frailty singly or in combination have different impact on health outcomes. Age (Dordr) 36:923–931. https://doi.org/10.1007/s11357-013-9590-3

Young JWS, Shear NH (2017) Cutaneous drug reactions in the elderly. Drugs Aging 34:655–672. https://doi.org/10.1007/s40266-017-0483-5

Zingale LC, Beltrami L, Zanichelli A, Maggioni L, Pappalardo E, Cicardi B, Cicardi M (2006) Angioedema without urticaria: a large clinical survey. Can Med Assoc J 175:1065–1070. https://doi.org/10.1503/cmaj.060535

Cutaneous Adverse Drug Reactions in Human Immunodeficiency Virus Infection

13

Rannakoe J. Lehloenya and Jonny Peter

Abbreviations

AHR	Abacavir hypersensitivity reaction
ART	Antiretroviral therapy
cADR	Cutaneous adverse drug reactions
DRESS	Drug rash with eosinophilia and systemic symptoms
FDE	Fixed drug eruption
HIV	Human immunodeficiency virus
IRIS	Immune reconstitution inflammatory syndrome
MDE	Morbilliform drug eruption
MDH	Multiple drug hypersensitivity
OIs	Opportunistic infections
PT	Patch tests
SJS/TEN	Stevens-Johnson syndrome/toxic epidermal necrolysis

R. J. Lehloenya (✉)
Division of Dermatology, Department of Medicine, University of Cape Town and Groote Schuur Hospital, Cape Town, South Africa

Groote Schuur Hospital, Cape Town, South Africa
e-mail: rannakoe.lehloenya@uct.ac.za

J. Peter
Division of Allergy and Clinical Immunology, Department of Medicine, University of Cape Town, Cape Town, South Africa

Allergy and Immunology Unit, University of Cape Town Lung Institute, Cape Town, South Africa

N. H. Shear, R. P. Dodiuk-Gad (eds.), *Advances in Diagnosis and Management of Cutaneous Adverse Drug Reactions*, https://doi.org/10.1007/978-981-13-1489-6_13

Key Points

- The incidence of cutaneous adverse drug reactions (CADR) is higher in persons infected with the human immunodeficiency virus (HIV).
- Stevens-Johnson syndrome/toxic epidermal necrolysis, drug rash with eosinophilia and systemic symptoms (DRESS), and maculopapular eruption are more common in HIV-infected persons, while other forms of CADR like fixed drug eruption, lichenoid drug reaction, drug-induced vasculitis, urticaria, and angioedema are not more common in this population.
- The management of CADR in HIV-infected persons is similar to that in the general population. However, initiation of multiple drugs at the same time, overlapping toxicity profile of antiretroviral drugs and drugs used to treat HIV-associated opportunistic infections (OIs), temporal overlap between CADR and HIV-related immune reconstitution inflammatory syndrome (IRIS), and the limited number of effective antiretrovirals and drugs used to treat OIs make the management of HIV and related OIs post-CADR a major challenge.

13.1 Introduction

In populations with a high prevalence of infection, the human immunodeficiency virus (HIV) has profoundly changed the disease profile, the clinical presentation of common diseases, the incidence of previously rare diseases, and consequently the pattern of drug use. The incidence of cutaneous adverse drug reactions (CADR) has similarly been affected by the pandemic (Selik et al. 2002; Adih et al. 2011).

13.2 Epidemiology of CADR in HIV

It is well established that CADR is more common in HIV-infected persons, although the exact incidence is unknown. The incidence is estimated to be as high as 100 times higher than in the general population (Coopman et al. 1993; Mittmann et al. 2012). Severe CADR associated with HIV continues to decline as safer regimen for treatment of HIV and associated opportunistic infections (OIs) are developed (Takaki et al. 2017). This is exemplified by the reduction in the incidence of Stevens-Johnson syndrome (SJS) and toxic epidermal necrolysis (TEN) associated with antituberculosis therapy since removal of thioacetazone from the regimen (Salami et al. 2010). However, in resource-constraint settings, cost-related limitations in formularies offset these potential reductions in the incidence of CADR. Early initiation of antiretroviral therapy (ART) in recent years has led to a decrease in HIV-associated OIs and a decline in the use of prophylactic drugs (Murphy et al. 2007). This has also considerably reduced exposure of HIV-infected persons to antimicrobials, the commonest group of drugs causing HIV-associated CADR (Cohen et al. 2011).

It is not clear if the incidence of HIV-associated CADR is higher in some ethnic populations. The incidence of CADR to some drugs is linked to the prevalence of specific HLA alleles in a population. These associations seem to be population specific, and the alleles are not necessarily expressed with the same frequency in all populations (Su et al. 2016). A good example is the lower incidence of abacavir hypersensitivity syndrome in persons of African descent as a result of a much lower expression of class I major histocompatibility complex allele HLA-B*57:01 (Small et al. 2017). There is currently no data to suggest that special populations like children, pregnant women, and the elderly with HIV have a different predisposition to CADR. Interestingly despite the neonatal use of nevirapine in the prevention of mother to child transmission of HIV, nevirapine-associated CADR has rarely been reported in neonates in comparison to pregnant women. The reasons for this are not clear.

13.3 Mechanism of CADR in HIV

The pathophysiology of CADR in HIV, like that of CADR in general, is not fully understood. It is thought to be multifactorial, an interplay between metabolic, immunologic, host, and viral factors. Persistent injury of HIV-infected cells, immune dysregulation, increased oxidative stress, depletion of immunoregulatory cells, and consumption of protective antioxidant molecules are thought to predispose to excessive "danger signals" resulting in a cascade of immune responses, cytokine release, and hypersensitivity reactions (Coopman et al. 1993; Rieder et al. 1995; Smith et al. 1997; Naisbitt et al. 2002). CD4 count has a limited utility as a marker of immune dysregulation and the subsequent risk of developing CADR (Boonyagars et al. 2017).

Genetic predisposition to CADR is being elucidated for many drugs used in HIV. Abacavir and HLA-B*5701 is the best known and now used in clinical practice for patient selection before initiating the drug in populations with a high prevalence of the allele (Phillips and Mallal 2009). On occupying the peptide-binding groove of the HLA protein, the abacavir is thought to change the stereochemistry of the binding cleft in the peptide-binding groove and the peptide specificity of HLA binding. Peptides that are then presented in this context are recognized as "foreign" and elicit a T-cell response (Peter et al. 2017). Other associations include HLA-C*04:01 and nevirapine-induced SJS/TEN and nevirapine-associated DRESS with HLA-DRB1*01:01 and HLA-Cw*04 (Littera et al. 2006; Gao et al. 2012; Carr et al. 2017).

13.4 Spectrum and Presentation of HIV-Associated CADR

All phenotypes of CADR have been reported in HIV-infected persons. Morbilliform drug eruption, drug rash with eosinophilia and systemic symptoms (DRESS), and SJS/TEN have a higher incidence in HIV compared to non-HIV-infected persons after a similar drug exposure (Saka et al. 2013). Other phenotypes like urticaria, angioedema, drug-induced vasculitis, lichenoid drug eruption, fixed drug eruption, and acute generalized exanthematous pustulosis do not seem to have a higher incidence in HIV neither do they present differently (Lehloenya and Kgokolo 2014). Some drugs seem to induce a specific constellation of symptoms and signs. Abacavir hypersensitivity reaction is characterized by fever, constitutional symptoms, gastrointestinal disturbances, and respiratory symptoms. The rash is reported in 70% of cases and is often a late symptom (Hernandez et al. 2000; Hughes et al. 2008). Efavirenz has been associated with a photodistributed annular erythema without systemic features (Isaacs et al. 2013). The presentation, severity, and clinical course of CADR do not seem to be different from that of the general population, in respect of clinical features and severity.

13.5 Drugs Associated with CADR in HIV

There are more than 100 drugs that have been reported to cause CADR in HIV. Limitations in case definitions, rarity of CADR, inaccurate reporting, and lack of confirmatory tests make it difficult to confirm the ascribed drug causality in many cases. There are only a few drugs, e.g., trimethoprim-sulfamethoxazole and first-line antituberculosis drugs that have a definite higher incidence in HIV (Lehloenya and Kgokolo 2014). Others like nevirapine and abacavir, although common causes of CADR in HIV, are used almost exclusively in HIV making it difficult to determine if they cause CADR just as frequently in non-HIV-infected persons (Centers for Disease Control and Prevention (CDC) 2001). As a general principle, a drug can cause any phenotype of CADR although some drugs have stronger association with some phenotypes (Lehloenya and Kgokolo 2014). Drugs that are commonly reported to cause treatment-limiting CADR in HIV are listed in Table 13.1.

Although infrequent, cross-reactivity has been reported between structurally related drugs including trimethoprim-sulfamethoxazole and dapsone (Holtzer et al. 1998), efavirenz and nevirapine (Soriano et al. 2000; Manosuthi et al. 2006), emtricitabine and lamivudine (Suarez-Lorenzo et al. 2016), and darunavir and trimethoprim-sulfamethoxazole (Lin and Hung 2015).

13.6 Management

The treatment of acute CADR in HIV does not seem to differ from that in the general population. However, there are some unique challenges in HIV. These include similar clinical features of CADR and many HIV-associated diseases; initiation of multiple drugs with overlapping toxicities at the same time; drug-drug interactions; immune reconstitution inflammatory syndrome (IRIS); multiple drug hypersensitivity (MDH), defined as a predilection to react to different chemically and structurally unrelated drugs with no evidence of cross-reactivity; and pressure to re-initiate therapy quickly in life-threatening conditions (Lehloenya and Kgokolo 2014). Thus, there is often clinical, diagnostic, and management uncertainty as well as

Table 13.1 Drugs that commonly cause severe cutaneous adverse reaction in HIV

Drug	Associated CADR	Incidence	Management	References
Nevirapine	MDE, DRESS SJS/ TEN, urticaria	15–32% DRESS: 5% SJS/TEN: 0.3–14%	If severe, discontinue the drug. If mild, monitor closely. Treat through unless severe, very low cross-reactivity with nevirapine	(Yunihastuti et al. 2014; Budamakuntla et al. 2015; Sarfo et al. 2014; Stewart et al. 2016)
Efavirenz	MDE, SJS/ TEN, DRESS, annular erythema	MDE: up to 20% SJS/TEN: 0.1%	If severe CADR continue and mild disease monitor closely. Very low cross-reactivity with nevirapine	(Isaacs et al. 2013; Yunihastuti et al. 2014)
Abacavir	AHR, SJS/ TEN	AHR: up to 8% depending on population SJS/TEN: rare	HLA screening Patch testing Alternative drugs	(Yunihastuti et al. 2014; Cutrell et al. 2004)
Anti-TB drugs	DRESS, SJS/TEN	5–20%	Discontinue treatment Alternative regimen if available Rechallenge	(Lehloenya and Dheda 2012; Yunihastuti et al. 2014)
Trimethoprim-sulfamethoxazole	MPE, SJS/ TEN, DRESS, FDE and urticaria	30–40% SJS/TEN: 8% DRESS: 6%	Alternative drug Desensitization Cross-reactivity with dapsone	(Yunihastuti et al. 2014; Lin et al. 2007; Chantachaeng et al. 2011)
Fluconazole	FDE, DRESS, SJS/TEN	Rare	Alternative drug Desensitization Low, if any cross-reactivity with other azoles	(Yunihastuti et al. 2014; Rankin and Jariwala 2012; Pasmatzi et al. 2011; George et al. 2012; Pinto and Chan 2009)

Abbreviations: *MDE* morbilliform drug eruption, *DRESS* drug rash with eosinophilia and systemic symptoms, *SJS/TEN* Stevens-Johnson syndrome and toxic epidermal necrolysis, *AHR* abacavir hypersensitivity reaction, *FDE* fixed drug eruption

unnecessary interruption of therapy. In diseases where there are few safe and effective drugs, e.g., tuberculosis and *Pneumocystis jiroveci* pneumonia, this poses further management challenges that are accentuated in resource-limited settings (Lehloenya and Kgokolo 2014; Lehloenya and Dheda 2012). For these reasons, a rational and pragmatic approach is required when managing HIV-associated CADR. Important considerations include:

- Is this really CADR or is there another diagnosis? It is important to exclude alternative diagnoses if possible. Scoring systems like the Algorithm for Assessment of Drug Causality in Stevens-Johnson Syndrome and Toxic Epidermal Necrolysis (ALDEN) and Naranjo score are useful guides to ascribing drug causality (Sassolas et al. 2010; Naranjo et al. 1981).
- If it is CADR, is it warranted to interrupt therapy? This decision has to be balanced against the severity of CADR, impact of treatment interruption on outcome of the disease being treated, and availability of alternative treatment. For example, life-threatening OIs being treated may imminently pose a greater danger to the patient than CADR. It is important to remember that initially severe reaction like SJS/TEN or DRESS may present as a morbilliform eruption.
- Is the withdrawal of the drug(s) going to impact on other comorbid conditions and pharmacokinetics of other drugs and increase the risk of drug resistance as a result of suboptimal drug combinations or monotherapy?
- If therapy is interrupted, is an alternative necessary? In HIV, prophylactic treatment to OIs is often initiated, e.g., trimethoprim-sulfamethoxazole for *P. jiroveci* prophylaxis, or treatment is initiated empirically, e.g., antituberculosis therapy. Usually prophylaxis does not need to be reinitiated. In cases of empiric treatment, confirmation of diagnosis or expert recommendation is needed to justify exposing the patient to alternative drug(s) or re-exposing them to the offending drug(s) (Lehloenya and Dheda 2012).
- Is desensitization possible? There are published protocols for desensitization of drugs commonly implicated in HIV-associated CADR. Among others, the list includes trimethoprim-sulfamethoxazole, nevirapine, efavirenz, first-line antituberculosis drugs, and fluconazole (Yunihastuti et al. 2014). Recurrence of OIs in HIV is not uncommon. If treatment with the same drug(s) that caused CADR is necessary, it is important to remember that once treatment is interrupted, even for short periods, the patient has to be desensitized again. For this reason, patient counselling on treatment compliance is critical (Todd 2006; Pascopella et al. 2011).
- In cases of limited therapeutic options, polypharmacy, and a pressing need to continue therapy, rechallenge with the offending drugs to eliminate the offender from the regimen has been shown to be safe if performed in hospital following protocols, even in severe CADR like SJS/TEN. There are limited data on the utility of patch tests (PT) in HIV. It has been used successfully for abacavir hypersensitivity. However, in HIV-associated tuberculosis, PT seems to induce systemic rechallenge reactions of similar severity as oral rechallenges and has limited utility (Lehloenya et al. 2011, 2016).
- How soon should the alternative drug(s) be initiated or rechallenge performed? The natural history of the specific CADR, half-life of the offending drug(s), and concurrent viral infections all need to be considered when initiating new drug(s) or rechallenging. Premature initiation of new drug(s) can make it difficult to differentiate between ongoing CADR; cross-reactivity between related drugs, e.g., trimethoprim-sulfamethoxazole and dapsone; and MDH to bridging therapy to minimize monotherapy-associated drug resistance. Rechallenge and introduction of new drugs should be delayed until CADR and associated laboratory

parameters have normalized or are on a downward trend (Lehloenya and Dheda 2012; Lehloenya et al. 2011, 2012).

- Retrospective genetic testing to identify the offending drug is a possibility for drugs and populations for which this is established.
- Adverse drug reactions lead to lower treatment compliance, already a major challenge in HIV (Bezabhe et al. 2015).

13.7 Outcomes

Mortality and morbidity associated with CADR in HIV is not clear. Some studies suggest increased mortality while others dispute this. What is clear is that comorbidities, especially opportunistic infections, are associated with higher mortality (Saka et al. 2013; Knight et al. 2014; Kannenberg et al. 2012).

13.8 Summary

CADR is more common in HIV, although the incidence is falling. However, a majority of reactions are benign, and treatment interruption is often unnecessary. When interruption is warranted, other diagnoses have to be excluded, a careful drug ascription undertaken, the need for continuing therapy established, benefits vs. risks of treatment interruption assessed, and the option of using alternative drug(s), desensitization, or a rechallenge explored.

References

Adih WK, Selik RM, Hu X (2011) Trends in diseases reported on US death certificates that mentioned HIV infection, 1996–2006. J Int Assoc Physicians AIDS Care (Chic) 10(1):5–11

Bezabhe WM et al (2015) Adverse drug reactions and clinical outcomes in patients initiated on antiretroviral therapy: a prospective cohort study from Ethiopia. Drug Saf 38(7):629–639

Boonyagars L, Hirunwiwatkul P, Hurst CP (2017) CD4 count and risk of anti-tuberculosis drug-associated cutaneous reactions in HIV-infected Thai patients. Int J Tuberc Lung Dis 21(3):338–344

Budamakuntla L et al (2015) A retrospective study of spectrum of nevirapine induced cutaneous drug reactions in HIV positive patients. J US-China Med Sci 12:85–89

Carr DF et al (2017) Genome-wide association study of nevirapine hypersensitivity in a sub-Saharan African HIV-infected population. J Antimicrob Chemother 72(4):1152–1162

Centers for Disease Control and Prevention (CDC) (2001) Serious adverse events attributed to nevirapine regimens for postexposure prophylaxis after HIV exposures: worldwide, 1997–2000. MMWR Morb Mortal Wkly Rep 49:1153–1156

Chantachaeng W et al (2011) Cutaneous adverse reactions to sulfonamide antibiotics. Asian Pac J Allergy Immunol 29(3):284–289

Cohen MS et al (2011) Prevention of HIV-1 infection with early antiretroviral therapy. N Engl J Med 365(6):493–505

Coopman SA et al (1993) Cutaneous disease and drug reactions in HIV infection. N Engl J Med 328(23):1670–1674

Cutrell AG et al (2004) Updated clinical risk factor analysis of suspected hypersensitivity reactions to abacavir. Ann Pharmacother 38(12):2171–2172

Gao S et al (2012) HLA-dependent hypersensitivity reaction to nevirapine in Chinese Han HIV-infected patients. AIDS Res Hum Retrovir 28(6):540–543

George J et al (2012) Toxic epidermal necrolysis caused by fluconazole in a patient with human immunodeficiency virus infection. J Pharmacol Pharmacother 3(3):276–278

Hernandez J et al (2000) The rate of hypersensitivity reactions to abacavir is similar in under-represented populations and incarcerated subjects. AIDS 14:569

Holtzer CD, Flaherty JF Jr, Coleman RL (1998) Cross-reactivity in HIV-infected patients switched from trimethoprim-sulfamethoxazole to dapsone. Pharmacotherapy 18(4):831–835

Hughes CA et al (2008) Abacavir hypersensitivity reaction: an update. Ann Pharmacother 42(3):387–396

Isaacs T et al (2013) Annular erythema and photosensitivity as manifestations of efavirenz-induced cutaneous reactions: a review of five consecutive cases. J Antimicrob Chemother 68(12):2871–2874

Kannenberg SM et al (2012) Toxic epidermal necrolysis and Stevens-Johnson syndrome in South Africa: a 3-year prospective study. QJM 105(9):839–846

Knight L et al (2014) Factors associated with increased mortality in a predominantly HIV-infected population with Stevens Johnson syndrome and toxic epidermal necrolysis. PLoS One 9(4):e93543

Lehloenya RJ, Dheda K (2012) Cutaneous adverse drug reactions to anti-tuberculosis drugs: state of the art and into the future. Expert Rev Anti-Infect Ther 10(4):475–486

Lehloenya RJ, Kgokolo M (2014) Clinical presentations of severe cutaneous drug reactions in HIV-infected Africans. Dermatol Clin 32(2):227–235

Lehloenya RJ et al (2011) Outcomes of reintroducing anti-tuberculosis drugs following cutaneous adverse drug reactions. Int J Tuberc Lung Dis 15(12):1649–1657

Lehloenya RJ et al (2012) Multiple drug hypersensitivity reactions to anti-tuberculosis drugs: five cases in HIV-infected patients. Int J Tuberc Lung Dis 16(9):1260–1264

Lehloenya RJ et al (2016) Diagnostic patch testing following tuberculosis-associated cutaneous adverse drug reactions induces systemic reactions in HIV-infected persons. Br J Dermatol 175(1):150–156

Lin KY, Hung CC (2015) Clinical relevance of cross-reactivity between darunavir and trimethoprim-sulfamethoxazole in HIV-infected patients. AIDS 29(16):2213–2214

Lin D, Li WK, Rieder MJ (2007) Cotrimoxazole for prophylaxis or treatment of opportunistic infections of HIV/AIDS in patients with previous history of hypersensitivity to cotrimoxazole. Cochrane Database Syst Rev 2:CD005646

Littera R et al (2006) HLA-dependent hypersensitivity to nevirapine in Sardinian HIV patients. AIDS 20(12):1621–1626

Manosuthi W et al (2006) Incidence and risk factors of rash associated with efavirenz in HIV-infected patients with preceding nevirapine-associated rash. HIV Med 7(6):378–382

Mittmann N et al (2012) Incidence of toxic epidermal necrolysis and Stevens-Johnson syndrome in an HIV cohort: an observational, retrospective case series study. Am J Clin Dermatol 13(1):49–54

Murphy RA et al (2007) Antiretroviral therapy-associated toxicities in the resource-poor world: the challenge of a limited formulary. J Infect Dis 196(Suppl 3):S449–S456

Naisbitt DJ et al (2002) Covalent binding of the nitroso metabolite of sulfamethoxazole leads to toxicity and major histocompatibility complex-restricted antigen presentation. Mol Pharmacol 62(3):628–637

Naranjo CA et al (1981) A method for estimating the probability of adverse drug reactions. Clin Pharmacol Ther 30(2):239–245

Pascopella L et al (2011) When tuberculosis comes back: who develops recurrent tuberculosis in California? PLoS One 6(11):e26541

Pasmatzi E et al (2011) Short-term and low-dose oral fluconazole treatment can cause Stevens-Johnson syndrome in HIV-negative patients. J Drugs Dermatol 10(12):1360

Peter JG et al (2017) Severe delayed cutaneous and systemic reactions to drugs: a global perspective on the science and art of current practice. J Allergy Clin Immunol Pract 5(3):547–563

Phillips E, Mallal S (2009) Successful translation of pharmacogenetics into the clinic: the abacavir example. Mol Diagn Ther 13(1):1–9

Pinto A, Chan RC (2009) Lack of allergic cross-reactivity between fluconazole and voriconazole. Antimicrob Agents Chemother 53(4):1715–1716

Rankin BT, Jariwala S (2012) Graded challenge protocol for fluconazole hypersensitivity in a patient with cryptococcal pneumonitis. Ann Allergy Asthma Immunol 108(6):466

Rieder MJ et al (1995) Toxicity of sulfonamide-reactive metabolites in HIV-infected, HTLV-infected, and noninfected cells. J Acquir Immune Defic Syndr Hum Retrovirol 8(2):134–140

Saka B et al (2013) Stevens-Johnson syndrome and toxic epidermal necrolysis in sub-Saharan Africa: a multicentric study in four countries. Int J Dermatol 52(5):575–579

Salami TA, Asalu AF, Samuel SO (2010) Prevalence of cutaneous drug eruptions in adult Nigerians with HIV/AIDS. Niger Postgrad Med J 17(2):160–163

Sarfo FS et al (2014) Incidence and determinants of nevirapine and efavirenz-related skin rashes in West Africans: nevirapine's epitaph? PLoS One 9(4):e94854

Sassolas B et al (2010) ALDEN, an algorithm for assessment of drug causality in Stevens-Johnson syndrome and toxic epidermal necrolysis: comparison with case-control analysis. Clin Pharmacol Ther 88(1):60–68

Selik RM, Byers RH Jr, Dworkin MS (2002) Trends in diseases reported on U.S. death certificates that mentioned HIV infection, 1987–1999. J Acquir Immune Defic Syndr 29(4):378–387

Small CB et al (2017) HLA-B*57:01 allele prevalence in HIV-infected North American subjects and the impact of allele testing on the incidence of abacavir-associated hypersensitivity reaction in HLA-B*57:01-negative subjects. BMC Infect Dis 17(1):256

Smith KJ et al (1997) Increased drug reactions in HIV-1-positive patients: a possible explanation based on patterns of immune dysregulation seen in HIV-1 disease. The Military Medical Consortium for the Advancement of Retroviral Research (MMCARR). Clin Exp Dermatol 22(3):118–123

Soriano V et al (2000) Is there cross-toxicity between nevirapine and efavirenz in subjects developing rash? AIDS 14(11):1672–1673

Stewart A et al (2016) Severe antiretroviral-associated skin reactions in South African patients: a case series and case-control analysis. Pharmacoepidemiol Drug Saf 25(11):1313–1319

Su SC et al (2016) Severe cutaneous adverse reactions: the pharmacogenomics from research to clinical implementation. Int J Mol Sci 17(11):E1890

Suarez-Lorenzo I et al (2016) Severe reaction to emtricitabine and lamiduvine: evidence of cross-reactivity. Contact Dermatitis 74(4):253–254

Takaki I, Quirelli L, Cuman RK (2017) Adverse drug reaction in HIV-infected people treated with HAART in Maringá, Southern Brazil. Trop J Pharm Res 16(4):939–945

Todd G (2006) Adverse cutaneous drug eruptions and HIV: a clinician's global perspective. Dermatol Clin 24(4):459–472 vi

Yunihastuti E, Widhani A, Karjadi TH (2014) Drug hypersensitivity in human immunodeficiency virus-infected patient: challenging diagnosis and management. Asia Pac Allergy 4(1):54–67

Cutaneous Adverse Drug Reactions from Antituberculosis Treatment

14

Jonny Peter and Rannakoe J. Lehloenya

Abbreviations

ADRs	Adverse drug reactions
AGEP	Acute generalized exanthematous pustolosis
DPT	Drug provocation testing
DRESS	Drug rash with eosinophilia and systemic symptoms
DS-TB	Drug-susceptible TB
FDE	Fixed drug eruption
FQ	Fluoroquinolones
HAART	Highly active antiretroviral therapy
LDE	Lichenoid drug eruption
MDR-TB	Multidrug-resistant TB
SCAR	Severe cutaneous adverse drug reaction
SJS/TEN	Stevens-Johnson syndrome and toxic epidermal necrolysis
TB	Tuberculosis
XDR-TB	Extensively drug-resistant TB

J. Peter (✉)
Division of Allergy and Clinical Immunology, Department of Medicine, University of Cape Town, Cape Town, South Africa

Allergy and Immunology Unit, University of Cape Town Lung Institute, Cape Town, South Africa
e-mail: Jonny.Peter@uct.ac.za

R. J. Lehloenya
Division of Dermatology, Department of Medicine, University of Cape Town and Groote Schuur Hospital, Cape Town, South Africa
e-mail: rannakoe.lehloenya@uct.ac.za

N. H. Shear, R. P. Dodiuk-Gad (eds.), *Advances in Diagnosis and Management of Cutaneous Adverse Drug Reactions*, https://doi.org/10.1007/978-981-13-1489-6_14

Key Points

- The spectrum of CADR phenotypes associated with one or more antituberculosis (TB) drug includes maculopapular eruption, DRESS/DHS, fixed drug eruption (including the more severe bullous form), lichenoid drug eruption, SJS/TEN, AGEP, and cutaneous vasculitis. Type 1 hypersensitivity reactions causing urticaria/angioedema and anaphylaxis are described but uncommon. In high TB/HIV burden settings, the majority of anti-TB drug-related CADR occurs in HIV co-infected patients.
- Individual anti-TB drugs can cause different CADR phenotypes, while individual phenotypes can be caused by a number of first- and second-line anti-TB drugs; this makes identification of the culprit drug a major challenge.
- The key challenges of managing anti-TB drug-related CADR, especially in the context of HIV coinfection, include avoiding lengthy treatment interruption in patients with active TB and high TB-associated mortality and the rapid and safe identification of the culprit drug(s) to ensure CADR patients are able to receive an optimal anti-TB drug regimen.

14.1 Introduction

Tuberculosis (TB) is a global epidemic with more than ten million active cases and 1.4 million deaths in 2015 (WHO 2016). An estimated 1.2 million TB cases were co-infected with HIV (11% of global incidence), and over 400,000 people died of TB/HIV coinfection (25% of global deaths); approximately 80% of these in Africa (WHO 2016; Dheda et al. 2016). Multidrug-resistant TB (MDR-TB) and extensively drug-resistant TB (XDR-TB) are increasing in at-risk populations, with almost half a million new cases of MDR-TB in 2015 (WHO 2016).

Multidrug therapy for TB requires ≥ four drugs for at least 6 months, irrespective of drug susceptibility. Figure 14.1 shows the anti-TB drugs in clinical practice, their chemical structure, and associated CADRs. In TB/HIV coinfection, highly active antiretroviral therapy (HAART) adds further drug-drug interactions and toxicities, further complicating therapy. Rifampicin and isoniazid are the backbone drugs for drug-susceptible TB (DS-TB). In MDR-TB the bacilli are resistant to these two drugs. MDR-TB treatment requires tailored drug regimens of four or more effective drugs for up to 24 months (Dheda et al. 2016). Fluoroquinolones (FQ) and second-line injectables, such as aminoglycosides or capreomycin, are the backbone drugs for initial MDR-TB regimens. Newer drug regimens, aiming for a single shortened combination therapy for both DS- and MDR-TB, are in clinical trials; almost all include a FQ together with novel drugs such as bedaquiline or delamanid (Dawson et al. 2015). TB-associated CADR that result in treatment interruption and necessitate regimen change cause substantial morbidity and mortality and are associated with significant healthcare costs (Lehloenya and Dheda 2012).

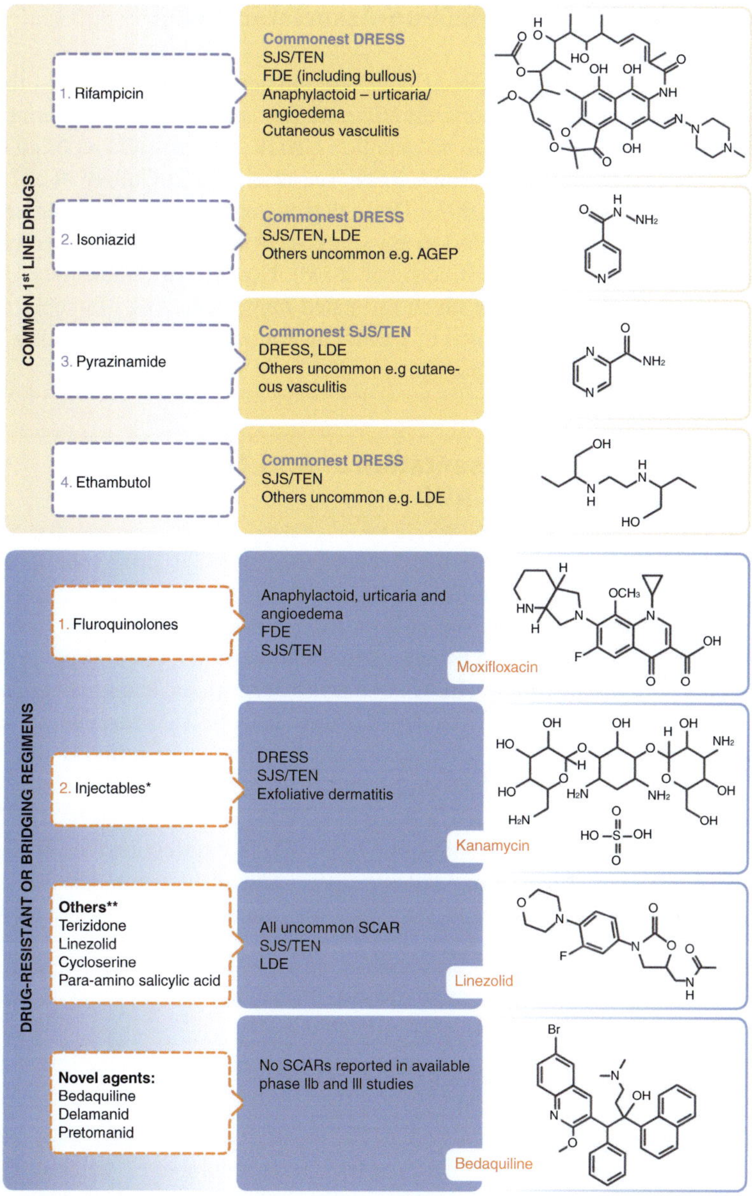

**Common injectable drugs include kanamycin, amikacin and streptomycin*
***This is not an exhaustive list of anti-tuberculosis drugs. These drugs used predominantly in the treatment of extremely-drug resistant TB*

Fig. 14.1 Antituberculosis drugs and CADRs. Abbreviations: *AGEP* acute generalized exanthematous pustulosis, *DRESS* drug rash with eosinophilia and systemic symptoms, *FDE* fixed drug eruption, *LDE* lichenoid drug eruption, *SCAR* severe cutaneous adverse drug reaction, *SJS/TEN* Stevens-Johnson syndrome and toxic epidermal necrolysis

14.2 Epidemiology of TB Drug-Associated CADR

Incidence figures for TB-associated CADR are unknown, as are details on the frequency of specific CADR phenotypes; some studies evaluating adverse drug reactions (ADRs) to anti-TB drugs do not mention CADR, whereas it is reported as the most common ADR in others (Todd 2006; Yee et al. 2003; Gulbay et al. 2006; Thong et al. 2003; Marra et al. 2007). Those that evaluate incidence and prevalence of TB-associated ADRs simply fail to classify CADR in any detail, often mentioning it as "rash" (Yee et al. 2003; Breen et al. 2006). However, available data suggest the incidence to be significant, with an estimated range of 5–23% (Tan et al. 2007; Kuaban et al. 1997); the incidence of treatment-limiting CADR is certainly much lower, but no epidemiological data is available.

14.3 Spectrum and Presentation of Anti-TB Drug-Associated CADR

All phenotypes of CADR have been reported to anti-TB drug therapies (see Fig. 14.1). Morbilliform drug eruptions or maculopapular exanthems account for most cases and in the majority are self-limiting. Severe cutaneous adverse drug reactions (SCAR) including DRESS, SJS/TEN, bullous fixed drug eruption (FDE), lichenoid drug eruption (LDE), and acute generalized exanthematous pustulosis (AGEP) are all reported to anti-TB drugs. The clinical presentation, severity, and clinical course of these reactions in the context of anti-TB drugs are similar to other known offending drugs and have been reviewed in detail elsewhere (Lehloenya and Dheda 2012; Peter et al. 2017). DRESS and SJS/TEN are by far the commonest SCAR in the context of TB/HIV coinfection (see section on "CADRs in HIV"). Urticaria/angioedema does occur to first-line anti-TB drugs, but our experience is that these reactions are uncommon as is anaphylaxis, although a recent Turkish study reported a prevalence of 3% in a HIV non-endemic setting (Buhari et al. 2015).

14.4 Anti-TB Drugs Associated with CADR

Figure 14.1 shows the spectrum of CADR phenotypes associated with specific anti-TB drugs. Although an anti-TB drug can cause a number of different CADR phenotypes, as we have improved our causality assessments, we see that specific drugs tend to have stronger association with certain phenotypes. A previous study suggested pyrazinamide to be the most common anti-TB drug associated with CADRs (Yee et al. 2003; Pozniak et al. 1992). However, our clinical and drug provocation testing experience suggests that although both pyrazinamide and isoniazid are common culprits, rifampicin is the most frequent offending drug (Lehloenya et al. 2011).

Among the SCAR phenotypes, isoniazid, rifampicin, ethambutol, pyrazinamide, and streptomycin have been associated most commonly with DRESS and SJS/TEN (Lehloenya et al. 2011, 2015). SJS/TEN has also been reported to second-line drugs including fluoroquinolones and cycloserine (Lehloenya and Dheda 2012). FDEs, although infrequently associated with anti-TB drugs, have been reported with rifamycins and fluoroquinolones (Lehloenya and Dheda 2012). LDEs have been reported with isoniazid, pyrazinamide, and ethambutol (Lehloenya and Dheda 2012). Although vasculitis to anti-TB therapy is rare, it has been reported with rifampicin and pyrazinamide (Lehloenya and Dheda 2012).

14.5 Pathogenesis

The immunopathogenesis of CADR to anti-TB drugs is likely to involve phenotype-specific mechanisms, and to date specific fundamental research is lacking. The majority of anti-TB drug CADRs have a delayed phenotype, consistent with T-cell-driven pathology. The central role of drug-specific T cells is supported by positive patch and lymphocyte proliferation testing to anti-TB drugs (Lehloenya et al. 2016; Schreiber et al. 1999). Furthermore, drug-specific CD4+ T-cell proliferation and cytokine production after stimulation with rifampicin and isoniazid in patients with anti-TB drug DRESS suggest a central role for these T cells in pathology (Ye et al. 2017). Unlike with a number of specific drug-SCAR combinations, including among HIV co-infected patients, no HLA risk allele has been identified for any of anti-TB drug CADR, although we are currently investigating a possible HLA risk allele for rifampicin-induced DRESS and SJS/TEN. An association between cytochrome p450 drug-metabolizing enzyme SNPs (CYP2C19 and CYP2C9) and increased TB-associated morbilliform eruption has been described, suggesting a role for differential pharmacokinetics in patients with anti-TB drug CADR (Kim et al. 2011).

The majority of SCAR to anti-TB drugs occurs within the context of HIV coinfection. As described in the section on "CADRs in HIV," the immune dysregulation in HIV with changes in homeostatic T-cell populations, immune activation states, immunometabolism, and concomitant viral and opportunistic infections may alter the thresholds for drug-specific T-cell activation, possibly negating the need for drug-specific HLA-T-clonotype pairs for the inductions of hypersensitivity reactions (Coopman et al. 1993; Rieder et al. 1995; Smith et al. 1997; Naisbitt et al. 2002). A key unanswered question is whether these reactions have immunological memory or whether patients will become tolerant to the offending drug after immune reconstitution.

Immediate hypersensitivity reactions occurring with anti-TB drugs are likely mediated by mast cell degranulation as supported by positive skin prick testing in patients with a history of anaphylaxis (Martinez et al. 1999). No drug-specific IgE antibodies have been published to any of the anti-TB drugs, suggesting the possibility of non-IgE reactions; however, details are lacking.

14.6 Management

Central to successful management of anti-TB drug CADR is avoidance of lengthy treatment interruption in patients with active TB disease, especially in advanced HIV-related immunosuppression. Treatment interruption increases TB-related mortality (Lehloenya and Dheda 2012). As outlined above, anti-TB drug SCAR introduces additional management complexities. For instance, through the need for early initiation of life-saving bridging therapy and oral drug challenge, we have noted ~25% of TB/HIV co-infected patients admitted with a SCAR will show multiple drug hypersensitivity, reacting to at least two chemically different first- or second-line drugs (Lehloenya et al. 2012). It is uncertain if these simply represent flare-up reactions or have long-lasting immunological memory, thus requiring long-term avoidance of all the implicated drugs (Pichler et al. 2017). Either way, they pose a major problem for short-term treatment success. Our clinical experience is that although general management considerations are similar to other drug reactions, based on clinical phenotype and severity, these comorbid complexities necessitate multidisciplinary specialist inputs, including from dermatologists, infectious diseases, allergologists, pharmacologists, and hepatologists. Our approach has been multidisciplinary input and a recent clinic, the first of its kind in Africa, to provide holistic care to these vulnerable patients in both in- and out-patient settings (Peter et al. 2015).

The key diagnostic focus in anti-TB drug CADR, especially SCAR, is rapid and safe identification of the offending drug(s). In vitro testing, such as lymphocyte transformation tests or ELISpot assays to anti-TB drug reactions, remains a research tool due to limited diagnostic accuracy and assay complexity (Lehloenya and Dheda 2012). In vivo testing, using either skin/intradermal or patch testing is useful, but specific drug concentrations and vehicles are not standardized or well validated across different populations. In addition, among HIV co-infected patients, both skin and patch testings with anti-TB drugs induce systemic reactions, similar to oral drug provocation, in >90% of cases (Lehloenya et al. 2016). Oral drug provocation testing (DPT) is considered the gold standard in establishing causality but carries the risk of inducing severe CADR. Thus, traditional contraindications to DPT include patients with severe or life-threatening reactions, pregnancy, and significant comorbidity (Aberer et al. 2003). However, in the context of active TB, and possible advanced immunosuppression, this risk needs to be balanced against the significant danger of suboptimal TB treatment (Lehloenya and Dheda 2012). We believe a safe DPT protocol to include (1) confirmation of active TB and the need for ongoing TB treatment, (2) resolution of skin and laboratory parameters resulting from the initial SCAR, (3) the use of an alternative three-drug bridging regimen (usually fluoroquinolones, aminoglycoside, and ethionamide), and (4) sequential oral rechallenge. In a retrospective review of DPT in Cape Town, 22 out of 23 reintroduction reactions occurred within 72 h of reintroducing the offending drug. Itch, hepatitis, and fever occurred in 48, 39, and 35% of patients (Lehloenya et al. 2011). Our yet to be published prospective data of 296 DPT of first-line anti-TB drugs performed in the context of an RCT to compare full versus incremental dose oral challenge confirms these earlier safety findings and proves incremental utility over in vivo diagnostics. Out of 296 DPTs, 48 (16%) had a positive challenge, 26 (52%) of which had negative patch and skin prick testing, and only six positive reactions had severe or life-threatening reactions. This protocol now needs to be validated in other high-burden TB/HIV endemic settings.

Type 1 hypersensitivity reactions can be treated successfully with rapid desensitization. In fact, Buhari et al. have shown the success of rapid systematic desensitization to FLTD over DPT to identify causative agent followed by desensitization (Buhari et al. 2015).

14.7 Outcomes

The majority of CADRs to anti-TB drugs are self-limiting and have a good prognosis (Lehloenya and Dheda 2012). Mortality and morbidity associated with specific phenotypes of anti-TB-associated SCAR are not clear.

14.8 Summary

TB requires complex, multiple drug therapy. CADRs during anti-TB drug therapy are common. The majority of reactions are benign and self-limiting, and treatment interruption is often unnecessary. TB disease severity, and frequent HIV comorbidity, drives a need to avoid unnecessary treatment interruptions or exclusion of effective drugs and means that rechallenge even in SCAR reactions may be justifiable. Increasing data shows the safety and utility of drug provocation testing performed in specialized centers. Multidisciplinary inputs are required to optimally care for these vulnerable patients.

References

Aberer W, Bircher A, Romano A, Blanca M, Campi P, Fernandez J et al (2003) Drug provocation testing in the diagnosis of drug hypersensitivity reactions: general considerations. Allergy 58(9):854–863

Breen RA, Miller RF, Gorsuch T, Smith CJ, Schwenk A, Holmes W et al (2006) Adverse events and treatment interruption in tuberculosis patients with and without HIV co-infection. Thorax 61(9):791–794

Buhari GK, Keren M, Dursun AB, Guler M, Dulkar G, Kalac N et al (2015) Immediate-type hypersensitivity reactions due to antituberculosis drugs: a successful readministration protocol. Ann Allergy Asthma Immunol 115(1):39–44

Coopman SA, Johnson RA, Platt R, Stern RS (1993) Cutaneous disease and drug reactions in HIV infection. N Engl J Med 328(23):1670–1674

Dawson R, Diacon AH, Everitt D, van Niekerk C, Donald PR, Burger DA et al (2015) Efficiency and safety of the combination of moxifloxacin, pretomanid (PA-824), and pyrazinamide during the first 8 weeks of antituberculosis treatment: a phase 2b, open-label, partly randomised trial in patients with drug-susceptible or drug-resistant pulmonary tuberculosis. Lancet 385(9979):1738–1747

Dheda K, Barry CE 3rd, Maartens G (2016) Tuberculosis. Lancet 387(10024):1211–1226

Gulbay BE, Gurkan OU, Yildiz OA, Onen ZP, Erkekol FO, Baccioglu A et al (2006) Side effects due to primary antituberculosis drugs during the initial phase of therapy in 1149 hospitalized patients for tuberculosis. Respir Med 100(10):1834–1842

Kim SH, Kim SH, Yoon HJ, Shin DH, Park SS, Kim YS et al (2011) NAT2, CYP2C9, CYP2C19, and CYP2E1 genetic polymorphisms in anti-TB drug-induced maculopapular eruption. Eur J Clin Pharmacol 67(2):121–127

Kuaban C, Bercion R, Koulla-Shiro S (1997) HIV seroprevalence rate and incidence of adverse skin reactions in adults with pulmonary tuberculosis receiving thiacetazone free anti-tuberculosis treatment in Yaounde, Cameroon. East Afr Med J 74(8):474–477

Lehloenya RJ, Dheda K (2012) Cutaneous adverse drug reactions to anti-tuberculosis drugs: state of the art and into the future. Expert Rev Anti-Infect Ther 10(4):475–486

Lehloenya RJ, Muloiwa R, Dlamini S, Gantsho N, Todd G, Dheda K (2015) Lack of cross-toxicity between isoniazid and ethionamide in severe cutaneous adverse drug reactions: a series of 25 consecutive confirmed cases. J Antimicrob Chemother 70(9):2648–2651

Lehloenya RJ, Todd G, Badri M, Dheda K (2011) Outcomes of reintroducing anti-tuberculosis drugs following cutaneous adverse drug reactions. Int J Tuberc Lung Dis 15(12):1649–1657

Lehloenya RJ, Todd G, Wallace J, Ngwanya MR, Muloiwa R, Dheda K (2016) Diagnostic patch testing following tuberculosis-associated cutaneous adverse drug reactions induces systemic reactions in HIV-infected persons. Br J Dermatol 175(1):150–156

Lehloenya RJ, Wallace J, Todd G, Dheda K (2012) Multiple drug hypersensitivity reactions to anti-tuberculosis drugs: five cases in HIV-infected patients. Int J Tuberc Lung Dis 16(9):1260–1264

Marra F, Marra CA, Bruchet N, Richardson K, Moadebi S, Elwood RK et al (2007) Adverse drug reactions associated with first-line anti-tuberculosis drug regimens. Int J Tuberc Lung Dis 11(8):868–875

Martinez E, Collazos J, Mayo J (1999) Hypersensitivity reactions to rifampin. Pathogenetic mechanisms, clinical manifestations, management strategies, and review of the anaphylactic-like reactions. Medicine 78(6):361–369

Naisbitt DJ, Farrell J, Gordon SF, Maggs JL, Burkhart C, Pichler WJ et al (2002) Covalent binding of the nitroso metabolite of sulfamethoxazole leads to toxicity and major histocompatibility complex-restricted antigen presentation. Mol Pharmacol 62(3):628–637

Peter JG, Dlamini S, Lehloenya RJ (2015) A South African multi-disciplinary drug hypersensitivity clinic. J Allergy Clin Immunol 28(4):270–274

Peter JG, Lehloenya R, Dlamini S, Risma K, White KD, Konvinse KC et al (2017) Severe delayed cutaneous and systemic reactions to drugs: a global perspective on the science and art of current practice. J Allergy Clin Immunol Pract 5(3):547–563

Pichler WJ, Srinoulprasert Y, Yun J, Hausmann O (2017) Multiple drug hypersensitivity. Int Arch Allergy Immunol 172(3):129–138

Pozniak AL, MacLeod GA, Mahari M, Legg W, Weinberg J (1992) The influence of HIV status on single and multiple drug reactions to antituberculous therapy in Africa. AIDS (London, England) 6(8):809–814

Rieder MJ, Krause R, Bird IA, Dekaban GA (1995) Toxicity of sulfonamide-reactive metabolites in HIV-infected, HTLV-infected, and noninfected cells. J Acquir Immune Defic Syndr Hum Retrovirol 8(2):134–140

Schreiber J, Zissel G, Greinert U, Schlaak M, Muller-Quernheim J (1999) Lymphocyte transformation test for the evaluation of adverse effects of antituberculous drugs. Eur J Med Res 4(2):67–71

Smith KJ, Skelton HG, Yeager J, Ledsky R, Ng TH, Wagner KF (1997) Increased drug reactions in HIV-1-positive patients: a possible explanation based on patterns of immune dysregulation seen in HIV-1 disease. The Military Medical Consortium for the Advancement of Retroviral Research (MMCARR). Clin Exp Dermatol 22(3):118–123

Tan WC, Ong CK, Kang SC, Razak MA (2007) Two years review of cutaneous adverse drug reaction from first line anti-tuberculous drugs. Med J Malaysia 62(2):143–146

Thong BY, Leong KP, Tang CY, Chng HH (2003) Drug allergy in a general hospital: results of a novel prospective inpatient reporting system. Ann Allergy Asthma Immunol 90(3):342–347

Todd G (2006) Adverse cutaneous drug eruptions and HIV: a clinician's global perspective. Dermatol Clin 24(4):459–472 vi

WHO (2016) Global tuberculosis report 2016. World Health Organisation, Geneva

Ye YM, Hur GY, Kim SH, Ban GY, Jee YK, Naisbitt DJ et al (2017) Drug-specific CD4+ T-cell immune responses are responsible for antituberculosis drug-induced maculopapular exanthema and drug reaction with eosinophilia and systemic symptoms syndrome. Br J Dermatol 176(2):378–386

Yee D, Valiquette C, Pelletier M, Parisien I, Rocher I, Menzies D (2003) Incidence of serious side effects from first-line antituberculosis drugs among patients treated for active tuberculosis. Am J Respir Crit Care Med 167(11):1472–1477

Part IV

Approach to the Patient with a Cutaneous Adverse Drug Reaction

15 Practical Approach to Diagnosis and Management of Cutaneous Adverse Drug Reactions

Cristina Olteanu, Neil H. Shear, and Roni P. Dodiuk-Gad

Abbreviations

ADR	Adverse drug reaction
AGEP	Acute generalized exanthematous pustulosis
cADR	Cutaneous adverse drug reaction
DERM	Drug eruptions and reactions manual
DRESS	Drug reaction with eosinophilia and systemic symptoms
HLA	Human leukocyte antigen
SJS	Stevens–Johnson syndrome
SSLR	Serum sickness-like reaction
TEN	Toxic epidermal necrolysis
UMC	Uppsala Monitoring Centre
WHO	World Health Organization

C. Olteanu
Division of Dermatology, Department of Medicine, University of Alberta, Edmonton, AB, Canada
e-mail: olteanu@ualberta.ca

N. H. Shear
Division of Dermatology, Department of Medicine, Sunnybrook Health Sciences Centre, University of Toronto, Toronto, ON, Canada

Division of Clinical Pharmacology and Toxicology, Department of Medicine, Sunnybrook Health Sciences Centre, Toronto, ON, Canada

R. P. Dodiuk-Gad (✉)
Division of Dermatology, Department of Medicine, Sunnybrook Health Sciences Centre, University of Toronto, Toronto, ON, Canada

Department of Dermatology, Emek Medical Center, Afula, Israel

Bruce Rappaport Faculty of Medicine, Technion-Institute of Technology, Haifa, Israel

N. H. Shear, R. P. Dodiuk-Gad (eds.), *Advances in Diagnosis and Management of Cutaneous Adverse Drug Reactions*, https://doi.org/10.1007/978-981-13-1489-6_15

Key Points

- Cutaneous adverse drug reactions are an important topic in dermatology because they can result in substantial morbidity and mortality.
- Diagnosing a drug eruption is challenging, and a systematic approach should be used.
- Physicians must differentiate between a simple drug eruption involving only the skin and a complex drug eruption with systemic involvement.
- The cutaneous morphology of a drug eruption does not always mirror the systemic involvement. Hence, internal organ involvement should be explored even in a mild simple drug eruption particularly in the presence of a high fever.
- There are validated diagnostic criteria for DRESS and AGEP that should be utilized, and SCORTEN, a validated prognostic tool for TEN, is to be used.

15.1 Introduction

An adverse drug reaction (ADR) has been defined by the World Health Organization as "a response to a drug that is noxious and unintended and occurs at doses normally used in man" (Edwards and Aronson 2000); this term has been in use for over 40 years. Exposure to drugs has been increasing over time as a consequence of longer patient survival and polymedication of an aging population. Cutaneous reactions are the most frequent adverse reaction in response to drugs (Knowles and Shear 2007; Verma et al. 2013). Up to 2% of cutaneous adverse drug reactions are severe and life-threatening, including Stevens–Johnson syndrome/toxic epidermal necrolysis, acute generalized exanthematous pustulosis (AGEP), and drug reaction with eosinophilia and systemic symptoms (DRESS) (Wolf et al. 2005). Adverse drug reactions are an important topic in dermatology because they can result in substantial morbidity and mortality (Bouvy et al. 2015).

It is important to differentiate between an "adverse reaction" and an "adverse effect." An "adverse reaction" is described from the point of view of the patient, while an "adverse effect" is described from the point of view of the medication (Edwards and Aronson 2000).

Cutaneous adverse drug reactions can range in clinical manifestations. They can range from a mild exanthem involving only the skin to a reaction including systemic symptoms in addition to the skin manifestations, which can be fatal such as in the cases of life-threatening drug reactions (Chung et al. 2016). The most common types of ADRs are common-mild and rare-severe. Common-severe reactions are not seen as they are not approved for clinical usage, and rare-mild reactions usually go unnoticed or are not reported by patients (Naldi and Crotti 2014).

15.2 Mechanisms of Cutaneous Adverse Drug Reactions

There are several types of reactions in the modern pharmacological classification of ADRs. Type A reactions, "augmented" or "on-target," are the most common (approximately 80–90% of all drug reactions are type A) and are described as predictable reactions and dose dependent on the pharmacology of the drug. Type B reactions are uncommon, referred to as "bizarre" or "off-target," and may be dose dependent in susceptible individuals, depending on their genetic and environmental predispositions. The other types of reactions are types C, D, E, and F. Type C reactions, also known as "chronic," are dose- and time-related. Type D, also known as delayed, is time-related. Type E is due to withdrawal effects. Type F reactions are known as unexpected failure of therapy (Knowles et al. 2000; Young and Shear 2017).

15.3 Morphological Subtypes of Cutaneous Adverse Drug Reactions

It is necessary to assess the morphology of the primary lesions when classifying cutaneous ADRs. The four main categories are exanthematous, urticarial, pustular, and blistering. There are two major steps in diagnosing drug eruptions: determine the morphology and assess systemic involvement (Nigen et al. 2003) Table 15.1.

15.4 Simple vs. Complex Cutaneous Adverse Drug Reactions

A cutaneous adverse drug reaction can be considered "simple" or "complex." A "simple" reaction only involves the skin, while a "complex" reaction includes systemic involvement of organs in addition to the skin involvement. We recommend that patients with cutaneous adverse drug reactions be assessed for systemic involvement because the severity of skin manifestations does not always mirror the severity of the systemic involvement. Clues to systemic involvement could include, but are not limited to, symptoms such as cough, malaise, fever, and myalgias (Young and

Table 15.1 Types of cutaneous adverse drug reactions

Type of reaction	Morphological characteristics			
	Exanthematous	Urticarial	Blistering	Pustular
Simple	Drug rash	Urticaria	Fixed drug eruption	Acneiform
Complex	Drug reaction with eosinophilia and systemic symptoms (DRESS)	Serum sickness-like reaction (SSLR)	Stevens–Johnson syndrome/toxic epidermal necrolysis (SJS/TEN or TENS)	Acute generalized exanthematous pustulosis (AGEP)

Shear 2017). Any further investigations should be done based on the patient's symptoms. If there is suspected systemic involvement, there should be a basic laboratory screen performed including a full blood count, liver and renal function tests, and urine analysis (Nigen et al. 2003).

15.5 Practical Approach to the Diagnosis and Management of Cutaneous Adverse Drug Reactions

Our suggested clinical assessment of drug-induced skin injury is called the 4 Ds by Dr. Shear: diagnosis of the adverse event, differential diagnosis, drug exposure, and determining probabilities (Dodiuk-Gad et al. 2017).

15.5.1 Diagnosis of the Adverse Event

Any patient taking medications with a cutaneous eruption should be evaluated for a cutaneous ADR to determine if the clinical signs are a result of the medication or related to a different cause. The diagnosis of a cutaneous ADR is based on three key steps Fig. 15.1. The first step is determining morphology, according to the four main categories: exanthematous, urticarial, pustular, and blistering. The second step is to determine if there is any systemic involvement in addition to the cutaneous involvement as this will help to distinguish between a "simple" and a "complex" reaction (Nigen et al. 2003). The third step is determining the histology. Drug eruptions elicit a variety of inflammatory disease patterns histologically and can be used to help differentiate between the various cutaneous adverse drug reactions. Hence, skin biopsies can be very useful in the process of diagnosing cutaneous adverse drug reactions (Orime 2017). In addition, it is valuable to use validated diagnostic criteria of specific types of drug eruptions, if available. Currently, only DRESS and AGEP have published validated diagnostic criteria, with DRESS having two. Please see Chap. 7 *DRESS* and Chap. 8 *AGEP*.

15.5.2 Differential Diagnosis

It is essential to establish a differential diagnosis, keeping in mind all the possible diagnoses. In addition, it is encouraged to rank the approximate likelihood of each condition (Dodiuk-Gad et al. 2017).

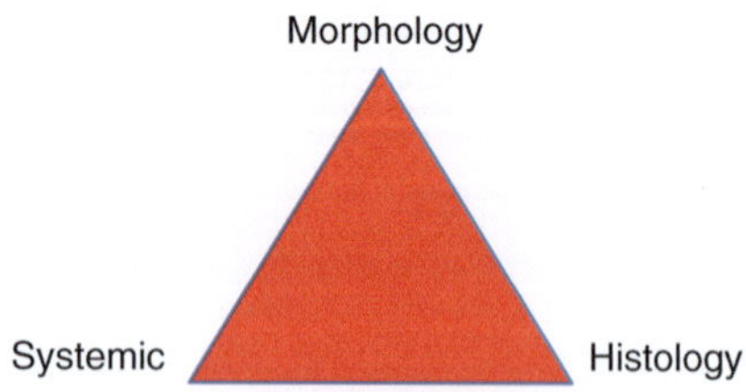

Fig. 15.1 Dr. Shear's diagnostic triangle of cutaneous adverse drug reactions (Dodiuk-Gad et al. 2017)

15.5.3 Drug Exposure (Drugs Taken and the Lag Period)

First and foremost, it is important to determine drug exposures. Physicians could consider obtaining the assistance of family members, pharmacists, and others that might know which medications the patient was taking prior to the adverse event. In addition, the lag period of a drug reaction is crucial to analyze carefully when determining the causative agent since different cutaneous drug reactions have different timelines. The lag period is the time between initiation of the drug and the onset of the first symptoms of the drug reaction. All medications, especially those taken in the 8 weeks prior to the cutaneous adverse drug reaction, must be considered as possible causative agents. Physicians should also ask patients about over-the-counter medications in addition to prescription drugs (Nigen et al. 2003). Physicians may want to consider creating a drug exposure timeline chart to visualize the chronology. The timeline could include relevant information including the first day of taking the medication, dosage, and the last day that the patient took the medication for each drug as well as adding the signs and symptoms throughout this time period (Nigen et al. 2003; Dodiuk-Gad et al. 2017). The time frame is very useful because it is influenced by the reaction pattern. For example, a drug eruption that is caused by an IgE-mediated mechanism will occur approximately minutes after a drug's initiation, while a reaction such as SJS/TEN (the term TENS may be used to describe the spectrum of SJS/TEN) will take several weeks to begin after a drug's initiation (Young and Shear 2017).

15.5.4 Determine Probabilities

The biggest challenge in assessing drug-induced skin injury is establishing whether it was caused by a medication a patient was taking or another cause that is unrelated. In order to effectively assess a causal relationship, it is crucial to take a thorough and detailed history including asking patients if they had any history of cutaneous rashes themselves or in their family and whether withdrawing the drug improved the eruption. There are resources to help aid in determining the probability of a drug reaction including PubMed (http://www.ncbi.nlm.nih.gov/pubmed) and Litt's Drug Eruptions and Reactions Manual (DERM) and database (http://www.drugeruptiondata.com/). For more information on literature review, please see Chap. 17 *Drug Safety Literature*. Physicians may also rate the reaction based on Edwards et al.'s causality assessment criteria (Edwards and Aronson 2000) or Naranjo et al.'s adverse drug reaction probability scale, which classifies the drug reaction according to a probability category as definite, probable, possible, or doubtful (Dodiuk-Gad et al. 2017; Naranjo et al. 1981). There are also in vitro and in vivo diagnostic assessments including HLA genetic tests that could be performed. In the past few years there has been excellent progress in discovering the underlying mechanisms of drug eruptions. There have been multiple studies showing that ADRs can have a genetic predisposition in that there are associations between a specific HLA allele, a drug, an ethnic background, and a drug eruption. These HLA genetic tests are best

Table 15.2 Systematic approach for the diagnosis of cutaneous drug eruption

1	Determination of the morphology of the primary lesion based on four main categories: exanthematous, urticarial, bullous, and pustular
2	Assessment of systemic involvement based on patient's vital signs and symptoms and basic laboratory screen: full blood count, liver and renal function tests, and urine analysis
3	Skin biopsy for histopathology and if relevant direct immunofluorescence studies
4	The usage of validated diagnostic criteria, if available
5	Establishment of a working diagnosis and a differential diagnosis that takes into account all possible diagnoses
6	Drug exposure analysis—determination of the lag period and creation of a timeline
7	Determination of probabilities for the associations between the suspected drug and the clinical event according to patients' history, literature, and in vitro and in vivo diagnostic assessments including HLA genetic tests
8	Based on steps 6 and 7, identification of the suspected drugs
9	Communication with the patient, family, healthcare providers, and regulatory agencies
10	Proper follow-up for the patient in a timely and appropriate manner

utilized as genetic screening prior to drug prescription. However, these HLA genetic tests may also serve as a simple, safe, and reliable method for establishing causality in specific cases of drug eruptions such as toxic epidermal necrolysis induced by specific drugs such as carbamazepine and allopurinol (Fan et al. 2017). Please refer to Chap. 3 *Pharmacogenomics and CADRs*. Other in vitro tests may include lymphocyte transformation test and basophil activation test. Patch test is an important in vivo test that may be used in assessment of a drug eruption. Refer to Chap. 18 *In Vitro and In Vivo Tests in Cutaneous Adverse Drug Reactions* (*CADRs*). Caution should always be exercised regarding false-positive and false-negative results of these in vitro and in vivo tests. Table 15.2 summarizes the major steps in the systematic approach for the diagnosis of cutaneous drug eruptions.

15.6 Communication with the Patient and Family, Healthcare Providers, and Regulatory Agencies

Patient and family: It is very important to maintain communication with the patient and the family as this will strengthen the therapeutic relationship with the physician and assist the patient in dealing with the adverse drug reaction that could cause immediate and long-term psychological complications, especially following life-threatening drug reactions (Dodiuk-Gad et al. 2016; Lew et al. 2015). In addition, good communication decreases the chances of future lawsuits. Physicians are advised to keep in mind the "apology laws" when saying "sorry" in regard to the adverse cutaneous drug reaction. See the following website for more information: http://www.sorryworks.net. It is also prudent to have an honest and empathetic discussion with the patient and family (if the patient permits). We recommend providing disclosure in a meeting that has been arranged at a time convenient for all members and ensure that all of the necessary/required participants are able to attend. It would be helpful to start the meeting by explaining the aim of the meeting/

discussion. It is a good practice to state the facts while not mentioning that the cutaneous adverse drug event was an "error" or "mistake" because they can be multifactorial in origin. The patient would benefit from being provided all the information pertinent to the adverse drug reaction including the medications she or he should avoid and the ones that can be taken safely as alternatives, as well as if there is a genetic predisposition to develop the particular cutaneous adverse drug reaction. In addition, we recommend that all patients have their allergy written on a medic-alert bracelet. Regarding family consultation, first-degree family members should also be instructed to avoid the offending drug in cases of SJS/TEN (TENS) and DRESS (Dodiuk-Gad et al. 2017).

Other healthcare providers: Physicians should provide the patients' family physician with information regarding the adverse event to maintain proper communication between physicians and ensure that the patient receives proper follow-up (Dodiuk-Gad et al. 2017).

Regulatory agencies: Cutaneous ADRs should be reported to the manufacturer and regulatory agencies. The following are examples of international reporting systems: MedWatch, the FDA Safety Information and Adverse Event Reporting Program (http://www.fda.gov/safety/MedWatch/default.htm), and the WHO Uppsala Monitoring Centre (UMC) http://www.who-umc.org. (Dodiuk-Gad et al. 2017)

References

Bouvy JC, De Bruin ML, Koopmanschap MA (2015) Epidemiology of adverse drug reactions in Europe: a review of recent observational studies. Drug Saf 38(5):437–453

Chung WH, Wang CW, Dao RL (2016) Severe cutaneous adverse drug reactions. J Dermatol 43(7):758–766

Dodiuk-Gad RP, Olteanu C, Feinstein A, Hashimoto R, Alhusayen R, Whyte-Croasdaile S, Finkelstein Y, Burnett M, Sade S, Cartotto R et al (2016) Major psychological complications and decreased health-related quality of life among survivors of Stevens-Johnson syndrome and toxic epidermal necrolysis. Br J Dermatol 175(2):422–424

Dodiuk-Gad RP, Chung W-H, Shear NH (2017) Adverse medication reactions. In: Clinical and basic immunodermatology. Springer, Cham

Edwards IR, Aronson JK (2000) Adverse drug reactions: definitions, diagnosis, and management. Lancet 356(9237):1255–1259

Fan WL, Shiao MS, Hui RC, Su SC, Wang CW, Chang YC, Chung WH (2017) HLA association with drug-induced adverse reactions. J Immunol Res 2017:3186328

Knowles SR, Shear NH (2007) Recognition and management of severe cutaneous drug reactions. Dermatol Clin 25(2):245–253 viii

Knowles SR, Uetrecht J, Shear NH (2000) Idiosyncratic drug reactions: the reactive metabolite syndromes. Lancet 356(9241):1587–1591

Lew TT, Creamer D, Mackenzie J, Walsh SA (2015) Post-traumatic stress disorder following drug reaction with eosinophilia and systemic symptoms. Br J Dermatol 172(3):836–837

Naldi L, Crotti S (2014) Epidemiology of cutaneous drug-induced reactions. G Ital Dermatol Venereol 149(2):207–218

Naranjo CA, Busto U, Sellers EM, Sandor P, Ruiz I, Roberts EA, Janecek E, Domecq C, Greenblatt DJ (1981) A method for estimating the probability of adverse drug reactions. Clin Pharmacol Ther 30(2):239–245

Nigen S, Knowles SR, Shear NH (2003) Drug eruptions: approaching the diagnosis of drug-induced skin diseases. J Drugs Dermatol 2(3):278–299

Orime M (2017) Immunohistopathological findings of severe cutaneous adverse drug reactions. J Immunol Res 2017:6928363

Verma R, Vasudevan B, Pragasam V (2013) Severe cutaneous adverse drug reactions. Med J Armed Forces India 69(4):375–383

Wolf R, Orion E, Marcos B, Matz H (2005) Life-threatening acute adverse cutaneous drug reactions. Clin Dermatol 23(2):171–181

Young JWS, Shear NH (2017) Cutaneous drug reactions in the elderly. Drugs Aging 34(9):655–672

Histopathology of Severe Drug Eruptions

16

Mari Orime and Riichiro Abe

Abbreviations

AGEP	Acute generalized exanthematous pustulosis
cADR	Cutaneous adverse drug reactions
CMV	Cytomegalovirus
DIHS	Drug-induced hypersensitivity syndrome
DRESS	Drug reaction with eosinophilia and systemic symptoms
EM	Erythema multiforme
EuroSCAR	European severe cutaneous adverse reaction
GPP	Generalized pustular psoriasis
GVHD	Graft-versus-host disease
HHV-6	Human herpesvirus 6
HHV-7	Human herpesvirus 7
IgA	Immunoglobulin A
MPE	Maculopapular eruptions
SJS/TEN	Stevens–Johnson syndrome/toxic epidermal necrolysis
SSSS	staphylococcal scalded skin syndrome
TARC	Thymus and activation-regulated chemokine

M. Orime · R. Abe (✉)
Division of Dermatology, Niigata University Graduate School of Medical and Dental Sciences, Niigata, Japan
e-mail: orimem@med.niigata-u.ac.jp; aberi@med.niigata-u.ac.jp

N. H. Shear, R. P. Dodiuk-Gad (eds.), *Advances in Diagnosis and Management of Cutaneous Adverse Drug Reactions*, https://doi.org/10.1007/978-981-13-1489-6_16

Key Points

- Established SJS/TEN shows full-thickness, extensive keratinocyte necrosis that develops into the formation of subepidermal bullae. There is generally less dermal inflammation than in EM major.
- Although the histopathology of DRESS is non-specific, the association between two or more of four patterns—eczematous changes, interface dermatitis, AGEP-like patterns, and EM-like patterns—in a single biopsy specimen is suggestive of the diagnosis and of severe cutaneous manifestations. The presence of necrotic keratinocytes tends to be associated with greater liver and/or renal involvement. Cutaneous dendritic cells may be involved in the clinical course.
- AGEP typically exhibits spongiform subcorneal and/or superficial intraepidermal pustules in association with edema of the papillary dermis and abundant mixed perivascular infiltrates. The differential diagnosis between AGEP and GPP is usually difficult, despite AGEP having several characteristic aspects. The pathological similarities may be attributable to the mutually shared mutation in the *IL36RN* gene.

16.1 Introduction

Common cutaneous adverse drug reactions (cADRs), such as maculopapular eruptions (MPEs), often display various degrees of vacuolar interface dermatitis associated with non-specific eosinophilic and/or neutrophilic infiltrates (Weyers and Metze 2011). In contrast, the histopathology of severe cADRs is characteristic of the individual condition. This section reviews the histopathological features of several severe cADRs.

16.1.1 Stevens–Johnson Syndrome (SJS)/Toxic Epidermal Necrolysis (TEN)

The histologic findings of SJS/TEN are subepidermal bullae with overlying confluent necrosis of the epidermis and sparse perivascular lymphocytic infiltrates (Goldstein et al. 1987). In early lesions of SJS/TEN, necrotic keratinocytes are observed scattered in the basal layer of the epidermis, histologically resembling a feature of erythema multiforme (EM) major: necrotic keratinocytes scattered throughout the epidermis with vacuolar alteration at the dermoepidermal junction (Schwartz et al. 2013; Ackerman 1997). In established SJS/TEN, there is extensive, full-thickness keratinocyte necrosis, leaving the cytoplasm of keratinocytes eosinophilic, which eventuates in the formation of subepidermal bullae. In SJS/TEN, the epidermis displays major epidermal necrosis, whereas in EM major, the epidermis displays less necrosis and the change is predominantly in the basal layer. The Japanese criteria for SJS/TEN propose at least ten necrotic keratinocytes at a magnification of 200× for diagnosis. Perivascular inflammatory infiltrates in the upper dermis are minimal to absent, and exocytosis is slight or absent. SJS/TEN tends to show less dermal inflammation than is seen in the pronounced dermal infiltration and extravasation of erythrocytes in EM major (Cote et al. 1995; Rzany et al. 1996). In contrast, a previous study of 37 TEN patients showed that degree of inflammation correlates with a worse prognosis and that the quantification of dermal mononuclear cell infiltration is roughly as accurate as TEN-specific Severity Illness Score (SCORTEN) in predicting patient outcome (Quinn et al. 2005).

Skin specimens that are snap-frozen, immediately cryostat-sectioned, and stained with hematoxylin-eosin have been used to help the initial diagnosis and prediction of disease activity of SJS/TEN that shows EM-like lesions (Hosaka et al. 2010).

Differential diagnoses other than EM major include staphylococcal scalded skin syndrome (SSSS), linear immunoglobulin A (IgA) bullous dermatosis, and acute graft-versus-host disease (GVHD). SSSS shows only superficial, rather than full-thickness, epidermal necrosis, and it is caused by a staphylococcal exfoliative toxin that cleaves a specific peptide bond on desmoglein-1 (Amagai and Stanley 2012; Handler and Schwartz 2014). Linear IgA bullous dermatosis may clinically resemble TEN, although the former shows no epidermal necrolysis (Coelho et al. 2006; Dellavalle et al. 2003; Khan et al. 2009). Severe acute GVHD demonstrates complete epidermal necrosis that may be difficult to distinguish from TEN. The remarkable epidermal change of acute GVHD is satellite cell necrosis consisting of apoptotic keratinocytes accompanied by tightly adherent lymphocytes in the epidermis; however, discriminating between the two diseases may be difficult when the epidermal necrosis is prominent (Chavan and el-Azhary 2011). If erythematous follicular papules displaying folliculotropic infiltrates accompanied by basal vacuolation and satellite cell necrosis can be observed as the early exanthema of acute GVHD, they might provide clues for distinguishing severe acute GVHD from TEN (Friedman et al. 1988).

16.1.2 Drug-Induced Hypersensitivity Syndrome (DIHS)/Exanthema in Drug Reaction with Eosinophilia and Systemic Symptoms (DRESS)

Histopathological investigation is not crucial for the diagnosis of drug-induced hypersensitivity syndrome (DIHS) when we use the diagnostic criteria established by the Japanese consensus group (Kardaun et al. 2007; Shiohara et al. 2006), nor is it crucial for the diagnosis of exanthema in drug reaction with eosinophilia and systemic symptoms (DRESS) when we use the diagnostic criteria proposed by the European Severe Cutaneous Adverse Reaction to Drugs group (EuroSCAR/RegiSCAR) (Kardaun et al. 2007).

The histopathology of DRESS is heterogeneous and has no specific diagnostic hallmarks. Frequently reported features include spongiosis, various degrees of basal vacuolization, necrotic keratinocytes, dense and diffuse dermal-epidermal infiltrates with lymphocytic exocytosis, dermal edema, and superficial perivascular infiltrates of mostly lymphocytes with or without eosinophils (Bocquet et al. 1996; Chen et al. 2010; Chiou et al. 2008). Clinicopathological studies on DRESS diagnosis and prognosis have revealed that an association between two or more of four patterns—eczematous changes, interface dermatitis, acute generalized exanthematous pustulosis (AGEP)-like pattern, and EM-like pattern—in a single biopsy specimen is suggestive of the diagnosis and of severe cutaneous manifestations. These features are significantly more prominent in cases of DRESS than in cases of MPE (Ortonne et al. 2015). Furthermore, apoptotic keratinocytes tend to be more closely associated with liver and/or renal involvement (Chi et al. 2014; Ortonne et al. 2015; Skowron et al. 2015; Walsh et al. 2013). A possible correlation between the intensity of the dermal lymphocytic infiltrates and DRESS severity is suggested (Goncalo et al. 2016). In contrast, epidermal spongiosis is associated with the absence of renal involvement and with non-severe forms of DRESS (Skowron et al. 2015). Immunohistochemically, the number of plasmacytoid dendritic cells, a subset of leukocytes capable of producing interferon-α upon viral infection, is elevated in DIHS skin, and the number of these cells in the peripheral blood decreases around the viral reactivation period (Sugita et al. 2010). Thymus and activation-regulated chemokine (TARC), a family of CC chemokines known to play an important role in Th2-type immune response and to potentially reflect the activity of skin rash in DRESS, is expressed on CD11c-positive dendritic cells in the lesional dermis, which suggests that such cells may be the main source of TARC in patients with DRESS (Ogawa et al. 2013).

SJS/TEN and AGEP share some overlapping clinical features with DRESS (Matsuda et al. 2013; Teraki et al. 2010). However, the histopathology of DRESS is quite distinct from that of TEN and AGEP, and DRESS lacks full-thickness necrosis and sterile non-follicular subcorneal pustules (Halevy et al. 2010; Kardaun et al. 2010; Kardaun et al. 2013). In our personal experience of DRESS cases, none of the following have been found to correlate with the disease severity: interface dermatitis, the extent of necrotic keratinocytes, and spongiosis (unpublished data). In discussing the histopathology of DRESS, some differences among various case reports and clinical studies may be attributable to differences in case definitions and in the stages of evolution of the skin lesion (Goldstein et al. 1987). The wide variety of histopathological findings might be due to the various clinical manifestations, such as MPE-like and EM-like eruptions, observed in DRESS patients. When a biopsy is performed, it is recommended that a description be made of the type of lesion used for the biopsy, i.e., macular or confluent erythema, purpura, papule, or pustule, for more than one site and at several points in time. The relation between the onset of the lesion and the time of biopsy should be noted in terms of hours or days, instead of "early" or "late."

Several viruses, such as human herpesvirus (HHV)-6, HHV-7, cytomegalovirus (CMV), and Epstein–Barr virus, are reactivated in the prolonged clinical course (Tohyama and Hashimoto 2011). Cutaneous lesions emerging as late systemic manifestations of CMV tend to be rare, and these present as ulcerated erythematous papules that histopathologically display intranuclear inclusion (Asano et al. 2009). Since cutaneous manifestations are associated with fatal gastrointestinal complications, the early consideration and identification of CMV reactivation are crucial for establishing the diagnosis and improving the prognosis.

16.1.3 Acute Generalized Exanthematous Pustulosis (AGEP)

The typical histopathology of AGEP is spongiform subcorneal and/or superficial intraepidermal pustules in association with edema of the papillary dermis and abundant mixed perivascular infiltrates (Beylot et al. 1996; Burrows and Russell Jones 1993). From a large series of AGEP cases, several unique findings were demonstrated: a higher prevalence of necrotic keratinocytes (67%), which was stated as a major epidermal feature, and a strikingly high prevalence of dermal infiltrates (93–100%) containing neutrophils (100%) as well as eosinophils (81%) (Halevy et al. 2010). The evaluation of leukocytoclastic vasculitis varies by report from 20% to less than 1% (Roujeau et al. 1991). This difference might be attributable to the misinterpretation of erythrocyte extravasation as vasculitis (Halevy et al. 2010).

AGEP and generalized pustular psoriasis (GPP) share common clinicopathological features, characterized by widespread pustules with systemic symptoms such as high fever and hyperleukocytosis with neutrophils predominating (Roujeau et al. 1991). The morphology of the spongiotic pustules is often indistinguishable between those seen in AGEP and those particularly seen in the acute phase of GPP. In one study of 43 cases of AGEP and 24 cases of GPP, several histological features were documented for the successful differential diagnosis (Kardaun et al. 2010). AGEP is differentiated from GPP by the following characteristic features: the presence of eosinophils in the pustules or dermis, necrotic keratinocytes, mixed neutrophil-rich interstitial and mid-dermal perivascular infiltrates, and the absence of tortuous or dilated blood vessels. Moreover, chronic GPP with pustules on prolonged existing lesions shows significant epidermal psoriasiform changes, such as hyperkeratosis and parakeratosis (Kardaun et al. 2010). These pathological similarities between AGEP and GPP might derive from a mutually occurring mutation in the *IL36RN* gene encoding the interleukin-36 receptor antagonist. There are several reports of AGEP cases with homozygous or heterozygous *IL36RN* mutations, particularly in patients with intraoral involvement, and this involvement might underlie the mutation in some forms of AGEP (Navarini et al. 2013; Nakai et al. 2015; Navarini et al. 2015) (Fig. 16.1).

The histologic features and differential diagnoses of severe cADRs are summarized in Table 16.1.

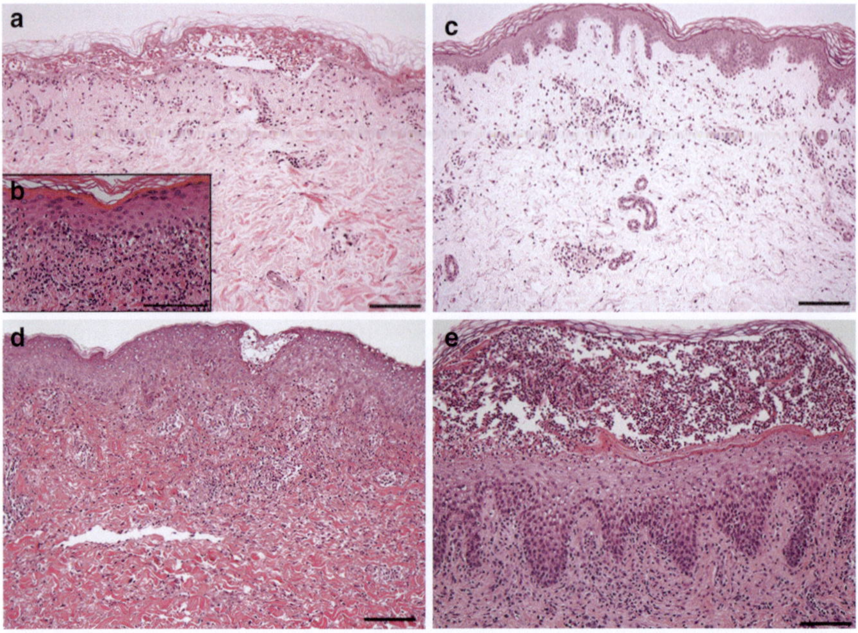

Fig. 16.1 Hematoxylin-eosin sections of several cutaneous adverse reactions. (**a**) Toxic epidermal necrolysis. Subepidermal bullae under full-thickness epidermal necrosis. Note the cell-poor dermal inflammation. (**b**) Erythema multiforme. An interface reaction pattern with infiltrates of lymphocytes and scattered necrotic keratinocytes. (**c, d**) Drug-induced hypersensitivity syndrome/exanthema in drug reaction with eosinophilia and systemic syndrome. Two cases that are associated with liver function deficiency show different histopathologies: intermittent interface change, few necrotic keratinocytes and slight spongiosis in (**c**); diffuse interface change, several necrotic keratinocytes and considerable spongiosis with a spongiotic bulla in (**d**). (**e**) Acute generalized exanthematous pustulosis. Spongiform superficial intraepidermal pustules and polymorphous perivascular infiltrates containing mainly neutrophils. Bar = 100 μm

Table 16.1 The histologic features and differential diagnoses of severe cADRs

Disease	Histology	Differential diagnoses
SJS/TEN	Epidermis In the early lesions: scattered necrotic keratinocytes in the basal layer of the epidermis In the established lesions: subepidermal bullae with overlying full-thickness keratinocyte necrosis Dermis Minimal to absent perivascular inflammatory infiltrates, slight or absent exocytosis	1. EM major: scattered necrotic keratinocytes, vacuolar alteration of the dermoepidermal junction 2. SSSS: necrosis only in the superficial epidermis 3. Linear IgA bullous dermatosis: no epidermal necrolysis 4. Acute GVHD: folliculotropic infiltrates with basal vacuolation and satellite cell necrosis

Table 16.1 (continued)

Disease	Histology	Differential diagnoses
DIHS/ DRESS	An association between several patterns in a single biopsy specimen Epidermis Spongiosis, basal vacuolization, necrotic keratinocytes Dermis Dermal-epidermal infiltrates with lymphocytic exocytosis, dermal edema, superficial perivascular infiltrates	1. MPE: subtle non-specific change 2. SJS/TEN: full-thickness epidermal necrosis 3. AGEP: sterile subcorneal pustules
AGEP	Epidermis Spongiform subcorneal and/or superficial intraepidermal pustules, necrotic keratinocytes Dermis Dermal edema, perivascular infiltrates with neutrophils and eosinophils, leukocytoclastic vasculitis or erythrocyte extravasation	1. GPP: epidermal hyperkeratosis and parakeratosis, fewer necrotic keratinocytes, fewer eosinophils in the pustules, dermal tortuous or dilated blood vessels

SJS/TEN Stevens–Johnson syndrome, *TEN* toxic epidermal necrolysis, *EM* erythema multiforme, *SSSS* staphylococcal scalded skin syndrome, *IgA* immunoglobulin A, *GVHD* acute graft-versus-host disease, *DIHS/DRESS* drug-induced hypersensitivity syndrome/exanthema in drug reaction with eosinophilia and systemic symptoms, *AGEP* acute generalized exanthematous pustulosis, *MPE* maculopapular eruptions, *GPP* generalized pustular psoriasis

References

Ackerman AB (1997) Histologic diagnosis of inflammatory skin diseases: an algorithmic method based on pattern analysis, 2nd edn. Williams & Wilkins, Baltimore, MD

Amagai M, Stanley JR (2012) Desmoglein as a target in skin disease and beyond. J Invest Dermatol 132(3 Pt 2):776–784. https://doi.org/10.1038/jid.2011.390

Asano Y, Kagawa H, Kano Y, Shiohara T (2009) Cytomegalovirus disease during severe drug eruptions: report of 2 cases and retrospective study of 18 patients with drug-induced hypersensitivity syndrome. Arch Dermatol 145(9):1030–1036. https://doi.org/10.1001/archdermatol.2009.195

Beylot C, Doutre MS, Beylot-Barry M (1996) Acute generalized exanthematous pustulosis. Semin Cutan Med Surg 15(4):244–249

Bocquet H, Bagot M, Roujeau JC (1996) Drug-induced pseudolymphoma and drug hypersensitivity syndrome (Drug Rash with Eosinophilia and Systemic Symptoms: DRESS). Semin Cutan Med Surg 15(4):250–257

Burrows NP, Russell Jones RR (1993) Pustular drug eruptions: a histopathological spectrum. Histopathology 22(6):569–573

Chavan R, el-Azhary R (2011) Cutaneous graft-versus-host disease: rationales and treatment options. Dermatol Ther 24(2):219–228. https://doi.org/10.1111/j.1529-8019.2011.01397.x

Chen YC, Chiu HC, Chu CY (2010) Drug reaction with eosinophilia and systemic symptoms: a retrospective study of 60 cases. Arch Dermatol 146(12):1373–1379. https://doi.org/10.1001/archdermatol.2010.198

Chi MH, Hui RC, Yang CH, Lin JY, Lin YT, Ho HC, Chung WH, Kuo TT (2014) Histopathological analysis and clinical correlation of drug reaction with eosinophilia and systemic symptoms (DRESS). Br J Dermatol 170(4):866–873. https://doi.org/10.1111/bjd.12783

Chiou CC, Yang LC, Hung SI, Chang YC, Kuo TT, Ho HC, Hu S, Hong HS, Chung WH (2008) Clinicopathological features and prognosis of drug rash with eosinophilia and systemic symptoms: a study of 30 cases in Taiwan. J Eur Acad Dermatol Venereol 22(9):1044–1049. https://doi.org/10.1111/j.1468-3083.2008.02585.x

Coelho S, Tellechea O, Reis JP, Mariano A, Figueiredo A (2006) Vancomycin-associated linear IgA bullous dermatosis mimicking toxic epidermal necrolysis. Int J Dermatol 45(8):995–996. https://doi.org/10.1111/j.1365-4632.2006.02752.x

Cote B, Wechsler J, Bastuji-Garin S, Assier H, Revuz J, Roujeau JC (1995) Clinicopathologic correlation in erythema multiforme and Stevens-Johnson syndrome. Arch Dermatol 131(11):1268–1272

Dellavalle RP, Burch JM, Tayal S, Golitz LE, Fitzpatrick JE, Walsh P (2003) Vancomycin-associated linear IgA bullous dermatosis mimicking toxic epidermal necrolysis. J Am Acad Dermatol 48(5 Suppl):S56–S57. https://doi.org/10.1067/mjd.2003.116

Friedman KJ, LeBoit PE, Farmer ER (1988) Acute follicular graft-vs-host reaction. A distinct clinicopathologic presentation. Arch Dermatol 124(5):688–691

Goldstein SM, Wintroub BW, Elias PM, Wuepper KD (1987) Toxic epidermal necrolysis. Unmuddying the waters. Arch Dermatol 123(9):1153–1156

Goncalo MM, Cardoso JC, Gouveia MP, Coutinho I, Gameiro AR, Brites MM, Tellechea OE (2016) Histopathology of the exanthema in DRESS is not specific but may indicate severity of systemic involvement. Am J Dermatopathol 38(6):423–433. https://doi.org/10.1097/dad.0000000000000439

Halevy S, Kardaun SH, Davidovici B, Wechsler J (2010) The spectrum of histopathological features in acute generalized exanthematous pustulosis: a study of 102 cases. Br J Dermatol 163(6):1245–1252. https://doi.org/10.1111/j.1365-2133.2010.09967.x

Handler MZ, Schwartz RA (2014) Staphylococcal scalded skin syndrome: diagnosis and management in children and adults. J Eur Acad Dermatol Venereol 28(11):1418–1423. https://doi.org/10.1111/jdv.12541

Hosaka H, Ohtoshi S, Nakada T, Iijima M (2010) Erythema multiforme, Stevens-Johnson syndrome and toxic epidermal necrolysis: frozen-section diagnosis. J Dermatol 37(5):407–412. https://doi.org/10.1111/j.1346-8138.2009.00746.x

Kardaun SH, Sidoroff A, Valeyrie-Allanore L, Halevy S, Davidovici BB, Mockenhaupt M, Roujeau JC (2007) Variability in the clinical pattern of cutaneous side-effects of drugs with systemic symptoms: does a DRESS syndrome really exist? Br J Dermatol 156(3):609–611. https://doi.org/10.1111/j.1365-2133.2006.07704.x

Kardaun SH, Kuiper H, Fidler V, Jonkman MF (2010) The histopathological spectrum of acute generalized exanthematous pustulosis (AGEP) and its differentiation from generalized pustular psoriasis. J Cutan Pathol 37(12):1220–1229. https://doi.org/10.1111/j.1600-0560.2010.01612.x

Kardaun SH, Sekula P, Valeyrie-Allanore L, Liss Y, Chu CY, Creamer D, Sidoroff A, Naldi L, Mockenhaupt M, Roujeau JC (2013) Drug reaction with eosinophilia and systemic symptoms (DRESS): an original multisystem adverse drug reaction. Results from the prospective RegiSCAR study. Br J Dermatol 169(5):1071–1080. https://doi.org/10.1111/bjd.12501

Khan I, Hughes R, Curran S, Marren P (2009) Drug-associated linear IgA disease mimicking toxic epidermal necrolysis. Clin Exp Dermatol 34(6):715–717. https://doi.org/10.1111/j.1365-2230.2008.03011.x

Matsuda H, Saito K, Takayanagi Y, Okazaki T, Kashima K, Ishikawa K, Kai Y, Takeo N, Hatano Y, Okamoto O, Fujiwara S (2013) Pustular-type drug-induced hypersensitivity syndrome/drug reaction with eosinophilia and systemic symptoms due to carbamazepine with systemic muscle involvement. J Dermatol 40(2):118–122. https://doi.org/10.1111/1346-8138.12028

Nakai N, Sugiura K, Akiyama M, Katoh N (2015) Acute generalized exanthematous pustulosis caused by dihydrocodeine phosphate in a patient with psoriasis vulgaris and a heterozygous IL36RN mutation. JAMA Dermatol 151(3):311–315. https://doi.org/10.1001/jamadermatol.2014.3002

Navarini AA, Valeyrie-Allanore L, Setta-Kaffetzi N, Barker JN, Capon F, Creamer D, Roujeau JC, Sekula P, Simpson MA, Trembath RC, Mockenhaupt M, Smith CH (2013) Rare variations in IL36RN in severe adverse drug reactions manifesting as acute generalized exanthematous pustulosis. J Invest Dermatol 133(7):1904–1907. https://doi.org/10.1038/jid.2013.44

Navarini AA, Simpson MA, Borradori L, Yawalkar N, Schlapbach C (2015) Homozygous missense mutation in IL36RN in generalized pustular dermatosis with intraoral involvement compatible with both AGEP and generalized pustular psoriasis. JAMA Dermatol 151(4):452–453. https://doi.org/10.1001/jamadermatol.2014.3848

Ogawa K, Morito H, Hasegawa A, Daikoku N, Miyagawa F, Okazaki A, Fukumoto T, Kobayashi N, Kasai T, Watanabe H, Sueki H, Iijima M, Tohyama M, Hashimoto K, Asada H (2013) Identification of thymus and activation-regulated chemokine (TARC/CCL17) as a potential marker for early indication of disease and prediction of disease activity in drug-induced hypersensitivity syndrome (DIHS)/drug rash with eosinophilia and systemic symptoms (DRESS). J Dermatol Sci 69(1):38–43. https://doi.org/10.1016/j.jdermsci.2012.10.002

Ortonne N, Valeyrie-Allanore L, Bastuji-Garin S, Wechsler J, de Feraudy S, Duong TA, Delfau-Larue MH, Chosidow O, Wolkenstein P, Roujeau JC (2015) Histopathology of drug rash with eosinophilia and systemic symptoms syndrome: a morphological and phenotypical study. Br J Dermatol 173(1):50–58. https://doi.org/10.1111/bjd.13683

Quinn AM, Brown K, Bonish BK, Curry J, Gordon KB, Sinacore J, Gamelli R, Nickoloff BJ (2005) Uncovering histologic criteria with prognostic significance in toxic epidermal necrolysis. Arch Dermatol 141(6):683–687. https://doi.org/10.1001/archderm.141.6.683

Roujeau JC, Bioulac-Sage P, Bourseau C, Guillaume JC, Bernard P, Lok C, Plantin P, Claudy A, Delavierre C, Vaillant L et al (1991) Acute generalized exanthematous pustulosis. Analysis of 63 cases. Arch Dermatol 127(9):1333–1338

Rzany B, Hering O, Mockenhaupt M, Schroder W, Goerttler E, Ring J, Schopf E (1996) Histopathological and epidemiological characteristics of patients with erythema exudativum multiforme major, Stevens-Johnson syndrome and toxic epidermal necrolysis. Br J Dermatol 135(1):6–11

Schwartz RA, McDonough PH, Lee BW (2013) Toxic epidermal necrolysis: Part I. Introduction, history, classification, clinical features, systemic manifestations, etiology, and immunopathogenesis. J Am Acad Dermatol 69(2):173.e171–173.e113. https://doi.org/10.1016/j.jaad.2013.05.003; quiz 185-176.

Shiohara T, Inaoka M, Kano Y (2006) Drug-induced hypersensitivity syndrome (DIHS): a reaction induced by a complex interplay among herpesviruses and antiviral and antidrug immune responses. Allergol Int 55(1):1–8. https://doi.org/10.2332/allergolint.55.1

Skowron F, Bensaid B, Balme B, Depaepe L, Kanitakis J, Nosbaum A, Maucort-Boulch D, Berard F, D'Incan M, Kardaun SH, Nicolas JF (2015) Drug reaction with eosinophilia and systemic symptoms (DRESS): clinicopathological study of 45 cases. J Eur Acad Dermatol Venereol 29(11):2199–2205. https://doi.org/10.1111/jdv.13212

Sugita K, Tohyama M, Watanabe H, Otsuka A, Nakajima S, Iijima M, Hashimoto K, Tokura Y, Miyachi Y, Kabashima K (2010) Fluctuation of blood and skin plasmacytoid dendritic cells in drug-induced hypersensitivity syndrome. J Allergy Clin Immunol 126(2):408–410. https://doi.org/10.1016/j.jaci.2010.06.004

Teraki Y, Shibuya M, Izaki S (2010) Stevens-Johnson syndrome and toxic epidermal necrolysis due to anticonvulsants share certain clinical and laboratory features with drug-induced hypersensitivity syndrome, despite differences in cutaneous presentations. Clin Exp Dermatol 35(7):723–728. https://doi.org/10.1111/j.1365-2230.2009.03718.x

Tohyama M, Hashimoto K (2011) New aspects of drug-induced hypersensitivity syndrome. J Dermatol 38(3):222–228. https://doi.org/10.1111/j.1346-8138.2010.01176.x

Walsh S, Diaz-Cano S, Higgins E, Morris-Jones R, Bashir S, Bernal W, Creamer D (2013) Drug reaction with eosinophilia and systemic symptoms: is cutaneous phenotype a prognostic marker for outcome? A review of clinicopathological features of 27 cases. Br J Dermatol 168(2):391–401. https://doi.org/10.1111/bjd.12081

Weyers W, Metze D (2011) Histopathology of drug eruptions - general criteria, common patterns, and differential diagnosis. Dermatol Pract Concept 1(1):33–47. https://doi.org/10.5826/dpc.0101a09

Evaluation of Drug Safety Literature: A Guide for the Practicing Dermatologist

17

Sandra R. Knowles and Jackie Campbell

Abbreviations

ADR	Adverse drug reactions
AGEP	Acute generalized exanthematous pustulosis
CARE	Case report
CBC	Complete blood count
CCB	Calcium channel blockers
CRD	Centre for reviews and dissemination
DARE	Database of reviews of effects
FAERS	US FDA Adverse Event Reporting System
FDA	US Food and Drug Administration
LFTs	Liver function tests
MeSH	Medical subject headings
NHSEED	NHS economic evaluation database
TRIP	Turning research into practice
VAERS	US CDC Vaccine Adverse Event Reporting System

A literature search is an integral part of the evaluation of a patient with a suspected adverse drug reaction and can provide information on clinical presentation and diagnosis, time course, dose relationship, reversibility, cross-reactivity, treatment

S. R. Knowles (✉)
Department of Pharmacy, Sunnybrook Health Sciences Centre, Toronto, ON, Canada

Faculty of Pharmacy, University of Toronto, Toronto, ON, Canada
e-mail: sandra.knowles@sunnybrook.ca

J. Campbell
Department of Pharmacy, Sunnybrook Health Sciences Centre, Toronto, ON, Canada
e-mail: jackie.campbell@sunnybrook.ca

N. H. Shear, R. P. Dodiuk-Gad (eds.), *Advances in Diagnosis and Management of Cutaneous Adverse Drug Reactions*, https://doi.org/10.1007/978-981-13-1489-6_17

and prognosis, mechanism and pathogenesis, and testing. Using a case example, we will demonstrate the components of a literature search, using a systematic approach to identify relevant information (Aoki et al. 2013). This summary is not meant to be an exhaustive review, but rather provides the practicing dermatologist with the necessary skills to conduct a literature search.

Case Example: A 48-year-old man was started on diltiazem 240 mg once daily for treatment of hypertension. After 10 days of treatment, he developed fever and malaise, and a diffuse facial erythema and edema with coalescing nonfollicular pustules on the upper trunk and flanks. Laboratory testing revealed increased complete blood count (CBC) with neutrophilia and a slight (2× normal) elevation in liver function tests (LFTs). Based on the symptom presentation, you suspect that this is a case of acute generalized exanthematous pustulosis (AGEP). The diltiazem is discontinued and the patient's symptoms resolve (Knowles et al. 1998*).*

Step 1: Research question. Firstly, the research question must be formulated to perform a comprehensive literature search. In our case example, there are three questions:

(a) Have there been previous reports of diltiazem causing AGEP?
(b) What testing, if any, is available to aid in the diagnosis?
(c) Can other calcium channel blockers (CCB) be used in this patient?

For the purposes of this chapter, we will consider only the first question.

Step 2: Literature sources. Secondly, sources to search need to be identified. Sources can include books (e.g., *Meyler's Side Effects of Drugs*), databases (e.g., Litt's Drug Eruption and Reaction Database), and journal articles. Various databases such as PubMed or EMBASE, Google Scholar, and government websites can be searched. PubMed (https://www.ncbi.nlm.nih.gov/pubmed/) is a free database from the US National Center for Biotechnology Information that provides access to the MEDLINE database and includes links to full-text content when available (through PubMed Central and publisher websites). EMBASE is a biomedical and pharmacological database produced by Elsevier. Although there is some duplication between EMBASE and MEDLINE, EMBASE has a more European emphasis and includes more non-English language articles. EMBASE is a subscription-only database (Ng and Peh 2010). Google Scholar is a search engine for a wide range of academic fields. It generally provides a broader range of articles than traditionally found in academic databases, including theses, books, and abstracts from professional societies, preprint sources, and universities (Anders and Evans 2010; Nourbakhsh et al. 2012). Searching on Google may also provide additional information such as grey literature. Grey literature refers to material that may not be commercially published (e.g., unpublished studies, dissertations, conference abstracts). For most drug-induced cutaneous eruptions, searching PubMed (MEDLINE), Google Scholar, and/or Google will result in a comprehensive literature review.

Drug Hypersensitivity
- Drug Eruptions
  - Acute generalized exanthematous pustulosis
  - Drug hypersensitivity syndrome
  - Erythema nodosum
  - Hand-foot syndrome
  - Nicolau syndrome
  - Serum sickness
  - Stevens-Johnson syndrome

Skin-diseases/ci (Note: important to use subheading "chemically induced")

Fig. 17.1 MeSH categories applicable for searching for cutaneous adverse drug reactions

Step 3: Select keywords. Thirdly, keywords need to be established. Many databases use a "thesaurus" that reconciles different spellings and terminology for a topic under the same subject heading. MeSH (Medical Subject Headings) terms used in MEDLINE, an example of a thesaurus, are used to index articles. Using a hierarchical structure, each MeSH term is located in one or more trees, going from more general terms to more specific ones (Fig. 17.1). A detailed description of the uses of MeSH vocabulary for searching is beyond the scope of this chapter but can be found on the National Library of Medicine website. (See PubMed Tutorial at https://www.nlm.nih.gov/bsd/disted/pubmedtutorial/cover.html.) The PubMed database automatically explodes all MeSH terms (Baumann 2016).

A number of MeSH categories may be applicable for cutaneous adverse reactions (see Fig. 17.1). "Drug eruptions" is a more general term; when this term is "exploded," then all articles in the tree (e.g., drug hypersensitivity syndrome, Stevens–Johnson syndrome, acute generalized exanthematous pustulosis) will be included.

Although the use of MeSH terms improves the accuracy of the search, free-text searching is helpful for newer topics, differences in spelling (e.g., anaemia, anemia), acronyms (e.g., AGEP, SDRIFE), or synonyms (e.g., generic and brand names, lay and medical terminology). A combination of MeSH and text-word searches is recommended (Jenuwine and Floyd 2004; Chang et al. 2006). Use of truncated or wildcard words will also help expand the search (see Fig. 17.2).

In our example, MeSH terms that could be used are "acute generalized exanthematous pustulosis," "diltiazem," "skin tests," "patch tests," "immunologic activation," "calcium channel blockers," and "cross reactions." Free-text terms that could be included are AGEP and Cardizem (it is useful to add in brand names, especially with newer drugs).

Step 4: Search. The next step is implementing the search. Combine different combinations of keywords using the Boolean operators (AND/OR/NOT). Use of subheadings for MeSH terms is optional, as they will narrow the search results. Often the initial search will not include subheadings, especially for rare cutaneous adverse reactions, but these can be added to subsequent searches if the initial search results in too many hits.

Truncated words: using the base of the word to find any word containing that base (depending on the database the most commonly used symbol is either * or $) e.g., derm$ = dermatologist, dermatology, dermatitis

Wildcard words: replacing one or more characters in a word (often used for different spellings or plurals) e.g., wom?n = woman or women

Boolean operators: used for combining search terms

- AND: narrows the search
- OR: broadens the search
- NOT: excludes specific information from the search

Subheadings: used with MeSH headings to describe specific aspects of the article e.g., AE = adverse effects, CI = chemically induced (useful for drug-induced effects), TU = therapeutic use

Limits: to filter results from databases and include publication types (e.g., case studies, review articles), date of publication, age group, language

Phrase searching: use of a specific phrase or title by including in quotation marks e.g., "symmetrical drug related intertriginous and flexural exanthema"

Fig. 17.2 Glossary of terms

An example of a search strategy using a combination of MeSH terms and free-text words for the first research question is as follows: (diltiazem OR Cardizem) AND (acute generalized exanthematous pustulosis OR AGEP). This results in 22 articles and includes review articles on AGEP as well as individual case reports. In order to narrow the search further, filters can be applied (i.e., limit to English results in 15 articles). Use of publication filters to identify case reports only may miss some relevant articles and is generally not recommended. Rather, the abstracts of each article can be reviewed, and only those that include individual case reports would be retrieved. It is important to retrieve the articles whenever possible as case reports may not include an abstract, or the abstract may contain only limited information, or even misleading information.

When the key literature has been identified from the initial search, the search should be repeated using a different database or search engine; if the same references appear, then this validates that the initial search strategy was comprehensive. Additionally, it is vital to search the bibliographies of the individual articles to verify that all relevant literature has been identified.

Step 5: Evaluate the literature. Evidence-based medicine integrates clinical expertise with the best available external evidence in order to solve clinical problems (Sackett et al. 1996; Young and Solomon 2009). Ideally, the literature available to answer any clinical question would consist of the highest-quality evidence, i.e., systematic reviews of randomized controlled trials, meta-analyses, or randomized controlled trials (Murad et al. 2016). However, the best available evidence regarding most adverse drug reactions seen in dermatology practice will often be from case series or case-control studies or (most commonly) case reports. Although these sources are usually considered to provide the lowest quality of evidence, case reports are particularly important in that they often describe a new disease or intervention or identify rare adverse drug reactions associated with a particular drug (Aschermann 2014; Scott 2009).

Continuing with our example, there were 22 articles retrieved in the search (dating from 1993 to March 2017) and include the following, which were available online either free of charge or through a subscription service:

- *A 2007 multinational case-control study* that evaluates risk factors for AGEP identifies drugs found to be "highly" associated with it (this includes diltiazem) and discusses risks with different drug classes, including CCB (Sidoroff et al. 2007).
- *Review articles on AGEP.* Good-quality review articles may provide an overview of the reaction, including incidence, risk factors, etiology, pathogenesis, diagnosis and treatment, drugs reported to cause the reaction (e.g., diltiazem), and type of confirmatory testing used (Fernando 2012).
- *Case reports that implicate diltiazem in causing AGEP*. Some case reports also review literature to date, including earlier case reports (Knowles et al. 1998; Fernandez-Ruiz et al. 2009), while others refer to diagnostic testing and cross-reactivity with other CCBs (Saenz de Santa Maria Garcia et al. 2016). It is particularly useful to review case reports/reviews that are published several years apart in order to capture as many case reports as possible and determine if testing methodology has advanced. For example, as of 1998 only 5 cases of AGEP associated with diltiazem had been reported (Knowles et al. 1998) yet by 2009 at least 13 cases had been reported in the English and Spanish literature (Fernandez-Ruiz et al. 2009). A review of the bibliographies of these two articles yields references to additional case reports not identified by our search. This is not uncommon and highlights the value of retrieving the full text of each case report identified in a search.

  Of note, 7 of the 22 articles pulled from our search were case reports written in languages other than English. Such case reports often include English abstracts, bibliographies, tables, photographs, and/or additional information that will help in the analysis (Barcik et al. 2009; Serrao et al. 2008). As well, some reports are published in more than one language (Fernandez-Ruiz et al. 2009).

Next, each article identified should be reviewed to determine the strengths and weaknesses of the evidence it provides and whether this information can be used to answer the clinical question.

In our example, at least two of the articles located in our search (review article, multinational case-control study) quickly confirm the answer to our first question—that diltiazem has been reported to cause AGEP in a number of case reports. However, it is important to review each individual case report, in order to identify gaps in information provided, and other possible causative drugs that may have been missed by the authors.

Key elements to consider when appraising a case report include the following (Gagnier et al. 2013):

- Relevant patient demographics and history are provided in sufficient detail.
- A timeline that organizes important information from the patient history is set out—e.g., timing of drug administration, occurrence of the reaction, and any interventions.

- Description of the reaction and how it was treated.
- Whether the diagnosis of AGEP is supported (e.g., by clinical features, blood tests, biopsy, patch testing).
- Sufficient details of diagnostic methods used are given.
- Possible confounding factors (e.g., other drugs or medical conditions) are identified.
- A discussion of relevant literature is included.

A comprehensive checklist that highlights how to review case reports is available from CARE—Case Report Guidelines (Anon n.d.). Although this is primarily for authors, it is an excellent resource to use to evaluate case reports.

It is important to note that some of the articles pulled during our search for the response to the first clinical question will also be useful in answering the other questions, i.e., availability of testing and cross-reactivity among CCB with respect to AGEP. However, rather than relying solely on these articles, it is important to conduct separate searches for each clinical question.

Additional resources that are available free online and may be helpful during a literature search are provided in Table 17.1.

Table 17.1 Selected online resources (free of charge)

Name of resource	Resource type	Location (URL)	Comments
Adverse drug reactions (ADRs)			
Canada Vigilance Adverse Reaction Online Database	Database	http://www.hc-sc.gc.ca/dhp-mps/medeff/databasdon/index-eng.php	Voluntary reports submitted to Health Canada of suspected adverse reactions submitted by consumers, health professionals, product manufacturers, and distributors
FAERS—US FDA Adverse Event Reporting System	Database	https://open.fda.gov/data/faers/	FAERS is a database that contains information on adverse event and medication error reports submitted to the US Food and Drug Administration (FDA)
US CDC Vaccine Adverse Event Reporting System (VAERS)	Information resource	https://wonder.cdc.gov/vaers.html https://vaers.hhs.gov/index	VAERS is a US vaccine safety surveillance program co-sponsored by the Centers for Disease Control and Prevention and the FDA
Medicines Safety Update (Australia)	Database	https://www.tga.gov.au/publication/medicines-safety-update	Provides practical information and advice on drug safety and information about emerging safety issues
European Database of Suspected Adverse Drug Reaction Reports	Database	http://www.adrreports.eu/en/	Online access to data on suspected adverse drug reaction reports for authorized medicines in the European Economic Area

Table 17.1 (continued)

Name of resource	Resource type	Location (URL)	Comments
Dermatology-based resources			
DermNet New Zealand	Dermatology-based resource	http://www.dermnetnz.org	Includes lots of information about drug-related reactions, by both drug and condition
RegiSCAR	Information resource	http://www.regiscar.org	Project dedicated to severe cutaneous adverse reactions (SCARs), with a focus on linking those interested in SCARs. May not be kept current
Chemical structures			
DrugBank	Database	https://www.drugbank.ca	Provides chemical, pharmacological, pharmaceutical information. Updated daily
PubChem	Database	https://pubchem.ncbi.nlm.nih.gov	US National Center for Biotechnology Information. Provides chemical structures, biological properties
Toxicology			
Toxnet—Toxline US National Library of Medicine	Database	https://toxnet.nlm.nih.gov/newtoxnet/toxline.htm	Resource to search databases on toxicology, hazardous chemical, environmental health, and toxic releases; maintained through the US National Library of Medicine (NLM)
LiverTox	Database	https://livertox.nih.gov/	Resource for clinical and research information on drug-induced liver injury; administered through the US NLM
Drug information			
Drug Information Portal	Information resource	https://druginfo.nlm.nih.gov/drugportal/	Provides a gateway for selected drug information including consumer health information, use in breastfeeding, ongoing and completed clinical trials, US product monograph
Others			
CRD (Centre for Reviews and Dissemination)	Information resource	https://www.crd.york.ac.uk/CRDWeb/HomePage.asp	Abstracts systematic reviews. University of York (UK). Includes comprehensive guide on basic and advanced searching. Formerly DARE (Database of Reviews of Effects) and NHSEED (NHS Economic Evaluation Database)
TRIP (formerly Turning Research Into Practice)	Search engine	https://www.tripdatabase.com	Clinical search engine, focuses on evidence-based medicine content. Permits search of several resources at a time. Includes place on evidence hierarchy for each article

- After an initial search, review citations of key articles to identify MeSH headings that were used to ensure that all relevant search terms are included
- Use the "related citation" button to identify articles with similar keywords
- If there are too many search results, limit the search (e.g., language, age) or include the use of subheadings
- Google and Google Scholar are helpful to identify grey literature
- Do not rely on abstracts only for information on the published case; the full article is often needed for additional detail
- Review and cross-references bibliographies of key articles to identify references that may have been missed

Fig. 17.3 Tips for searching the literature for cutaneous adverse drug reactions

17.1 Summary

A literature search is an integral part of the evaluation of a patient with a cutaneous adverse drug reaction (Shear 1990). Tips set out in Fig. 17.3 illustrate some important components of this process.

References

Anders ME, Evans DP (2010) Comparison of PubMed and Google Scholar literature searches. Respir Care 55(5):578–583

Anon (2018) CARE: case report guidelines. http://www.care-statement.org/. Accessed September 2018.

Aoki NJ, Enticott JC, Phillips LE (2013) Searching the literature: four simple steps. Transfusion 53(1):14–17

Aschermann M (2014) Case reports in current medical literature. Cor Vasa 56:e377–e378

Barcik K, Protas-Drozd F, Weiss-Rostkowska W, Flis E, Placek W (2009) Acute generalised exanthematous pustulosis (AGEP) due to diltiazem--a case report. Kardiol Pol 67(8):887–891

Baumann N (2016) How to use the medical subject headings (MeSH). Int J Clin Pract 70:171–174

Chang AA, Heskett KM, Davidson TM (2006) Searching the literature using medical subject headings versus text word with PubMed. Laryngoscope 116(2):336–340

Fernandez-Ruiz M, Lopez-Medrano F, Garcia-Ruiz F, Rodriguez-Peralto JL (2009) Diltiazem-induced acute generalized exanthemic pustulosis: a case and review of the literature. Actas Dermosifiliogr 100(8):725–727

Fernando SL (2012) Acute generalised exanthematous pustulosis. Australas J Dermatol 53(2):87–92

Gagnier JJ, Kienle G, Altman DG, Moher D, Sox H, Riley D et al (2013) The CARE guidelines: consensus-based clinical case reporting guideline development. Headache 53(10):1541–1547

Jenuwine ES, Floyd JA (2004) Comparison of medical subject headings and text-word searches in MEDLINE to retrieve studies on sleep in healthy individuals. J Med Libr Assoc 92(3):349–353

Knowles S, Gupta AK, Shear NH (1998) The spectrum of cutaneous reactions associated with diltiazem: three cases and a review of the literature. J Am Acad Dermatol 38(2 Pt 1):201–206

Murad MH, Asi N, Alsawas M, Alahdab F (2016) New evidence pyramid. Evid Based Med 21(4):125–127

Ng KH, Peh WC (2010) Getting to know journal bibliographic databases. Singap Med J 51(10):757–760 quiz 61

Nourbakhsh E, Nugent R, Wang H, Cevik C, Nugent K (2012) Medical literature searches: a comparison of PubMed and Google scholar. Health Inf Libr J 29(3):214–222

Sackett DL, Rosenberg WM, Gray JA, Haynes RB, Richardson WS (1996) Evidence based medicine: what it is and what it isn't. BMJ 312(7023):71–72

Saenz de Santa Maria Garcia M, Noguerado-Mellado B, Rojas Perez-Ezquerra P, Hernandez-Aragues I, De Barrio Fernandez M (2016) Acute generalized exanthematous pustulosis due to diltiazem: investigation of cross-reactivity with other calcium channel blockers. J Allergy Clin Immunol Pract 4(4):765–766

Scott JR (2009) In defense of case reports. Obstet Gynecol 114(2 Pt 2):413–414

Serrao V, Caldas Lopes L, Campos Lopes JM, Lobo L, Ferreira A (2008) Acute generalized exanthematous pustulosis associated with diltiazem. Acta Medica Port 21(1):99–102

Shear NH (1990) Diagnosing cutaneous adverse reactions to drugs. Arch Dermatol 126(1):94–97

Sidoroff A, Dunant A, Viboud C, Halevy S, Bavinck JN, Naldi L et al (2007) Risk factors for acute generalized exanthematous pustulosis (AGEP)-results of a multinational case-control study (EuroSCAR). Br J Dermatol 157(5):989–996

Young JM, Solomon MJ (2009) How to critically appraise an article. Nat Clin Pract Gastroenterol Hepatol 6(2):82–91

In Vitro and In Vivo Tests in Cutaneous Adverse Drug Reactions

18

Annick Barbaud

Abbreviations

AGEP	Acute generalized exanthematous pustulosis
AO	Angioedema
BAT	Basophil activation test
CADR	Cutaneous adverse drug reactions
DPTs	Drug patch tests
DRESS	Drug reaction with systemic symptoms
ELISpot	Enzyme-Linked Immunosorbent Spot
FDE	Fixed drug eruption
HS	Hypersensitivities
IDTs	Intradermal Drug Tests
IHS	Immediate HS
NMBA	Neuromuscular blocking agents
PBMC	Peripheral blood mononuclear cells
RCM	Radiocontrast media
SDRIFE	Symmetrical drug-related intertriginous and flexural exanthema
SJS/TEN	Stevens–Johnson syndrome/toxic epidermal necrolysis
UV	Ultraviolet

A. Barbaud (✉)
Department of Dermatology and Allergy, Faculty of Medicine, Tenon Hospital, Sorbonne University, Paris, France
e-mail: annick.barbaud@aphp.fr

N. H. Shear, R. P. Dodiuk-Gad (eds.), *Advances in Diagnosis and Management of Cutaneous Adverse Drug Reactions*, https://doi.org/10.1007/978-981-13-1489-6_18

Key Points

- Drug patch tests are useful in cutaneous adverse drug reactions (CADR) related to a delayed hypersensitivity. In severe CADR, they are well tolerated and have a good sensitivity in drug reactions with eosinophilia and systemic symptoms and acute generalized exanthematous pustulosis.
- Intradermal testing has to be done with injectable forms of the drugs, under hospital surveillance and after prick tests giving negative results. Intradermal tests can be useful with immediate readings in investigating immediate hypersensitivity and with readings done after 1 or 2 days in non-severe delayed hypersensitivity. In order to avoid false-positive results, they have to be done with concentrations respecting the thresholds given in literature.
- In immediate hypersensitivity, the measurement of tryptase levels in serum has to be done 30 min to 2 h after the onset of the reaction. In delayed HS, no test has a good sensitivity but combine three different cellular assays may help to overcome or bypass the assumed refractoriness of PBMC of SJS/TEN patients.

Drug skin tests, which are increasingly used, are very useful for the diagnosis of drug hypersensitivities. In literature, there are large variations in their modalities of realization, which make comparisons between centers difficult. Moreover, there are differences in the approach of drug hypersensitivity (HS) reactions between Europe and North America (Torres et al. 2017).

According to recent publications, we propose in this chapter to summarize knowledge of the value of these methods and some guidelines for a good practice of these tests to avoid false-positive and false-negative results and to be able to compare the results reported in literature.

18.1 When to Test?

Drug skin tests can be performed several years after a cutaneous adverse drug reaction (CADR) including urticaria or angioedema (AO), but it is recommended to perform them at least 4 weeks and within 1 year after the event. The extinction of cutaneous reactivity in delayed HS is unknown but seems to be long-lasting. In immediate HS (IHS) to penicillins, skin reactivity decreases rapidly after the onset of the iatrogenic accident. Concerning beta-lactam antibiotics, 50% of patients lose their skin reactivity when they are retested 1 year after the first evaluation (Blanca et al. 1999). Romano et al. (2014) showed that of 72 subjects with positive tests after a cephalosporin IHS, 45/72 (62.5%) lost their skin reactivity when they were retested 1 year later, 3 years, and 5 years after initial positive results.

18.2 Drug Patch Tests

It is recommended to do drug patch tests (DPTs) at least 4 weeks after the disappearance of CADR and discontinuation of systemic corticosteroids or immunosuppressive drugs and ultraviolet (UV) exposure on the skin area tested and 1 week after discontinuation of topical corticosteroids on the site tested (Barbaud et al. 2001; Brockow et al. 2002). In drug reaction with systemic symptoms (DRESS), they must be done at least 6 months after the disappearance of the CADR and in the absence of high virus replication (Barbaud et al. 2013; Barbaud 2014).

They are performed as patch tests with haptens used for the investigation of contact dermatitis.

It is possible to use ready-to-use products in which most drugs are diluted at 10% in petrolatum; unfortunately only a limited number of molecules marketed by Chemotechnique (Vellinge, Sweden) are available in ready-to-use material. In most of the cases, it is necessary to prepare the test material in diluting the drugs in their marketed form provided by the patients themselves. This patch test material has to be prepared just before testing.

There are numerous recommendations on the dilution to be used (Barbaud et al. 2001; Brockow et al. 2002). Two sets of European guidelines have been published for clinicians to conduct DPTs with the drug in its commercially available form with each drug diluted to 30% (Barbaud et al. 2001) or 20% (Brockow et al. 2002) in pet. Ideally, a concentration of 10% of active ingredient should be obtained. Brajon et al. (2014) showed that the exact amount of the active ingredient in diluted commercial forms of drugs prepared at 30% in pet. Varied from 0.05 to 30% and that 25% of the DPTs had an active ingredient's concentration of less than 2%. We prefer the concentration of 30% (Barbaud et al. 2001) instead of 20% (Brockow et al. 2002) because it is the only one in which there is a significant number of controls in literature (Brajon et al. 2014). From a practical point of view, as it is difficult to obtain a 10% active ingredient's concentration for every drug tested, we suggest that published DPT results should give the exact concentration of active ingredient, so that results among centers may be compared. In multicenter studies of DPTs, it would be convenient to either use the same generic forms of drugs or consider only active ingredient concentrations to enable standardization of methods among centers.

When the active ingredient is in pure form, e.g., in lyophilisate, it is recommended to dilute it at 10% in pet (Barbaud et al. 2001).

Drug patch tests must be conducted with caution, as some drugs, such as carbamazepine, pseudoephedrine, and aciclovir, can re-induce a cutaneous adverse drug reaction. With these drugs, it is advisable to start with low concentrations, e.g., 1%, and if negative at higher concentrations up to 10% (Barbaud et al. 2001; Barbaud 2014).

To avoid false-positive results, some drugs have to be tested with lower concentrations. The content of the capsules of celecoxib should be tested at 5% or at 10% in petrolatum and not with higher concentrations (Kleinhans et al. 2002). Colchicine at 10% induces false-positive results, and its threshold of specificity is unknown. Captopril in commercialized forms diluted at 1% and chloroquine in commercialized forms diluted at 30% in petrolatum induce sometimes false-positive results; misoprostol in commercialized forms has to be diluted at 1% in petrolatum (Barbaud et al. 2001).

Analysis of literature does not permit to specify the best vehicle for preparing drug patch test material. There are sometimes discrepancies between the results obtained by diluting in water or in petrolatum, tending to favor petrolatum

(A. Barbaud, personal data, unpublished). For corticosteroids and steroid hormones, if drug patch tests are negative in using petrolatum, for dilution, it is advisable to dilute steroids in ethyl alcohol (Barbaud et al. 2001). For patch tests used for the investigation of contact dermatitis, some recommend the use of 20 μL of material prepared in pet (40 mg/cm^2) and 15 μL for liquid preparations (Johansen et al. 2015). To date, there is no recommendation to apply a given volume of drug preparation into the patch test chambers.

The patch tests are applied on the upper back using chambers, according to the methods used in patch testing for contact dermatitis. They are left for 2 days and then read at Day 2 (30 min after taking off the test's material) and Day 4 or 5, with a weekly reading for corticosteroids. In fixed drug eruption, drug patch tests are applied in duplicate, on the back but also on the residual skin site ("in situ DPTs") (Andrade et al. 2011). Reading result's criteria are identical to those used for contact allergy (i.e., negative, irritant, + to +++). In case of anaphylactic shock, drug patch tests are contraindicated as they have a poor value in IHS but, moreover, because they can be dangerous in re-inducing the shock. Anaphylactic shocks induced by patch tests have been reported with beta-lactams, neomycin, gentamicin, bacitracin, and diclofenac. If there is doubt about a history of severe IHS, if drug patch tests are done, it is necessary to read them at 20 min to ensure that there is no immediate reaction.

A control patch test has to be done with the vehicle used for dilution as sensitization to pet (Ulrich et al. 2004) or ethyl alcohol does exist. The relevance of a positive DPT must always be checked, as a DPT might be positive because the patient has had a previous contact dermatitis to the drug tested or to one of its excipient without any relevance to the investigated CADR (Barbaud et al. 2001).

In case of a positive DPT done with a drug product in its commercial form, the manufacturer must be contacted in order to furnish all the components and allowing to test them separately, in order to specify which active ingredient or excipient is responsible for the positive reaction. The dilution used to test the excipient is chosen according to data from literature (De Groot 2008).

In investigating a photosensitivity reaction induced by a drug, both drug patch tests and drug photopatch tests with the responsible drug have to be performed. It is recommended to test with a 1% concentration of active ingredient or 0.1% for phenothiazines (Gonçalo et al. 2013). The irradiation for drug photopatch tests is performed 1 or 2 days after applying the DPT with a 5 J/cm^2 UVA irradiation (Gonçalo et al. 2013).

A nonirradiated control patch is also applied. The reading is done 2 days after the irradiation. Criteria for positive results are identical to those used for patch tests with haptens, IR, + to +++. It has been demonstrated that photoscratch patch tests are more irritating and do not have a better value than photopatch tests (Conilleau et al. 2000).

A summary of good practice for drug patch testing is given in Table 18.1.

Drug patch tests have a rather low sensibility but are well tolerated. They are of value for the investigations of maculopapular exanthema, systemic contact dermatitis, baboon syndrome, symmetrical drug-related intertriginous and flexural exanthema (SDRIFE) or flexural exanthema, eczematous reactions at injection sites, acute generalized exanthematous pustulosis (AGEP), DRESS, and toxic epidermal necrolysis or Stevens-Johnson syndrome (SJS/TENs) (Table 18.2). They have no

Table 18.1 Recommendations for drug patch tests

1. Precautions
No skin lesions on site tested
At least 1 month after discontinuation of systemic corticosteroids and immunosuppressants
At least 1 month after stopping exposure to ultraviolet light on the test area
At least 1 week after discontinuation of application of topical corticosteroids on the site tested
The site tested should not be wet during the entire investigation period
2. Contraindication
Anaphylactic shock with tested drug
3. When to test
Test more than 4 weeks and as soon as possible after the disappearance of the CADR. In case of DRESS, test at least 6 months after the DRESS ensuring that there is no intercurrent relapse or a high viral reactivation
4. Prepare patch test material
Use a commercially available patch test preparation (Chemotechnique, Vellinge, Sweden)
Or prepare the material from a drug product in its marketed form
Note the tradename and dosage of the drug being tested
Reduce the tablet to fine powder, recover the contents of a capsule, collect a liquid medication
Dilute the material at 30% in petrolatum (or alcohol *) and note the final concentration of active ingredient
OR for lyophilisate, dilute the material to a final concentration of 10%
With acyclovir, carbamazepine, pseudoephedrine: start at 1% active ingredient
For the envelope of a capsule: moisten it and then test it
5. Ensure the absence of irritation induced by the patch test material
Check the recommended concentrations in literature and the existence of at least ten controls (from the literature or personal) Test desloratadine to a maximum of 10% and colchicine to 1% Pay attention to the presence of sodium lauryl sulfate in the formulation of certain drugs (Brajon et al. 2014; Andrade et al. 2011)
6. Apply the material
Under Finn Chamber on Scanpor® 8 mm (SmartPractice) or IQ chamber® or IQ Ultra chamber® (Chemotechnique)
On the skin of the back. In case of fixed drug eruption applied in addition in situ
Test the excipient used for dilutions (petrolatum, alcohol)
7. First reading at 48 h
Material left in place for 2 days
Remove the material, mark the location of the tests with a skin pencil
Make the first reading 30 min after the withdrawal of the material
Report results in negative (0); irritant (IR); positive with erythema and papule (+); erythema, papule, and vesicles (++); or erythema, papule, numerous confluent vesicles (+++)
8. Second reading
Indispensable after 96 h or if not possible at 120 h
For corticosteroids make an extra reading at 1 week
Report results in 0, IR, +, ++ or +++
9. Determining the relevance of the test
Ensure that positivity is not due to a contact allergy to any of the components of the preparation unrelated to the exploration of the CADR

(continued)

Table 18.1 (continued)

10. In case of positive patch test: detail
Recover the different components of the drug product in its commercialized form used to prepare the material, and then, test them separately to clarify whether it is a sensitization to an active ingredient or to an excipient
11. A negative patch tests does not exclude the responsibility of a drug
Dilution in alcohol is recommended for progesterone and estrogens and for corticosteroids if dilutions in petrolatum lead to negative results

Table 18.2 The value of drug skin tests according to the clinical features of the cutaneous adverse drug reactions (adapted from Barbaud A. 2014)

	Patch tests	Prick tests	Intradermal drug tests (IDTs)
Urticaria or angioedema	Not useful. If done, have to be read at 20 min, then at 48 h and 96 h	With dilutions	In beginning with high dilutions of the drug
Anaphylactic shock	Dangerous. Forbidden, can re-induce the shock	With dilutions, e.g., at 10-3 of the usual concentrations for beta-lactams	In beginning with high dilutions of the drug
Vasculitis	No value	No value	No value and forbidden as they can re-induce the vasculitis
Maculopapular rash	Useful (positive in 10 to 40% of the series)	+ before IDT and can be positive with delayed readings at 24 h	With immediate but especially delayed readings at 24 h and later if negative
Localized eczema due to heparins	Can be positive	No value but done before IDT	With immediate but especially delayed readings at 24 h and later if negative (frequently positive only after 3 days)
SDRIFE and systemic drug-induced Baboon syndrome	Useful (maybe 52% to 82%?)	One case with delayed positivity with amoxicillin	Unknown value
FDE	Useful on the residual area (positive in 40% of the cases)	Unknown value	Unknown value
AGEP	Useful (positive in 50 to 58% of the cases)	Unknown value	Unknown value could be useful. Tolerance unknown

Table 18.2 (continued)

	Patch tests	Prick tests	Intradermal drug tests (IDTs)
DRESS	Useful (positive in 32 to 64% of the cases). Done at least 6 months after the disappearance of the rash and biological disturbances. With highly reactive drugs, e.g., carbamazepine or pseudoephedrine, begin with at 1% and then if negative continue with higher concentrations. Multiple drug reactivities to different drug classes may occur	Unknown value, probably very low value, some cases with delayed reactions	Unknown value. Has to be cautiously applied (relapses have been reported) and done only for absolutely necessary drugs, with a low drug causality assessment
SJS/TEN	Can be done but are rarely positive in 9 to 23.5% of the cases	No value	Could be dangerous (flare-up reactions). Forbidden with any highly suspected drug

SDRIFE symmetrical drug-related intertriginous and flexural exanthema, *FDE* fixed drug eruption, *AGEP* acute generalized exanthematous pustulosis, *DRESS* drug reaction with eosinophilia and systemic symptoms, *SJS/TEN* Stevens-Johnson syndrome/toxic epidermal necrolysis

value in urticaria, angioedema, vasculitis, or pruritus induced by drugs. Many drugs have been reported to have positive results when explored by DPTs (Barbaud 2014; Brajon et al. 2014). On the other hand, the DPTs performed with allopurinol, salazopyrin, or paracetamol are mostly or ever negative in literature and in our experience (Barbaud et al. 2013; Santiago et al. 2010).

18.3 Drug Prick Tests

They can be done with any form of commercialized drug, usually, in undiluted form: pills reduced to very fine powder, capsule contents, liquid, or injectable solutions. In moderate and severe IHS, especially with beta-lactam antibiotics, drug preparations for prick tests should be highly diluted. Concentrations should be initiated at least at 10^{-3} of the usual concentrations to avoid systemic reactions.

As done for aeroallergens, drug prick tests are performed after stopping antihistamines 1 for at least 3 days, but 7 days for desloratadine and loratadine, and without immunosuppressive drugs (Blanca et al. 2009). Stopping beta-blockers has always to be discussed in terms of risk/benefit. If stopped, this therapeutic interruption has to be restricted to the day of the tests, and the antihypertensive drugs have to be readministered 3 h after the end of the skin test procedure. Prick tests are carried out on the volar surface of the forearm by putting a drop of drug product or a small amount of powder, then in perforating the epidermis with a special lancet and not with a needle (Barbaud et al. 2001; Brockow et al. 2002; Bousquet et al. 2012). The results are compared to those obtained with a negative control (0.9% serum saline) and a positive control (histamine). They can be performed with all drugs except codeine. Nonspecific degranulations are observed at the usual concentrations with certain antibiotics such as spiramycin (maximum concentration up to 37,500 IU/mL), erythromycin (maximum up to 5 mg/mL), and pefloxacin (maximum up to 0.32 mg/mL). Reading of prick tests is done at 20 min. At 20 min, the prick test is positive if the papule (wheal) is greater than or equal to those measured on the negative control plus 3 mm and if there is a surrounding erythema. Prick tests are of value for investigating IHS. Of 236 investigations for drug allergy in children, prick tests had a low sensitivity of 6.9%, an average positive predictive value of 50%, but very good specificity (98.8%) and negative predictive value (85.7%) (Indradat et al. 2016).

In CADR supposed to be due to delayed HS, it is necessary to draw a persistent marking of the site of the prick test, because delayed positive results after 24 h can occur. Even if rare, they can reveal a delayed HS even in case of negative patch tests done with the same drug.

A prick test has a delayed positive reaction when there is erythema and infiltration at its skin location (Barbaud et al. 2013; Barbaud 2014). Seldom late positivities of prick tests have been reported in MPR, DRESS, or AGEP (Barbaud et al. 2013; Barbaud 2014).

18.4 Intradermal Drug Tests (IDTs)

The IDTs are performed after ensuring the negativity of the prick tests performed with the drug to be tested. In most of the cases, but platinum salts, dilutions for intradermal testing are done in serum saline, phenolated or non-phenolated. A negative control has to be done with the solvent used for dilution. The dilution used to start the IDTs will depend on the severity of the initial CADR. In immediate reactions, IDTs should be performed after ensuring that there is no reaction on the prick tests. IDTs are then started with low concentrations. For most of the drugs, in case of immediate reaction, it is necessary to start with a concentration at 1/1000 of the usage concentration or lower. We emphasize that for anaphylactic shock to beta-lactam antibiotics, the reactivity can be very severe and that it is necessary firstly to start the tests with prick tests with highly diluted solutions and then to continue with IDT also done with very low concentrations, which will be gradually increased if the IDTs with low concentrations have negative results on the 20-min reading.

Many teams base their technique for performing IDTs on the diameter of the injection papule or initial wheal (Wi), trying to obtain a certain diameter of the Wi and not injecting a given volume of drug allergen (Gomes et al. 2004). This technique, which is often considered as the easiest, has many disadvantages. Firstly, the diameter chosen for Wi may vary from one team to another (from 2 to 10 mm in the ENDA survey). It is then easy to imagine that the amount of allergen administered to the patient also varies greatly from one center to another. Secondly, such IDTs are operator dependent and therefore not very reproducible. Thirdly, the risk of reinitiating the initial accident in doing IDT is thus difficult to evaluate because the amount of drug allergen administered to the patient is unknown. Fourth, the amount of drug allergen administered can vary according to the patient's age and hence the resistivity of his skin.

To compare the risks of induction of relapse of CADR by IDTs and to determine the thresholds of their specificity, it is therefore essential that each operator injects the same amount of allergen and then reads the tests at the same time and with the same criteria for positivity.

The previous two publications of European recommendations contained inaccuracies (Barbaud et al. 2001; Brockow et al. 2002). After a survey (Gomes et al. 2004) and then a 6-year multicenter study of ENDA members whose results have not yet been published, some recommendations can be summarized as follows.

IDT can only be done under hospital supervision and with drugs commercialized for injectable use. In severe CADR supposed to be due to delayed HS, IDT cannot be done with the drugs highly suspected. The recommended volume for injection is 0.02 mL. The diameter of the injection papule (wheal) should be measured immediately after injection (Wi).The reaction is then measured at 20 min. At 20 min, the IDT is considered positive if the diameter of the measured wheal (W20) is greater than or equal to the diameter of the Wi + 3 mm and if there is a surrounding erythema that has also to be measured. In case of delayed HS, IDT can be positive on delayed readings. The IDT is considered having a delayed positive result if an erythema and infiltration occur at the site of injection at 24 or 48 h readings.

IDT can induce false-positive, irritant results. From a literature survey, specific thresholds for drug IDT have been published (Brockow et al. 2013). These thresholds were determined according to literature studies in which IDTs were performed using numerous different techniques. The most widely studied drug classes are beta-lactams, iodinated radiocontrast media (RCM) agents, general anesthetics, and heparins (Table 18.3).

Amoxicillin, amoxicillin-clavulanic acid, or ampicillin can be tested up to 20 mg/mL and cephalosporins up to 2 mg/mL (Blanca et al. 2009; Brockow et al. 2013; Hjortlund et al. 2013). IDT with diluted solutions is of interest with other antibiotics (Brockow et al. 2013; Kuyucu et al. 2014; Brož et al. 2012) such as glycopeptides (Perrin-Lamarre et al. 2010), macrolides (Araujo and Demoly 2008; Mori et al. 2010) or quinolones (Lobera et al. 2010), RCM (Brockow et al. 2009; Lerondeau et al. 2016), insulins (Waton 2011), proton pump inhibitors (Bonadonna et al. 2012), and corticosteroids (Soria et al. 2011; Patel and Bahna 2015; Barbaud and Waton 2016). With the latter, transient skin atrophies have been reported (Soria et al. 2011).

Heparin and heparinoids can be tested up to 1/10th of their usual concentration (Scherer et al. 2008). IDTs can be performed with heparins in the case of erythematous, edematous, localized reaction at the injection site or maculopapular exanthema. Nevertheless, they are formally contraindicated in case of necrosis at the site of injection of heparins. The late reading of IDTs with heparins should not take into account the very frequent hematoma at the injection site. Moreover, as the positive

Table 18.3 Maximum concentrations[a] recommended for **intradermal** testing

	Maximal concentration	References
Antibiotics		
Amoxicillin, ampicillin	20 mg/mL	Blanca et al. (2009); Brockow et al. (2013)
Cephalosporins	2 mg/mL	Blanca et al. (2009); Brockow et al. (2013)
Ciprofloxacin	6.66 μg/mL	Brož et al. (2012)
Clarithromycin	0.05 mg/mL	Brož et al. (2012)
Rifampicin	2 μg/mL	Brož et al. (2012)
Anesthetics		
atracurium	10 μg/mL	Mertes et al. (2011)
Cisatracurium	20 μg/mL	Mertes et al. (2011)
Mivacurium	2 μg/mL	Mertes et al. (2011)
Pancuronium	200 μg/mL	Mertes et al. (2011)
Rocuronium	50 μg/mL	Mertes et al. (2011)
Suxamethonium	100 μg/mL	Mertes et al. (2011)
Vecuronium	400 μg/mL	Mertes et al. (2011)
Etomidate	200 μg/mL	Mertes et al. (2011)
Midazolam	500 μg/mL	Mertes et al. (2011)
Propofol	1000 μg/mL	Mertes et al. (2011)
Thiopental	2500 μg/mL	Mertes et al. (2011)
Ketamine	1000 μg/mL	Mertes et al. (2011)
Alfentanil	50 μg/mL	Mertes et al. (2011)
Fentanyl	5 μg/mL	Mertes et al. (2011)
Morphine	10 μg/mL	Mertes et al. (2011)
Remifentanil	5 μg/mL	Mertes et al. (2011)
Sufentanil	0.5 μg/mL	Mertes et al. (2011)
Bupivacaine	250 μg/mL	Mertes et al. (2011)
Lidocaine	1000 μg/mL	Mertes et al. (2011)
Mepivacaine	1000 μg/mL	Mertes et al. (2011)
Ropivacaine	200 μg/mL	Mertes et al. (2011)
Anti-TNF		
infliximab	2 mg/mL	Benucci et al. (2008); Fréling et al. (2015)
adalimumab	50 mg/mL	Benucci et al. (2008)
etanercept	5 mg/mL	Benucci et al. (2008)
Dyes		
Patent blue	2500 μg/mL	Mertes et al. (2011)
Methylene blue	100 μg/mL	Mertes et al. (2011)
Heparins	1/10th of the usage concentration	Brockow et al. (2013); Scherer et al. (2008)
Interferons	usage concentration	Poreaux et al. (2014)
Radiocontrast media derivatives	1/10th of the usage concentration	Brockow et al. (2013); Lerondeau et al. (2016)
Platinum salts	1 mg/mL	Leguy-Seguin et al. (2007)

[a]For **intradermal** testing in patients who had an anaphylactic reaction, much lower doses have to be done. The first injected concentration has to be 1/1000 from the concentrations given in this table

reaction is often delayed, readings have to be performed after 72 h or later. In our experience, IDTs at the concentrations of use also appear specific; it is sometimes only the concentration of use that reveals a delayed HS (A. Barbaud, unpublished data).

IDTs to platinum salts are specific for immediate reading with dilutions of 1 mg/mL (Leguy-Seguin et al. 2007). On the other hand, we have to keep in mind that a nonspecific erythematous infiltration can occur at 24 h with these IDTs. Therefore, their delayed readings do not appear to be specific as published with carboplatin at 1 mg/mL (Guyot-Caquelin et al. 2010) and also observed with oxaliplatin (A. Barbaud, unpublished data).

IDTs with biologicals and cytokines are of little use. Thresholds for specificity with antitumor necrosis factors have been reported at the following concentrations: infliximab ≤2 mg/mL, adalimumab ≤50 mg/mL, and etanercept ≤5 mg/mL (Benucci et al. 2008; Fréling et al. 2015). IDTs with interferons were thought to be nonspecific, but they appear to be interesting with good positive and negative predictive values (Poreaux et al. 2014) in generalized exanthemas due to these molecules. The thresholds for specific IDT are reported in Table 18.3.

For general anesthetics, it would be necessary for the same IDT methods to be adopted. The BSACI group recommends injection of 0.03 mL resulting in injection papules with a diameter of between 4 and 6 mm (Ewan et al. 2010). On the other hand, the injection of a volume of 0.03–0.05 mL recommended in another publication that would result in a 4 mm in diameter of the Wi deserves to be controlled (Mertes et al. 2005). The one advising an injection of a volume of 0.02–0.05 mL resulting in a Wi with a diameter of 4 mm is probably better but also deserves a control of the average diameter obtained and to propose a more limited volume variation (Mertes et al. 2011).

18.5 In Vitro Tests for Drug Allergy

18.5.1 Immediate Hypersensitivity to Drugs

Discomforts and shocks in the course of a drug administration may have different causes. It is very useful to know if they correspond to mast cell degranulation and shock due to histamine release.

In immediate HS, tryptase levels in serum are correlated with mast cell activation. Its measurement has to be done 30 min to 2 h after the onset of urticaria, angioedema, or anaphylactic shock. Its acute level has to be compared to the basal one measured at least 24 h after the resolution of symptoms. According to Mayorga et al. (Mayorga et al. 2016), the minimal clinically significant elevation of the acute total tryptase level would be ≥20% above baseline levels plus 2 mg/L, within 4 h after symptomatic features. Mast cell diseases influence basal tryptase levels.

Tryptase levels in serum during the acute phase of an IHS are useful for confirming mast cell-mediated reactions with a sensitivity ranging from 30 to 94% and a specificity from 92 to 94% with higher tryptase levels observed in more severe clinical drug reactions (Mayorga et al. 2016).

Specific IgE determination by ImmunoCAP is available for a limited number of drugs among beta-lactam antibiotics and neuromuscular blocking agents (NMBA) and has a good specificity but a low sensitivity.

18.5.2 Basophil Activation Test (BAT)

Based on flow cytometry, this test identifies basophils by various markers (anti-IgE, CCR3, CRTH2, or CD203c) and measures their activation after exposure to the suspected drug by the expression of CD63 or CD203c. BAT protocols are not standardized (Mayorga et al. 2016). Their results depend on the method and on the severity of the adverse effects. They could be interesting in investigating IHS related to beta-lactam antibiotics or NMBA and, depending on laboratories, to RCM and quinolones. Depending on the tested drugs, sensitivity of BAT ranges from 22% to 86% with a good specificity.

The expression of basophil activation markers depends on the clinical entity and the culprit drug. The best marker for basophil activation was obtained in using CD203c for moxifloxacin-allergic patients and CD63 for ciprofloxacin-allergic patients (Fernández et al. 2016).The technique must be done with great caution. For example, due to photodegradation, for the BAT with moxifloxacin, positivity is lower in light (17.9%) than in dark (35.7%) conditions (Mayorga et al. 2013).

18.5.3 Delayed HS to Drugs

Most in vitro tests for diagnosing delayed HS are not available for routine investigation and are not standardized.

18.5.3.1 Lymphocyte Transformation Test

Lymphocyte transformation test is based on the incubation of peripheral blood mononuclear cells (PBMC) with the incriminated drug, then in studying the proliferative response. Proliferation of specific T cells stimulated with the suspected drug is measured by the incorporation of [^{3}H] or carboxyfluorescein diacetate succinimidyl ester content using flow cytometry (Mayorga et al. 2016). Sensitivity and specificity depend on the clinical manifestations (higher in maculopapular exanthema or DRESS than in SJS/TENs). From literature, in SJS/TENs, the sensitivity of LTT response is low, ranged from 11 to 27%. Drug-specific CD8+ T cells are refractory to further stimulation in vitro, similar to "exhausted" CD8+ T cells in HIV or chronic infections. The role of Treg cells is widely discussed in the literature with discordant results from one study to another (Tang et al. 2012; Porebski et al. 2013).

18.5.3.2 Enzyme-Linked Immunosorbent Spot (ELISpot) Assay

ELISpot determines the number of spot forming cells that release cytokines or cytokine markers after activation of PBMC by the suspected drug. For CADR, ELISpot is used for studying the release of interferon, granulysin, and granzyme B (Mayorga et al. 2016). The value of ELISpot interferon gamma has been reported in maculopapular exanthemas due to beta-lactam antibiotics and abacavir hypersensitivity syndrome (Esser et al. 2012).

IFN-gamma ELISpot assay remains positive a long time after the remission of SJS/TEN. From eight patients analyzed in clinical remission of SJS/TENs, IFN-gamma ELISpot was positive. A substantial cultured IFN-g ELISpot response was observed as long as 3 years after TENs occurrence (Fu et al. 2012).

In a case of DRESS finally determined as due to salazopyrin, in a patient with a history of multiple drug use, Phatharacharukul and Klaewsongkram (2013) insisted on the potential interest of interferon-gamma ELISpot achieved during the outbreak, to determine the responsible drug.

18.5.3.3 Cytokine Release

After in vitro drug stimulation, T cells produce inflammatory mediators that can be detected by flow cytometry and ELISA (Mayorga et al. 2016). Interferon gamma, interleukin (IL)-5, and IL-10 have been measured in CADR.

sFasL ELISA was positive in six out of eight patients with SJS/TENs. Its release after restimulation of PBMC by the responsible drug is long-lasting as it has been reported as detectable 2–4 years after disease remission (Fu et al. 2012).

18.5.3.4 Combination of Tests

From PBMC of 19 patients with drug allergy (urticaria, angioedema, and delayed reactions due to miscellaneous drugs), intracellular interleukin (IL)-5, IL-10, and interferon gamma investigated by flow cytometry and their secretion analyzed using ELISA were evaluated. Drug-specific cytokine production was demonstrated in 75% of the patients using flow cytometry and in 79% using ELISA. Combining ELISA and flow cytometry increased the sensitivity to 100% (Martin et al. 2010).

Combine three different cellular assays may help to overcome or bypass the assumed refractoriness of PBMC of SJS/TEN patients. From PBMC of 15 patients with well-defined SJS/TEN (ALDEN score $\geq$ 6) versus 18 controls, 11 assay end points based on drug-induced cell proliferation, cytokine production, and measurement of cell-mediated, drug-induced cytotoxicity by measuring granzyme B secretion (ELISpot) or granulysin production (flow cytometry) were done. No single assay achieved a sufficient sensitivity (max. 53%), but combining three tests enabled to identify the causative drug in 80% (12/15) of patients with a high specificity (95%). To determine causality in SJS/TEN patients, the first choice could be the combination of granulysin expression in CD4 + T cells with granzyme B-ELISpot and interferon-gamma secretion in cell supernatant of LTT. Another combination could be also of value: granulysin in NKp46+ cells, granzyme B-ELISpot, and IFN-gamma secretion in cell supernatant (Porebski et al. 2013).

In conclusion, in order to determine the thresholds for specificity, to evaluate the tolerance, and to compare the results from one center to another, it is time to consider standardizing drug skin testing methods. Reporting results as a concentration of active ingredient for patch tests is essential. For IDT, the only way is to work on a known allergen dose and not on injection-wheal diameters. For drugs, the volume that is now recommended is 0.02 mL to be administered slowly intradermally.

Methods for in vitro testing should be standardized to determine their interest in the routine exploration of CADR. Tryptase levels have to be determined in anaphylactic reactions.

There are too many different methods available to adequately assess the interest of BATs in drug-induced immediate hypersensitivity. Even if standardized, BAT will have to be carried out in laboratories having a great experience of these techniques.

In delayed hypersensitivity, the standardization of in vitro tests is also essential to determine interest during the outbreak or at distance of the CADR of the interferon-gamma ELISpot. For the SJS/TENs, it may be through the combination of several methods that the low reactivity of the CD8 + T cells will be overcome.

References

Andrade P, Brinca A, Gonçalo M (2011) Patch testing in fixed drug eruptions--a 20-year review. Contact Dermatitis 65:195–201

Araujo L, Demoly P (2008) Macrolides allergy. Curr Pharm Des 14:2840–2862

Barbaud A (2014) Skin testing and patch testing in non-IgE-mediated drug allergy. Curr Allergy Asthma Rep 14:442–448

Barbaud A, Collet E, Milpied B, Assier H, Staumont D, Avenel-Audran M et al (2013) A multicenter study to determine the value and safety of drug patch tests for the three main classes of severe cutaneous adverse drug reactions. Br J Dermatol 168:555–562

Barbaud A, Gonçalo M, Bruynzeel D, Bircher A (2001) Guidelines for performing skin tests with drugs in the investigation of cutaneous adverse drug reactions. Contact Dermatitis 45:321–328

Barbaud A, Trechot P, Reichert-Penetrat S, Commun N, Schmutz JL (2001) Relevance of skin tests with drugs in investigating cutaneous adverse drug reactions. Contact Dermatitis 45:265–268

Barbaud A, Waton J (2016) Systemic allergy to corticosteroids: clinical features and cross reactivity. Curr Pharm Des 22:6825–6831

Benucci M, Manfredi M, Demoly P, Campi P (2008) Injection site reactions to TNF-alpha blocking agents with positive skin tests. Allergy 63:138–139

Blanca M, Romano A, Torres MJ, Férnandez J, Mayorga C, Rodriguez J, Demoly P, Bousquet PJ, Merk HF, Sanz ML, Ott H, Atanasković-Marković M (2009) Update on the evaluation of hypersensitivity reactions to betalactams. Allergy 64:183–193

Blanca M, Torres MJ, Garcia JJ, Romano A, Mayorga C, de Ramon E et al (1999) Natural evolution of skin test sensitivity in patients allergic to beta-lactam antibiotics. J Allergy Clin Immunol 103:918–924

Bonadonna P, Lombardo C, Bortolami O, Bircher A, Scherer K, Barbaud A et al (2012) Hypersensitivity to proton pump inhibitors: Diagnostic accuracy of skin tests compared to oral provocation test. J Allergy Clin Immunol 130:547–549

Bousquet J, Heinzerling L, Bachert C, Papadopoulos NG, Bousquet PJ, Burney PG et al (2012) Practical guide to skin prick tests in allergy to aeroallergens. Allergy 67:18–24

Brajon D, Menetre S, Waton J, Poreaux C, Barbaud A (2014) Non-irritant concentrations and amounts of active ingredient in drug patch tests. Contact Dermatitis 71:170–175

Brockow K, Garvey LH, Aberer W, Atanaskovic-Markovic M, Barbaud A, Bilo MB et al (2013) ENDA/EAACI Drug Allergy Interest Group. Skin test concentrations for systemically administered drugs -- an ENDA/EAACI Drug Allergy Interest Group position paper. Allergy 68:702–712

Brockow K, Romano A, Aberer W, Bircher AJ, Barbaud A, Bonadonna P et al (2009) Skin testing in patients with hypersensitivity reactions to iodinated contrast media - a European multicenter study. Allergy 64:234–241

Brockow K, Romano A, Blanca M, Ring J, Pichler W, Demoly P (2002) General considerations for skin test procedures in the diagnosis of drug hypersensitivity. Allergy 57:45–51

Brož P, Harr T, Hecking C, Grize L, Scherer K, Jaeger KA, Bircher AJ (2012) Nonirritant intradermal skin test concentrations of ciprofloxacin, clarithromycin, and rifampicin. Allergy 67:647–652

Conilleau V, Dompmartin A, Michel M, Verneuil L, Leroy D (2000) Photoscratch testing in systemic drug-induced photosensitivity. Photodermatol Photoimmunol Photomed 16:62–66

De Groot AC (2008) Patch testing. In: Test concentrations and vehicles for 4350 chemicals, 3rd edn. Acdegroot Publishing, Wapserveen, the Netherlands, p 456

Esser S, Jablonka R, Heinemann FM, Reuter S, Jaeger H, von Krosigk A, Schenk-Westkamp P, Schadendorf D, Horn PA, Lindemann M (2012) Detection of abacavir hypersensitivity by ELISpot method. Inflamm Allergy Drug Targets 11:227–234

Ewan PW, Dugué P, Mirakian R, Dixon TA, Harper JN, Nasser SM (2010) BSACI guidelines for the investigation of suspected anaphylaxis during general anaesthesia. Clin Exp Allergy 40:15–31

Fernández TD, Ariza A, Palomares F, Montañez MI, Salas M, Martín-Serrano A, Fernández R, Ruiz A, Blanca M, Mayorga C, Torres MJ (2016) Hypersensitivity to fluoroquinolones: The expression of basophil activation markers depends on the clinical entity and the culprit fluoroquinolone. Medicine (Baltimore) 95:e3679

Fréling E, Peyrin-Biroulet L, Poreaux C, Morali A, Waton J, Schmutz JL et al (2015) IgE antibodies and skin tests in immediate hypersensitivity reactions to infliximab in inflammatory bowel disease: impact on infliximab retreatment. Eur J Gastroenterol Hepatol 27:1200–1208

Fu M, Gao Y, Pan Y, Li W, Liao W, Wang G, Li C, Li C, Gao T, Liu Y (2012) Recovered patients with Stevens-Johnson syndrome and toxic epidermal necrolysis maintain long-lived IFN-γ and sFasL memory response. PLoS One 7:e45516

Gomes E, Pichler W, Demoly P et al (2004) The drug ambassador project: the diversity of diagnostic procedures for drug allergy around. Europe J World Allergy Organ 17:1–10

Gonçalo M, Ferguson J, Bonevalle A, Bruynzeel DP, Giménez-Arnau A, Goossens A et al (2013) Photopatch testing: recommendations for a European photopatch test baseline series. Contact Dermatitis 68:239–243

Guyot-Caquelin P, Granel F, Kaminsky MC, Trechot P, Schmutz JL, Barbaud A (2010) False positive results can occur on delayed reading of intradermal tests with cisplatin. J Allergy Clin Immunol 125:1410–1411

Hjortlund J, Mortz CG, Skov PS, Bindslev-Jensen C (2013) Diagnosis of penicillin allergy revisited: the value of case history, skin testing, specific IgE and prolonged challenge. Allergy 68:1057–1064

Indradat S, Veskitkul J, Pacharn P, Jirapongsananuruk O, Visitsunthorn N, Indradat S (2016) Provocation proven drug allergy in Thai children with adverse drug reactions. Asian Pac J Allergy Immunol 34:59–64

Johansen JD, Aalto-Korte K, Agner T, Andersen KE, Bircher A, Bruze M et al (2015) European Society of Contact Dermatitis guideline for diagnostic patch testing - recommendations on best practice. Contact Dermatitis 73:195–221

Kleinhans M, Linzbach L, Zedlitz S, Kaufmann R, Boehncke WH (2002) Positive patch test reactions to celecoxib may be due to irritation and do not correlate with the results of oral provocation. Contact Dermatitis 47:100–102

Kuyucu S, Mori F, Atanaskovic-Markovic M, Caubet JC, Terreehorst I, Gomes E et al (2014) Hypersensitivity reactions to non-betalactam antibiotics in children: an extensive review. Pediatr Allergy Immunol 25:534–543

Leguy-Seguin V, Jolimoy G, Coudert B, Pernot C, Dalac S, Vabres P et al (2007) Diagnostic and predictive value of skin testing in platinum salt hypersensitivity. J Allergy Clin Immunol 119:726–730

Lerondeau B, Trechot P, Waton J, Poreaux C, Luc A, Schmutz JL, Paris C, Barbaud A (2016) Analysis of cross-reactivity among radiocontrast media in 97 hypersensitivity reactions. J Allergy Clin Immunol 137:633–635

Lobera T, Audícana MT, Alarcón E, Longo N, Navarro B, Muñoz D (2010) Allergy to quinolones: low cross-reactivity to levofloxacin. J Investig Allergol Clin Immunol 20:607–611

Martin M, Wurpts G, Ott H, Baron JM, Erdmann S, Merk HF, Sachs B (2010) In vitro detection and characterization of drug hypersensitivity using flow cytometry. Allergy 65:32–39

Mayorga C, Andreu I, Aranda A, Doña I, Montañez MI, Blanca-Lopez N, Ariza A, Nuin E, Blanca M, Miranda MA, Torres MJ (2013) Fluoroquinolone photodegradation influences specific basophil activation. Int Arch Allergy Immunol 160:377–382

Mayorga C, Celik G, Rouzaire P, Whitaker P, Bonadonna P, Rodrigues-Cernadas J, Vultaggio A, Brockow K, Caubet JC, Makowska J, Nakonechna A, Romano A, Montañez MI, Laguna JJ, Zanoni G, Gueant JL, Oude Elberink H, Fernandez J, Viel S, Demoly P, Torres MJ, In vitro tests for Drug Allergy Task Force of EAACI Drug Interest Group (2016) In vitro tests for drug hypersensitivity reactions: an ENDA/EAACI Drug Allergy Interest Group position paper. Allergy 71:1103–1134

Mertes PM, Laxenaire MC, Lienhart A, Aberer W, Ring J, Pichler WJ, Demoly P (2005) Reducing the risk of anaphylaxis during anaesthesia: guidelines for clinical practice. J Investig Allergol Clin Immunol 15:91–101

Mertes PM, Malinovsky JM, Jouffroy L, Working Group of the SFAR and SFA, Aberer W, Terreehorst I, Brockow K, Demoly P, ENDA; EAACI Interest Group on Drug Allergy (2011) Reducing the risk of anaphylaxis during anesthesia: 2011 updated guidelines for clinical practice. J Investig Allergol Clin Immunol 21:442–453

Mori F, Barni S, Pucci N, Rossi E, Azzari C, de Martino M, Novembre E (2010) Sensitivity and specificity of skin tests in the diagnosis of clarithromycin allergy. Ann Allergy Asthma Immunol 104:417–419

Patel A, Bahna SL (2015) Immediate hypersensitivity reactions to corticosteroids. Ann Allergy Asthma Immunol 115:178–182

Perrin-Lamarre A, Petitpain N, Trechot P, Cuny JF, Schmutz JL, Barbaud A (2010) Toxidermies aux glycopeptides. Résultats du bilan immuno-allergologique dans une série de huit cas. Ann Dermatol Venereol 137:101–105

Phatharacharukul P, Klaewsongkram J (2013) A case of sulfasalazine-induced hypersensitivity syndrome confirmed by enzyme-linked immunospot assay. Allergy Asthma Immunol Res 5:415–417

Poreaux C, Bronowicki JP, Debouverie M, Schmutz JL, Waton J, Barbaud A (2014) Managing generalized interferon-induced eruptions and the effectiveness of desensitization. Clin Exp Allergy 44:756–764

Porebski G, Pecaric-Petkovic T, Groux-Keller M, Bosak M, Kawabata TT, Pichler WJ (2013) In vitro drug causality assessment in Stevens-Johnson syndrome - alternatives for lymphocyte transformation test. Clin Exp Allergy 43:1027–1037

Romano A, Gaeta F, Valluzzi RL, Zaffiro A, Caruso C, Quaratino D (2014) Natural evolution of skin-test sensitivity in patients with IgE-mediated hypersensitivity to cephalosporins. Allergy 69:806–809

Santiago F, Gonçalo M, Vieira R, Coelho S, Figueiredo A (2010) Epicutaneous patch testing in drug hypersensitivity syndrome (DRESS). Contact Dermatitis 62:47–53

Scherer K, Tsakiris DA, Bircher AJ (2008) Hypersensitivity reactions to anticoagulant drugs. Curr Pharm Des 14:2863–2873

Soria A, Baeck M, Goossens A, Marot L, Duveille V, Derouaux AS et al (2011) Patch, prick or intradermal tests to detect delayed hypersensitivity to corticosteroids? Contact Dermatitis 64:313–324

Tang YH, Mockenhaupt M, Henry A, Bounoua M, Naldi L, Le Gouvello S, Bensussan A, Roujeau JC (2012) Poor relevance of a lymphocyte proliferation assay in lamotrigine-induced Stevens-Johnson syndrome or toxic epidermal necrolysis. Clin Exp Allergy 42:248–254

Torres MJ, Romano A, Celik G, Demoly P, Khan DA, Macy E, Park M, Blumenthal K, Aberer W, Castells M, Barbaud A, Mayorga C, Bonadonna P (2017) Approach to the diagnosis of drug hypersensitivity reactions: similarities and differences between Europe and North America. Clin Transl Allergy 7:7. https://doi.org/10.1186/s13601-017-0144-0

Ulrich G, Schmutz JL, Trechot P, Commun N, Barbaud A (2004) Sensitization to petrolatum: an unusual cause of false-positive drug patch-tests. Allergy 59:1006–1009

Waton J (2011) L'allergie à l'insuline: mise au point. Rev Fr Allergologie 51:336–342

19 Pharmacovigilance of Cutaneous Adverse Drug Reactions

Lois La Grenade, Maja Mockenhaupt, and Elizabeth Phillips

Abbreviations

AGEP	Acute generalized exanthematous pustulosis
cADRs	Cutaneous adverse drug reactions
DRESS	Drug reaction with eosinophilia and systemic symptoms
ED	Emergency department
EEMM	Erythema exsudativum multiforme majus
EuroSCAR	European severe cutaneous adverse reaction
FAERS	FDA Adverse Event Reporting System
FDA	US Food and Drug Administration
iSAEC	International Serious Adverse Events Consortium
MedDRA	Medical Dictionary for Regulatory Activities
MGPS	Multi-item gamma poisson shrinker

L. La Grenade (✉)
Division of Pharmacovigilance, Office of Surveillance and Epidemiology, Center for Drug Evaluation and Research, US Food and Drug Administration, Silver Spring, MD, USA
e-mail: Lois.LaGrenade@fda.hhs.gov

M. Mockenhaupt
Department of Dermatology, Medical Center and Medical Faculty, Dokumentationszentrum schwerer Hautreaktionen (dZh), University of Freiburg, Freiburg, Germany
e-mail: dzh@uniklinik-freiburg.de

E. Phillips
Institute for Immunology and Infectious Diseases, Murdoch University, Murdoch, WA, Australia

Vanderbilt University Medical Center, Nashville, TN, USA
e-mail: elizabeth.j.phillips@vanderbilt.edu

N. H. Shear, R. P. Dodiuk-Gad (eds.), *Advances in Diagnosis and Management of Cutaneous Adverse Drug Reactions*, https://doi.org/10.1007/978-981-13-1489-6_19

NEISS-CADES	National Electronic Injury Surveillance System-Cooperative Adverse Drug Event Surveillance System
SCAR	Severe cutaneous adverse reactions
SJS/TEN	Stevens–Johnson syndrome/toxic epidermal necrolysis
WHO	World Health Organization

Key Points

- Pharmacosurveillance of cADRs involves both pharmacovigilance and pharmacoepidemiology.
- Pharmacovigilance involves monitoring for adverse events, usually via passive surveillance systems and assessing reports for diagnostic validity and causality criteria.
- Pharmacoepidemiology usually involves active surveillance and can provide population based data such as incidence and risk factors.
- The goal of pharmacosurveillance of cADRs is to reduce the incidence of cADRs.
- Publication and dissemination of analyses and studies help achieve this goal.

19.1 Introduction

Pharmacosurveillance of cutaneous adverse drug reactions (cADRs) involves monitoring for these events in populations exposed to therapeutic drugs and drug products and biologic agents. Pharmacosurveillance may be subdivided into two main categories: (1) pharmacovigilance, which involves the use of traditional surveillance systems—passive (also known as spontaneous) and active—and (2) pharmacoepidemiology, the application of epidemiologic methods to detecting and quantifying adverse reactions and their impact on populations (Fig. 19.1). The term pharmacosurveillance implies ongoing systematic collection and analysis of data and timely dissemination of the results, in order to reduce or prevent the occurrence of adverse drug reactions.

Cutaneous reactions are the most frequently occurring adverse drug reaction, and the most common ones are milder and generally detected early in the life of a drug—often during the clinical trials. Pharmacosurveillance for cADRs therefore primarily targets the more severe cADRs such as Stevens–Johnson syndrome/toxic epidermal necrolysis (SJS/TEN), acute generalized exanthematous pustulosis (AGEP), and drug reaction with eosinophilia and systemic symptoms (DRESS), collectively often referred to as severe cutaneous adverse reactions (SCAR). All three are rare and consequently not often detected during clinical trials, which tend to enroll relatively small numbers of people, usually from selected populations. The remainder of this section will therefore focus on pharmacosurveillance of SCAR.

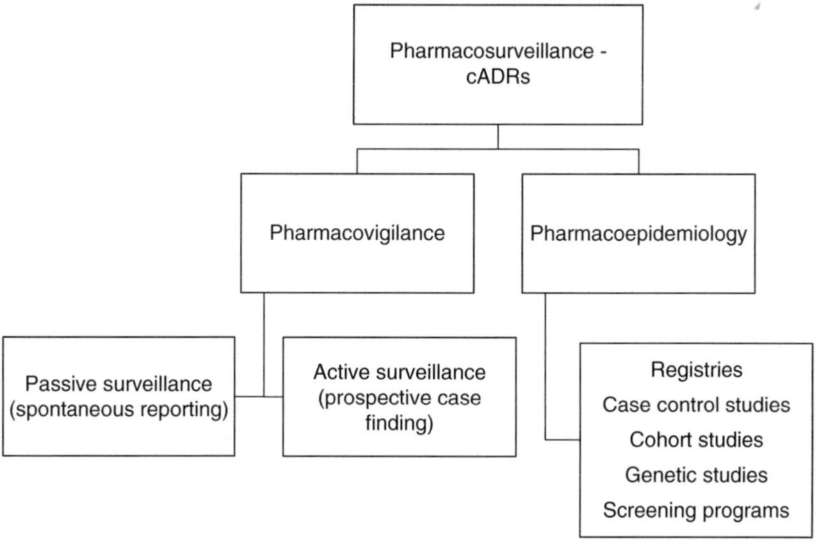

Fig. 19.1 Summary of pharmacosurveillance methods for cutaneous adverse drug reactions

19.2 Spontaneous Reporting Systems

Spontaneous reporting systems rely on voluntarily reported adverse events and are well suited for the detection of rare adverse reactions with a short latency period. Thus they are particularly well suited for detecting SCAR. It is worth noting that the term "event" rather than "reaction" is used to indicate reports submitted to a spontaneous database, before analysis and causality assessment. The term "reaction" is used once a causal relationship has been established. Another advantage of most spontaneous systems is that they are inclusive: all ages and all marketed drugs, for all indications, are included. The US Food and Drug Administration (FDA) Adverse Event Reporting System (FAERS) is an example of a spontaneous reporting system as also is the World Health Organization's (WHO) VigiBase® system. Adverse events in these systems are coded using the Medical Dictionary for Regulatory Activities (MedDRA) terminology, and the product names are standardized using the FAERS Product Dictionary or the WHO Drug Dictionary. The FDA has specially trained healthcare professionals dedicated to monitoring and analyzing the system, and signals for severe adverse events, including SCAR, have a very high priority. Detection of a SCAR signal immediately triggers a systematic search not only of FAERS itself but also of the medical literature and other similar databases including VigiBase®, which includes reports from participating national pharmacovigilance centers around the world. A careful analysis of all reports ensues with particular attention paid to the strength of evidence supporting the diagnosis and causality assessment. A review is then written with the results of the analysis. Further action by the agency depends on the results of all analyses and may include further monitoring, labeling changes including warnings in the more compelling instances, issuing drug safety communications, and sometimes publications in medical journals. Occasionally, the development of SCAR post marketing has even led to drug withdrawal from the market. Detection of SCAR during clinical trials may halt further drug development or if approved may result in the highest type of warning in the product's labeling—a boxed warning for SCAR.

Because FAERS and VigiBase® are large databases, containing more than 13 million reports each, additional methods may be used to assist in signal detection. Data mining is one such method. The data mining software used by FDA utilizes the Multi-item Gamma Poisson Shrinker (MGPS) data mining algorithm. Potential signals generated are then evaluated and analyzed with further action depending on the results. Although signals for SCAR are usually detected early, data mining may sometimes be useful for detecting other cADRs that are not as rare as SCAR.

But spontaneous reporting systems have limitations. Because reporting is voluntary, there is substantial underreporting, and there is no measure of the population exposed to drugs, so they cannot be used to estimate incidence as neither the numerator nor the denominator is known.

19.3 Active Surveillance

Pharmacoepidemiology methods, sometimes incorporating active surveillance, have therefore been used in some countries (Table 19.1). The best and earliest examples of this are the studies undertaken in European countries in the 1980s, retrospective studies on SJS and TEN in France and Germany (Roujeau et al. 1990; Schöpf et al. 1991), and, in the 1990s and 2000s, case-control studies like the SCAR and EuroSCAR study (Roujeau et al. 1995; Mockenhaupt et al. 2008). In parallel, the German registry on severe skin reactions was established, which due to its population-based approach was (and still is) able to calculate disease incidence (Sidoroff et al. 2007). As a prerequisite for these studies, a consensus definition of the clinical pattern of SJS and TEN was established.

The SCAR study was an international case-control study of SJS/TEN in which case ascertainment was prospective and as complete as possible, with the diagnosis adjudicated by an expert panel of dermatologists based on the consensus definition. Participating countries were France, Germany, Italy, and Portugal, and cases were collected over a 6-year period from 1989 to 1995. EuroSCAR was the following case-control surveillance study recruiting cases from 1997 to 2001. Case collection was expanded to include AGEP, and participating countries included Austria, France, Germany, Israel, Italy, and the Netherlands (Mockenhaupt et al. 2008; Rzany et al. 1996). RegiSCAR, the current study on SCAR, started in Europe but expanded also to countries outside Europe such as Taiwan and South Africa (International Registry on Severe Cutaneous Adverse Reactions to Drugs and Collection of Biological Samples) (Sekula et al. 2013). All cases ascertained by the German registry are included into RegiSCAR, and DRESS is investigated as a new entity of SCAR (Kardaun et al. 2013). The aims of RegiSCAR are to provide

Table 19.1 Key milestones in pharmacosurveillance of cutaneous adverse drug reactions

	Authors	Publication year	Journal	Article title
1	Roujeau JC, Guillaume JC, Fabre JP et al.	1990	*Archives of Dermatology*	Toxic epidermal necrolysis (Lyell syndrome). Incidence and drug etiology in France, 1981–1985
2	Schöpf E, Stühmer A, Rzany B et al.	1991	*Archives of Dermatology*	Toxic epidermal necrolysis and Stevens–Johnson syndrome. An epidemiologic study from West Germany
3	Roujeau JC, Kelly JP, Naldi L et al.	1995	*New England Journal of Medicine*	Medication use and the risk of Stevens–Johnson syndrome or toxic epidermal necrolysis
4	Mockenhaupt M, Viboud C, Dunant A et al.	2008	*Journal of Investigative Dermatology*	Stevens–Johnson syndrome and toxic epidermal necrolysis: assessment of medication risks with emphasis on recently marketed drugs. The EuroSCAR study
5	Sidoroff A, Dunant A, Viboud C et al.	2007	*British Journal of Dermatology*	Risk factors for acute generalized exanthematous pustulosis (AGEP)—results of a multinational case-control study (EuroSCAR)
6	Rzany B, Mockenhaupt M, Baur S et al.	1996	*Journal of Clinical Epidemiology*	Epidemiology of erythema exsudativum multiforme majus (EEMM), Stevens–Johnson syndrome (SJS) and toxic epidermal necrolysis (TEN) in Germany (1990–1992). Structure and results of a population-based registry
7	Sekula P, Dunant A, Mockenhaupt M et al.	2013	*Journal of Investigative Dermatology*	Comprehensive survival analysis of a cohort of patients with Stevens–Johnson syndrome and toxic epidermal necrolysis
8	Kardaun SH, Sekula P, Valeyrie-Allanore L, et al.	2013	*British Journal of Dermatology*	Drug reaction with eosinophilia and systemic symptoms (DRESS): an original multisystem adverse drug reaction. Results from the prospective RegiSCAR study
9	Chung WH, Hung SI, Hong HS, et al.	2004	*Nature*	Medical genetics: a marker for Stevens–Johnson syndrome
10	Sassolas B, Haddad C, Mockenhaupt M, Dunant A et al.	2010	*Clinical Pharmacology and Therapeutics*	ALDEN, an algorithm for assessment of drug causality in Stevens–Johnson syndrome and toxic epidermal necrolysis: comparison with case-control analysis
11	Chen P, Lin JJ, Lu CS et al., Taiwan SJS Consortium	2011	*New England Journal of Medicine*	Carbamazepine-induced toxic effects and HLA-B*1502 screening in Taiwan
12	Sukasem C, Chantratita W.	2016	*Pharmacogenomics*	A success story in pharmacogenomics: genetic ID card for SJS/TEN

continued pharmacosurveillance for SCAR, particularly for new drugs as they come on the market, and also to investigate genetic and other biologic risk factors. This research has contributed an enormous body of knowledge on the epidemiology of SCAR and provides a model for other researchers in the field. However, such active surveillance studies are expensive and time and resource intensive, so replication in other settings may not always be feasible.

A more practical approach may involve targeted active surveillance:

- Targeted to specific drugs, especially early in marketing, and particularly if other drugs in the class have been associated with the development of SCAR
- Targeted to a specific setting such as emergency units, hospitals, intensive care units, or burn units, where SCAR patients are more likely to be treated
- Targeted to specific populations, for example, children or the elderly
- Targeted to patients suffering from specific disorders

The literature abounds with examples of these types of studies (Hamilton and Fish 2013) not only done by active prospective collection of data but also by retrospective data ascertainment. Although prospective data collection is more accurate, retrospective studies do add information and should not be totally discounted.

The FDA also has access to active surveillance data for adverse drug events in the emergency department (ED) setting in the United States. It is the National Electronic Injury Surveillance System-Cooperative Adverse Drug Event Surveillance System (NEISS-CADES). It is a nationally representative survey of approximately 60 hospitals in the United States (Jhung et al. 2007) that has been ongoing since 2004 and is useful for estimating incidence and other characteristics of rare adverse events such as SCAR.

Targeted surveillance by North American groups aimed at quantifying the disease burden and identifying risk factors for SCAR is currently underway and beginning to yield results. The Canadian Pharmacogenomics Network for Drug Safety in 2011 confirmed HLA biomarkers for cADRs to carbamazepine in children (Castro-Pastrana et al. 2011) and is continuing work with other drugs and populations. In the United States, there have been two recent workshops on SCAR—the first in March 2015 organized by the National Institutes of Health's National Human Genome Research Institute (https://www.genome.gov/27560487/) and the second in March 2017 by Vanderbilt University (https://ww2.mc.vanderbilt.edu/sjsmeeting/). These have contributed to a resurgence of interest in SCAR research. Two associations so far are leading the way in targeted hospital surveillance and research: the American Burn Association and the Society of Dermatology Hospitalists. Members of both these groups are responsible for the management of the majority of US cases of SCAR.

19.4 Genetic Screening for Susceptibility to SCAR

Public health screening has long been a tool used to detect early disease or disease markers and to reduce or eliminate diseases. The discovery of genetic markers of susceptibility to SCAR starting in 2004 with the identification of the association between the HLA B*1502 allele and an increased risk of developing carbamazepine-induced SJS/TEN opened the door for the use of genetic screening in some populations (Chung et al. 2004; Chen et al. 2011). Since then several other alleles have been found to be risk factors for SJS/TEN and DRESS, with specific drugs. The highest prevalence of these alleles has so far been reported in Southeast Asian countries, which also have a relatively high incidence of SJS/TEN. The high prevalence of the HLA alleles and their strong association with carbamazepine-induced SJS/TEN have made the introduction in those countries of screening programs very cost-effective and successful in reducing the incidence of SJS/TEN with these drugs. In the United States, the FDA recommends pretreatment screening for specific alleles in patients of Southeast Asian ancestry. Genetic screening has not yet proven to be cost-effective in populations with low allele frequency but may become more useful in the future as other risk factors are identified.

The search for other genetic risk factors worldwide is already underway but is still in its infancy. One group currently working on this is the international Serious Adverse Events Consortium (iSAEC). It was formed in 2007 and comprises representatives from nine pharmaceutical companies in the United States, Europe, and Japan along with two information technology companies, a major US hospital network, and the Wellcome Trust. iSAEC's mission is to identify DNA variants that may be risk factors for developing drug-induced serious adverse events, including SJS/TEN. To date the group has published a paper establishing phenotype standardization criteria and collected samples from several hundred cases of SJS/TEN. Genome-wide association studies have begun, but sample sizes are still too small for valid analysis (Pirmohamed M, 2015, Research Directions in Genetically-Mediated Stevens–Johnson Syndrome/Toxic Epidermal Necrolysis—https://www.genome.gov/27560487/). The National Institutes of Health in the United States and other academic centers are also interested in undertaking genetic studies, and preliminary work in this area is underway.

19.5 Future of Pharmacosurveillance-Big Data Analysis

Advances in computer capabilities and the availability of large databases containing electronic medical and pharmacy data are currently being investigated for use in surveillance for ADRs, including cADRs. This may require more accurate use of current ICD codes for SCAR and/or the development of algorithms for text searching of narratives (Davis et al. 2015). The combined use of ICD codes and algorithms may also increase the accuracy of identifying SCAR in such databases. The FDA now has an active surveillance system using such electronic health systems—Sentinel. However, because it is based on electronic health and pharmacy records, it has not yet proven to be useful for SCAR and awaits the development of more accurate methods of identifying SCAR cases in such databases.

In summary, spontaneous reporting systems remain the cornerstone of pharmacosurveillance for early, rapid identification of SCAR. Active surveillance and other pharmacoepidemiology studies also have a role but are more important in the long-term characterization and prevention of SCAR.

References

Castro-Pastrana LI, Ghannadan R, Rieder MJ, Dahlke E, Hayden M, Carleton B (2011) Cutaneous adverse drug reactions in children: an analysis of reports from the Canadian Pharmacogenomics Network for Drug Safety (CPNDS). J Popul Ther Clin Pharmacol 18:e106–e120

Chen P, Lin JJ, Lu CS, Ong CT, Hsieh PF, Yang CC, Tai CT, Wu SL, Lu CH, Hsu YC, Yu HY, Ro LS, Lu CT, Chu CC, Tsai JJ, Su YH, Lan SH, Sung SF, Lin SY, Chuang HP, Huang LC, Chen YJ, Tsai PJ, Liao HT, Lin YH, Chen CH, Chung WH, Hung SI, Wu JY, Chang CF, Chen L, Chen YT, Shen CY, Taiwan SJS Consortium (2011) Carbamazepine-induced toxic effects and HLA-B*1502 screening in Taiwan. N Engl J Med 364(12):1126–1133

Chung WH, Hung SI, Hong HS, Hsih MS, Yang LC, Ho HC, Wu JY, Chen YT (2004) Medical genetics: a marker for Stevens-Johnson syndrome. Nature 428(6982):486

Davis RL, Gallagher MA, Asgari MM, Eide MJ, Margolis DJ, Macy E, Burmester JK, Selvam N, Boscarino JA, Cromwell LF, Feigelson HS, Kuntz JL, Pawloski PA, Penfold RB, Raebel MA, Sridhar G, Wu A, La Grenade LA, Pacanowski MA, Pinheiro SP (2015) Identification of Stevens-Johnson syndrome and toxic epidermal necrolysis in electronic health record databases. Pharmacoepidemiol Drug Saf 24(7):684–692

Hamilton GM, Fish J (2013) Pediatric toxic epidermal necrolysis: an institutional review of patients admitted to an intensive care unit. J Burn Care Res 34(6):e351–e358

Jhung MA, Budnitz DS, Mendelsohn AB, Weidenbach KN, Nelson TD, Pollock DA (2007) Evaluation and overview of the National Electronic Injury Surveillance System-Cooperative Adverse Drug Event Surveillance Project (NEISS-CADES). Med Care 45(10 Suppl 2):S96–S102

Kardaun SH, Sekula P, Valeyrie-Allanore L, Liss Y, Chu CY, Creamer D, Sidoroff A, Naldi L, Mockenhaupt M, Roujeau JC, RegiSCAR study group (2013) Drug reaction with eosinophilia and systemic symptoms (DRESS): an original multisystem adverse drug reaction. Results from the prospective RegiSCAR study. Br J Dermatol 169(5):1071–1080

Mockenhaupt M, Viboud C, Dunant A, Naldi L, Halevy S, Bouwes Bavinck JN, Sidoroff A, Schneck J, Roujeau JC, Flahault A (2008) Stevens-Johnson syndrome and toxic epidermal necrolysis: assessment of medication risks with emphasis on recently marketed drugs. The EuroSCAR-study. J Invest Dermatol 128(1):35–44

Roujeau JC, Guillaume JC, Fabre JP, Penso D, Fléchet ML, Girre JP (1990) Toxic epidermal necrolysis (Lyell syndrome). Incidence and drug etiology in France, 1981-1985. Arch Dermatol 126(1):37–42

Roujeau JC, Kelly JP, Naldi L, Rzany B, Stern RS, Anderson T, Auquier A, Bastuji-Garin S, Correia O, Locati F et al (1995) Medication use and the risk of Stevens-Johnson syndrome or toxic epidermal necrolysis. N Engl J Med 333(24):1600–1607

Rzany B, Mockenhaupt M, Baur S, Schröder W, Stocker U, Mueller J, Holländer N, Bruppacher R, Schöpf E (1996) Epidemiology of erythema exsudativum multiforme majus, Stevens-Johnson syndrome, and toxic epidermal necrolysis in Germany (1990-1992): structure and results of a population-based registry. J Clin Epidemiol 49(7):769–773

Schöpf E, Stühmer A, Rzany B, Victor N, Zentgraf R, Kapp JF (1991) Toxic epidermal necrolysis and Stevens-Johnson syndrome. An epidemiologic study from West Germany. Arch Dermatol 127(6):839–842

Sekula P, Dunant A, Mockenhaupt M, Naldi L, Bouwes Bavinck JN, Halevy S, Kardaun S, Sidoroff A, Liss Y, Schumacher M, Roujeau JC, RegiSCAR study group (2013) Comprehensive survival analysis of a cohort of patients with Stevens-Johnson syndrome and toxic epidermal necrolysis. J Invest Dermatol 133(5):1197–1204

Sidoroff A, Dunant A, Viboud C, Halevy S, Bavinck JN, Naldi L, Mockenhaupt M, Fagot JP, Roujeau JC (2007) Risk factors for acute generalized exanthematous pustulosis (AGEP)-results of a multinational case-control study (EuroSCAR). Br J Dermatol 157(5):989–996

Part V

Epilogue

Future Directions and Unmet Research Needs in Cutaneous Adverse Drug Reactions

20

Elizabeth Ergen, Jason Trubiano, Jonny Peter, and Elizabeth Phillips

Abbreviations

ADR	Adverse drug reactions
cADR	Cutaneous adverse drugs reactions
DIHS	Drug-induced hypersensitivity syndrome
DRESS	Drug reaction with eosinophilia and systemic symptoms
ELISpot	Enzyme-Linked Immunosorbent Spot
HLA	Human leukocyte antigen
IM-ADRs	Immunologically mediated ADRs
NNT	Number needed to test
NPV	Negative predictive value
PBMCs	Peripheral blood mononuclear cells
PPV	Positive predictive value
SCAR	Severe cutaneous adverse reactions
SJS/TEN	Stevens-Johnson syndrome/toxic epidermal necrolysis

E. Ergen
University of Alabama, Birmingham, AL, USA
e-mail: eergen@uabmc.edu

J. Trubiano
Austin Health, Heidelberg, VIC, Australia

J. Peter
University of Cape Town and Groote Schuur Hospital, Cape Town, South Africa
e-mail: jonny.peter@uct.ac.za

E. Phillips (✉)
Institute for Immunology and Infectious Diseases, Murdoch University, Murdoch, WA, Australia

Vanderbilt University Medical Center, Nashville, TN, USA
e-mail: elizabeth.j.phillips@vanderbilt.edu

N. H. Shear, R. P. Dodiuk-Gad (eds.), *Advances in Diagnosis and Management of Cutaneous Adverse Drug Reactions*, https://doi.org/10.1007/978-981-13-1489-6_20

Overview

- What breakthroughs have occurred in the last 10–20 years?
- What might the future look like?
- What are the present challenges in prevention, early diagnosis, and treatment?

Case Presentation

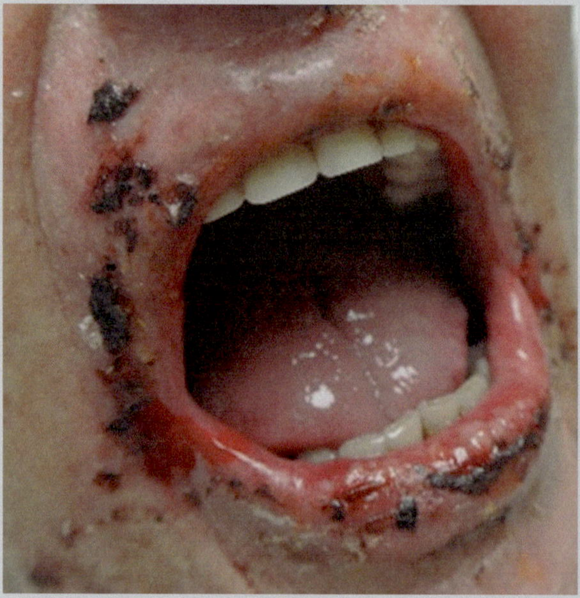

You are called about a 64-year-old female with a 3-day history of facial erythema and edema, conjunctival injection, blistering of her lips and oral mucosa, and a violaceous-erythematous exanthem on her trunk and extremities. She cannot tell you what medications she has been taking at home. Since being hospitalized, she has had intermittent fevers and was started on three new anti-infectives (vancomycin, piperacillin/tazobactam, and amphotericin B) in the past 2 weeks. She has acute myeloid leukemia and completed induction chemotherapy (doxorubicin and cytarabine) 1 week ago. She has a history of HSV-1 infection. Labs reveal normal liver and kidney function and expected cytopenias following induction chemotherapy. A chest X-ray reveals bilateral interstitial pulmonary infiltrates. Someone has already added vancomycin, piperacillin/tazobactam, and amphotericin to her list of allergies. The patient tells you she is afraid to ever take these medications again.

20.1 Pharmacogenomic Advances

In relation to the case above, a key question is: What knowledge about the genetic makeup of the individual could have prevented the reaction in question?

A key paradigm shift has been the discovery of strong associations between the human leukocyte antigen (HLA) and SCARs such as DRESS and SJS/TEN. Although some of the first associations between HLA and SCARs were described in the 1980s and 1990s such as HLA-B*58 and allopurinol (Chan and Tan 1989), the extremely strong association between HLA-B*57:01 and abacavir hypersensitivity by two independent groups in 2002 marked a new era of discovery that was facilitated by high-resolution HLA typing (Hetherington et al. 2002; Mallal et al. 2002). The utility of such findings and ultimate generalizability and widespread translation of HLA-B*57:01 into clinical practice was made possible by the use of adjunctive testing such as patch testing to define true immunologically mediated abacavir hypersensitivity (Saag et al. 2008; Mallal et al. 2008). The success of this was facilitated by the 100% negative predictive value (NPV) of HLA-B*57:01 screening but also by the fact that 55% of those carrying HLA-B*57:01 developed abacavir hypersensitivity meaning that only 30 patients would need to be screened to prevent one case, making this highly cost effective (Mallal et al. 2008). A key discovery following this in 2004 by Chung et al. was the association between HLA-B*15:02 and carbamazepine-induced SJS/TEN in Taiwanese, followed by studies that validated this association across other South and Southeast Asian populations (Chung et al. 2004). Since 2004, strong associations are being reported between other HLA alleles and other CADRs (Hung et al. 2005; Hung et al. 2006; Chung et al. 2014).

Not all CADR will be associated with genetic inheritance of HLA antigens. Non-IgE-mediated mast cell activation, with a clinical phenotype of flushing, urticaria, and angioedema, is now known to be due to inheritance of a specific mas-related G-protein coupled receptor on mast cells (MRGPRX2) which interacts with drugs containing a tetrahydroisoquinoline motif, like fluoroquinolones and neuromuscular blocking agents (McNeil et al. 2015). Other CADRs represent drug-infection interactions which may not occur on re-exposure to the drug. Yet other CADRs are associated with inheritance of specific alleles of drug-metabolizing enzymes (Tassaneeyakul et al. 2016). Still others represent off-target, non-immunologically mediated, effects of drugs with an undefined genetic basis.

A challenge for health systems will be deciding when and how to enact systems-wide programs to prevent CADR due to known genetic associations. Screening programs for HLA-B*15:02 led to near elimination of carbamazepine-SJS/TEN in Singapore (Toh et al. 2014). However, in Hong Kong the same testing resulted in an increase in phenytoin prescriptions and an increase in phenytoin-SJS/TEN with no net change in the incidence of SJS/TEN (Chen et al. 2014). Genetic screening has not been routinely implemented to prevent allopurinol-DRESS and allopurinol-SJS/TEN (due to HLA-B*58:01). Some barriers include the lack of a widely available, affordable, safe, and effective alternative agent for gout and a high number of individuals needing to be screened (200–1000) to prevent one case. Since patients with renal failure are at significantly higher risk of allopurinol SCAR, it has been suggested that implementation of screening should be targeted to patients with impaired renal function.

After accounting for all known genetic risk factors, it is still not possible to predict who will develop a CADR when exposed to a certain drug. This **positive predictive gap** (Table 20.1) might mean there are other genetic associations to be discovered or that there are other important cofactors that account for individual risk.

20.2 An Integrated Omics Approach

A more comprehensive approach to CADR would look how an individual's unique combination of genome, epigenome, transcriptome, proteome, metabolome, phenome, and exposome impacts their risk of CADR.

Epigenomic changes contribute to the variability in drug disposition, response, and toxicity. For example, Pan et al. in 2013 published data linking hsa-miR-1291-directed downregulation on ABCC1 to an increase in the intracellular accumulation of doxorubicin and an increase in chemosensitivity to the drug (Pan et al. 2013). In the case presented, it could be hypothesized that such an epigenetic modification, present in affected skin and mucosa (but not unaffected tissues), accounts for the tissue specificity of her adverse drug reaction. In the future, epigenome-wide association studies done on CADR cases and drug-tolerant controls, as well as affected and unaffected tissue, might provide information on all epigenetic modifications associated with CADR. In the subcategory of immunologically mediated ADRs (IM-ADRs), it would not be surprising if some of these modifications regulate immune responses. Finally, because epigenetic changes can be induced and reversed with drugs (decitabine, azacitidine), this research might provide a therapeutic target.

Transcriptomic, proteomic, and metabolomic changes in cells, tissues, and organs affected by CADR can yield new biomarkers for diagnosis/prognosis and give insight into mechanisms of disease pathogenesis. In 2008 a gene microarray study on blood and blister fluid from patients with SJS/TEN suggested that high-level transcription of a cytolytic protein called granulysin might be a signature of SJS/TEN (Chung et al. 2008). This is now being translated into development of a serum granulysin assay for clinical use in distinguishing SJS/TEN from other benign exanthems. In 2010, work by Bellon et al. characterized gene expression profiles in peripheral blood mononuclear cells (PBMCs) during the acute and resolution phase of CADRs and found that non-bullous and bullous reactions clustered separately (Bellon et al. 2010). We can imagine a future when mRNA extracted from a skin biopsy or blood of a CADR patient will be analyzed and matched with the signature of a specific CADR phenotype induced by a certain drug, aiding in earlier diagnosis and treatment. A challenge for researchers will be to define mRNA signatures for all CADRs. These patterns could ultimately provide insights into mechanisms.

Ecology and exposome, including drug exposures and infectious exposures, remote and proximal, are also important risk factors for CADR. It is possible

Table 20.1 Characteristics of HLA testing for CADR and implementation

Drug	HLA allele	HLA carriage rate	Disease prevalence	OR	NPV	PPV	NNT to prevent "1"	Clinical implementation	Single allele assay available
Abacavir Hypersensitivity syndrome	B*57:01	5–8% Caucasian <1% African/Asia 2.5% African American	8% (3% true HSR and 2–7% false positive diagnosis)	960	100% for patch test confirmed	55%	13	Guideline-based screening since 2008[a,b] (White et al. 2015)	Yes
Allopurinol SJS/TEN and DRESS/DIHS	B*58:01	9–11% Han Chinese 1–6% Caucasian	1/250–1/1000	>800	100% in Han Chinese	3%	250	Not routine/under consideration	Yes
Carbamazepine SJS/TEN	B*15:02	10–15% Han Chinese <0.1% Caucasian	1–4% (Han Chinese	>1000	100% in Han Chinese (with other B75 serotype)	3%	1000	Implemented in many Southeast Asian countries[b] (Leckband et al. 2013)	Yes
Dapsone DRESS/DHIS	B*13:01	2–20% Chinese 28% Papuans/Australian Aboriginals 0% European/African 1.5% Japanese	1–4% Han Chinese	20	99.8%	7.8%	84	Under consideration	Yes

NNT number needed to test
NPV negative predictive value, *PPV* positive predictive value
[a]Screening not routine in developing world or African/Southeast Asian countries where prevalence of HLA-B*57:01 < 1%
[b]When screening introduced and implemented successfully, there has been near elimination or measurable reduction of the drug-specific CADR

that the sequence and response to early infectious diseases, which determine an individual's immune repertoire (library of memory T-cells and B-cells), may be significant risk factors for CADR. In the heterologous immunity model of CADR, pathogen-specific T-cell responses generate either migratory or resident memory T-cells which cross-react with drug-modified self-peptide epitopes when the drug is introduced later in life. This induces pathology at the anatomic site of the resident memory T-cells (e.g., skin and mucosa) but not elsewhere. The presence of a shared dominant T-cell receptor clonotype for some CADR such as HLA-B*15:02 associated carbamazepine SJS/TEN which is absent in carbamazepine tolerant controls supports this model (White et al. 2015; Leckband et al. 2013). The composition of the microbiome, known to play an important role in the development of autoimmune and inflammatory diseases, may be associated with CADR.

Phenome, phenotypes, and retaxonimization. From a phenotypic perspective the key question is: What phenotype/CADR diagnosis does this case fit best with and what does that indicate about prognosis and treatment?

With many well-described CADRs and many more emerging in the literature, categorizing cases can be challenging even for the most experienced clinicians. There will always be cases missing key features and cases with overlapping features of multiple phenotypes. The situation is even more challenging for researchers seeking to verify cases using only what is available in the electronic health record. In the future in vivo patch testing and ex vivo/in vitro ELISpot, lymphocyte transformation test, etc. may be very useful in providing precise phenotyping.

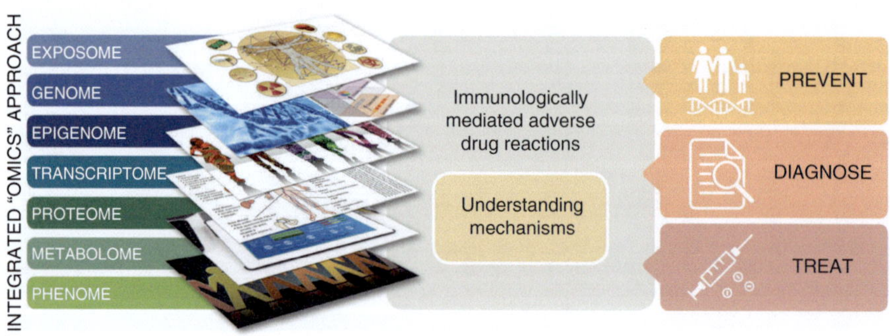

Fig. 20.1 The **exposome** is an organism's universe of exposures (medications, toxins, infections, etc.) during its lifetime, including during prenatal development. The **genome** is all of an organism's DNA. The **epigenome** is the array of modifications to DNA which regulate gene expression without altering the DNA sequence (methylation, acetylation, micro RNA). These modifications can differ between cells and tissues and at different developmental stages/time points. The **transcriptome** is all messenger RNA (mRNA) expressed by a cell, tissue, or organism at a given point in time. The **proteome** is all of the proteins expressed. The complete biochemical composition of a cell, organ, or organism is also known as its **metabolome**. The **phenome** is the set of observable characteristics of a cell, tissue, or organism

20.3 Conclusions

We can imagine a future when a rapid and affordable blood test might provide comprehensive information on all drugs likely to cause cutaneous adverse drug reactions in an individual. This information could be available in the patient's medical record and link to prescribing software, warning prescribers about potential CADRs.

The rate-limiting factor for advancements will likely be the accrual of large enough collections of human samples from diverse patient populations and drug-exposed but tolerant controls to do sufficiently powered genetic, transcriptomic, proteomic, epigenomic, metabolomic, and cellular studies.

Acknowledgments The authors would like to acknowledge Karen Adamson for contributing the graphic design of Fig. 20.1.

References

Bellon T, Alvarez L, Mayorga C, Morel E, Torres MJ, Martin-Diaz MA et al (2010) Differential gene expression in drug hypersensitivity reactions: induction of alarmins in severe bullous diseases. Br J Dermatol 162:1014–1022

Chan SH, Tan T (1989) HLA and allopurinol drug eruption. Dermatologica 179(1):32–33

Chen Z et al (2014) Effects of a HLA-B*15:02 screening policy on antiepileptic drug use and severe skin reactions. Neurology 83(22):2077–2084

Chung WH, Hung SI, Hong HS et al (2004) Medical genetics: a marker for Stevens-Johnson syndrome. Nature 428(6982):486

Chung WH, Hung SI, Yang JY et al (2008) Granulysin is a key mediator for disseminated keratinocyte death in Stevens-Johnson syndrome and toxic epidermal necrolysis. Nat Med 14(12):1343–1350

Chung WH, Chang WC, Lee YS et al (2014) Genetic variants associated with phenytoin-related severe cutaneous adverse reactions. JAMA 312(5):525–534

Hetherington S et al (2002) Genetic variations in HLA-B region and hypersensitivity reactions to abacavir. Lancet 359(9312):1121–1122

Hung SI, Chung WH, Liou LB et al (2005) HLA-B*5801 allele as a genetic marker for severe cutaneous adverse reactions caused by allopurinol. Proc Natl Acad Sci U S A 102(11):4134–4139

Hung SI, Chung WH, Jee SH et al (2006) Genetic susceptibility to carbamazepine-induced cutaneous adverse drug reactions. Pharmacogenet Genomics 16(4):297–306

Leckband SG, Kelsoe JR, Dunnenberger HM, George AL Jr, Tran E, Berger R, Müller DJ, Whirl-Carrillo M, Caudle KE, Pirmohamed M, Clinical Pharmacogenetics Implementation Consortium (2013) Clinical Pharmacogenetics Implementation Consortium guidelines for HLA-B genotype and carbamazepine dosing. Clin Pharmacol Ther 94(3):324–328

Mallal S et al (2002) Association between presence of HLA-B*5701, HLA-DR7, and HLA-DQ3 and hypersensitivity to HIV-1 reverse-transcriptase inhibitor abacavir. Lancet 359(9308):727–732

Mallal S et al (2008) HLA-B*5701 screening for hypersensitivity to abacavir. N Engl J Med 358(6):568–579

McNeil BD et al (2015) Identification of a mast-cell-specific receptor crucial for pseudo-allergic drug reactions. Nature 519(7542):237–241

Pan Y-Z, Zhou A, Hu Z, Yu A-M (2013) Small nucleolar RNA-derived MicroRNA hsa-miR-1291 modulates cellular drug disposition through direct targeting of ABC transporter ABCC1. Drug Metab Dispos 41(10):1744–1751. https://doi.org/10.1124/dmd.113.052092

Saag M et al (2008) High sensitivity of human leukocyte antigen-b*5701 as a marker for immunologically confirmed abacavir hypersensitivity in white and black patients. Clin Infect Dis 46(7):1111–1118

Tassaneeyakul W, Prabmeechai N, Sukasem C et al (2016) Associations between HLA class I and cytochrome P450 2C9 genetic polymorphisms and phenytoin-related severe cutaneous adverse reactions in a Thai population. Pharmacogenet Genomics 26(5):225–234

Toh DS, Tan LL, Aw DC et al (2014) Building pharmacogenetics into a pharmacovigilance program in Singapore: using serious skin rash as a pilot study. Pharmacogenomics J 14(4):316–321

White KD, Chung WH, Hung SI, Mallal S, Phillips EJ (2015) Evolving models of the immunopathogenesis of T cell-mediated drug allergy: The role of host, pathogens, and drug response. J Allergy Clin Immunol 136(2):219–234

Atlas of Cutaneous Adverse Drug Reactions

21

Alina G. Bridges and Kevin Brough

Acute Generalized Exanthematous Pustulosis

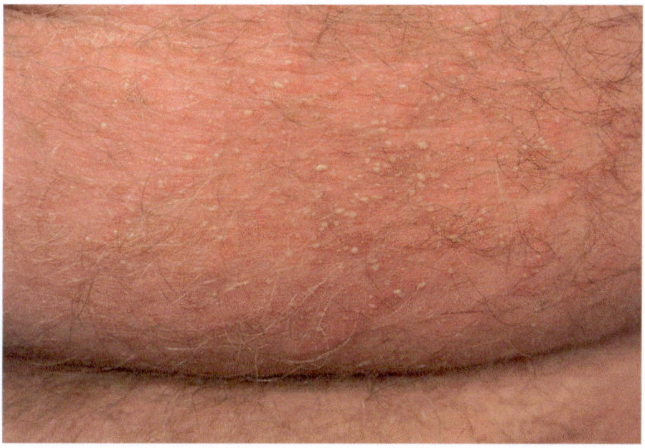

A. G. Bridges (✉)
Department of Laboratory Medicine and Pathology, Mayo Clinic, Rochester, MN, USA

Division of Dermatopathology and Cutaneous Immunopathology, Department of Dermatology, Mayo Clinic, Rochester, MN, USA
e-mail: bridges.alina@mayo.edu

K. Brough
Department of Dermatology, Mayo Clinic, Rochester, MN, USA

N. H. Shear, R. P. Dodiuk-Gad (eds.), *Advances in Diagnosis and Management of Cutaneous Adverse Drug Reactions*, https://doi.org/10.1007/978-981-13-1489-6_21

Acute Generalized
Exanthematous Pustulosis

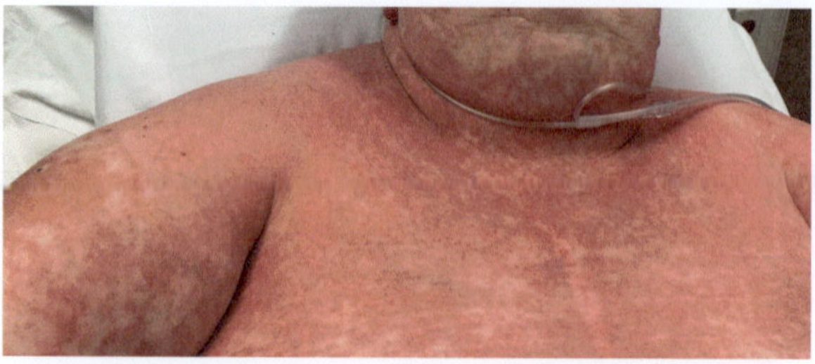

Acute Generalized
Exanthematous Pustulosis

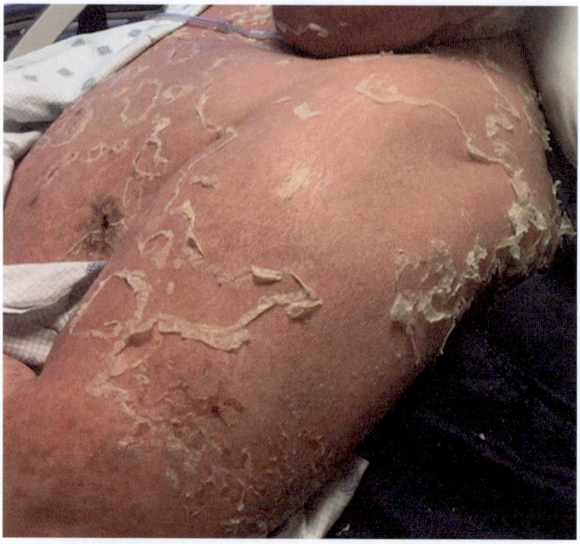

Azathioprine induced
Sweet syndrome

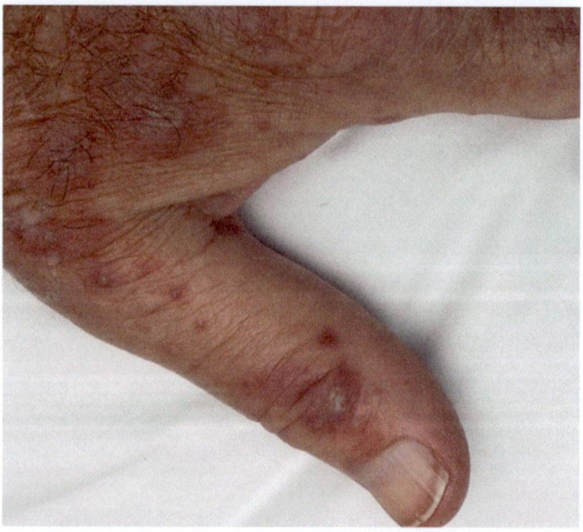

BRAF Inhibitor
Panniculitis

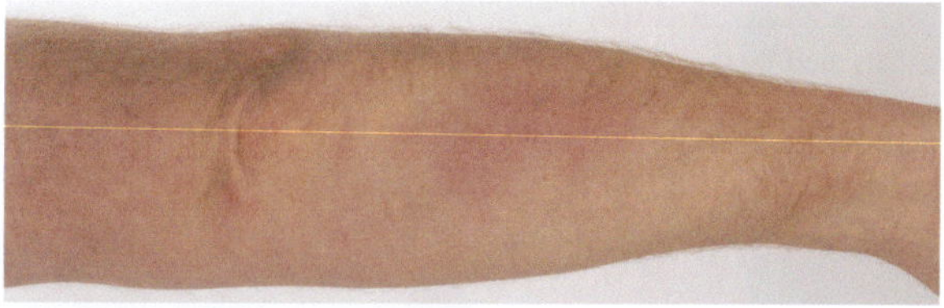

BRAF Inhibitor
Panniculitis

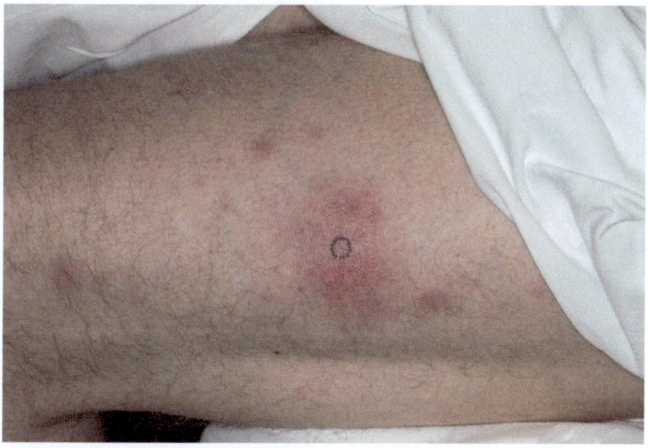

Chemotherapy induced
inflammation of Actinic
Keratosis

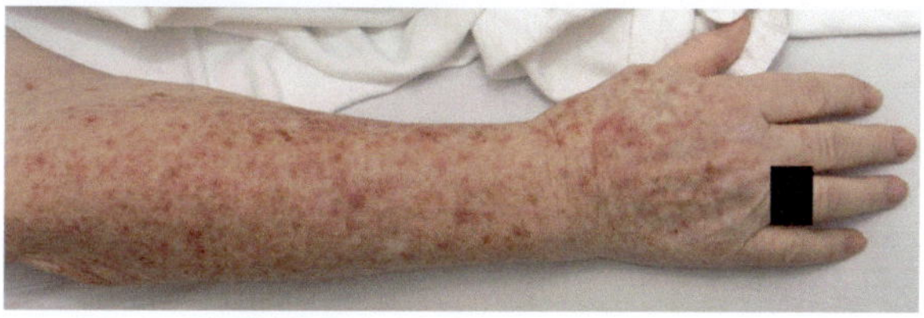

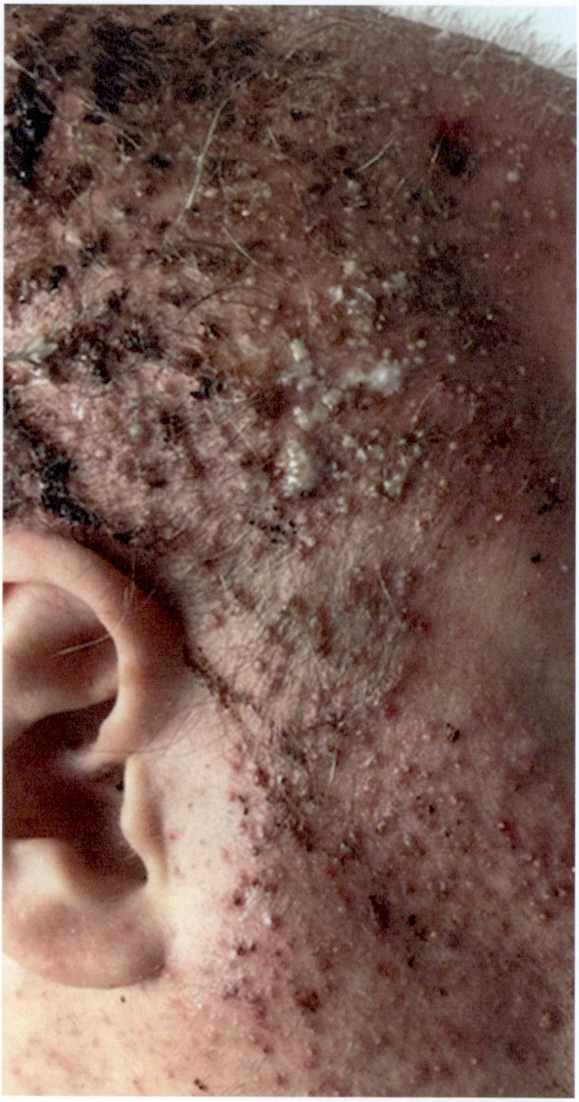

Drug reaction with eosinophilia and systemic symptoms

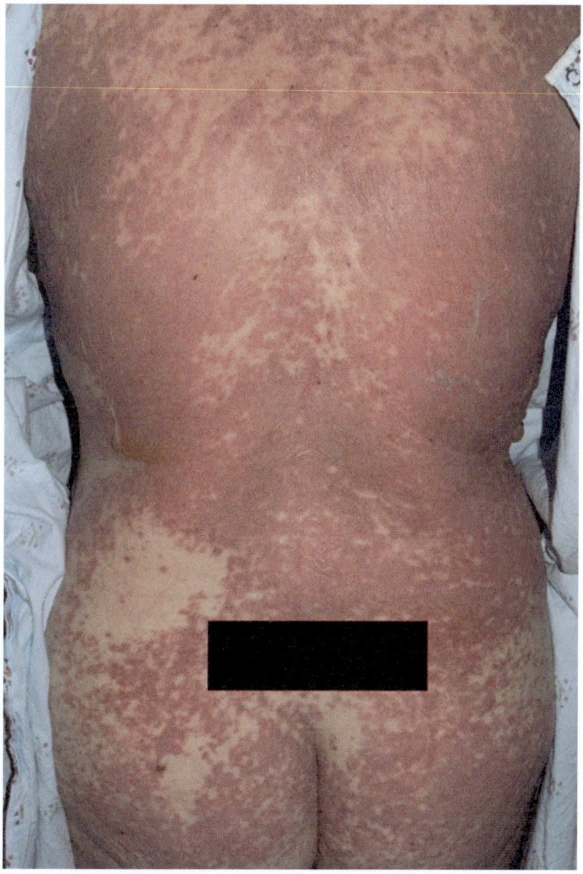

Drug Reaction with Eosinophilia and Systemic Symptoms

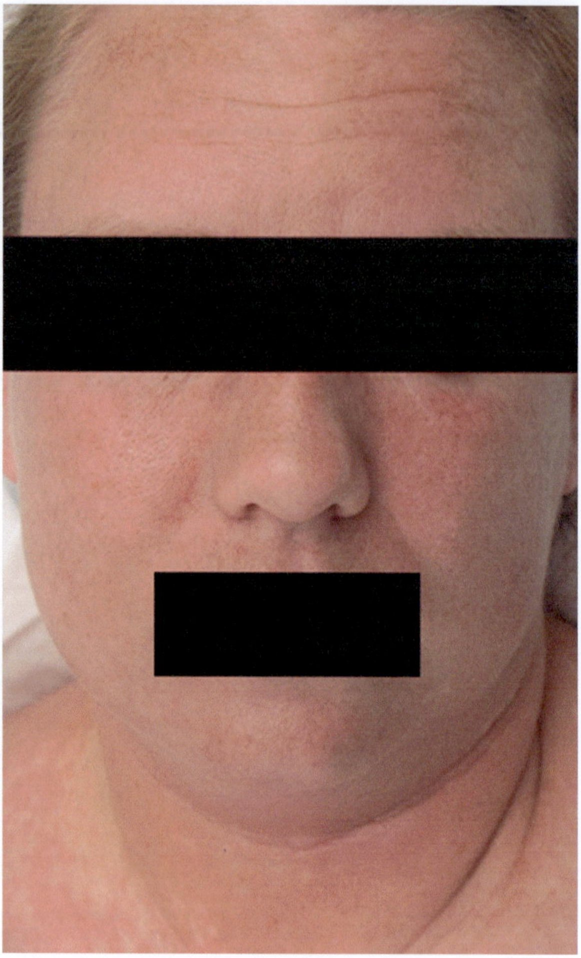

Drug Induced Bullous Pemphigoid

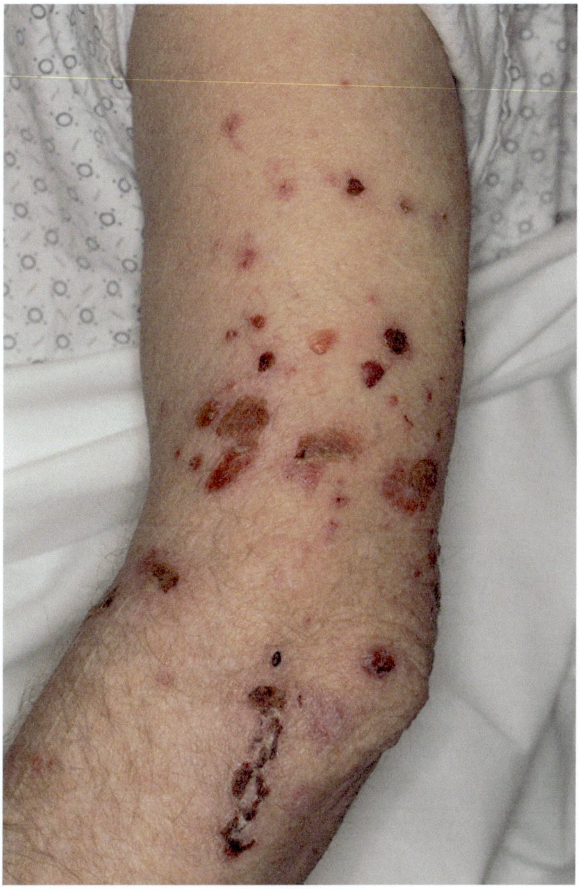

Drug-induced Linear IgA bullous dermatosis

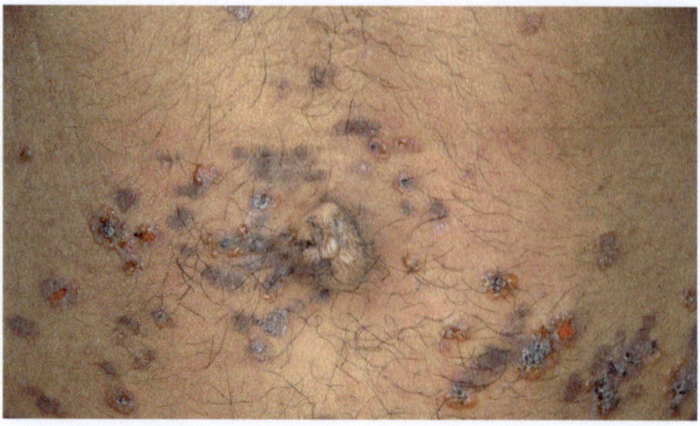

Drug-induced Linear IgA bullous dermatosis

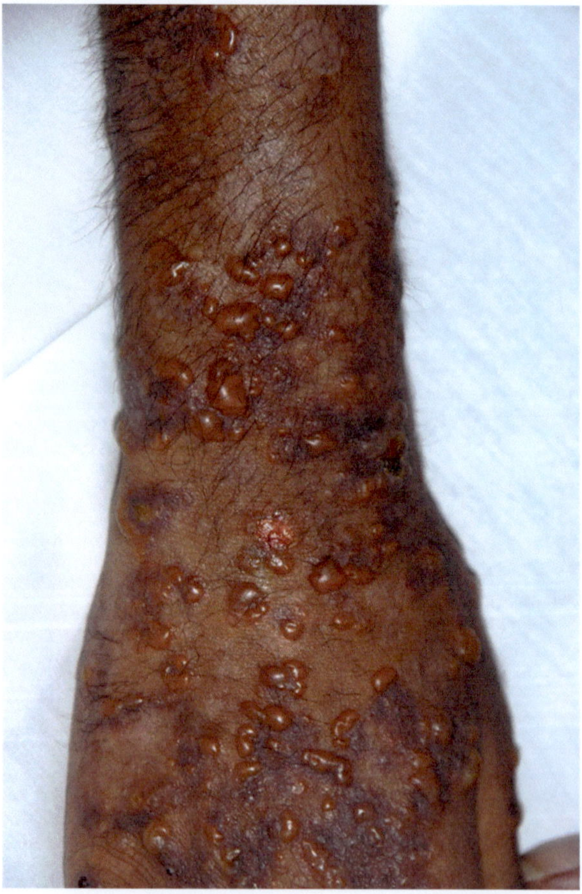

Drug-induced Linear IgA bullous dermatosis

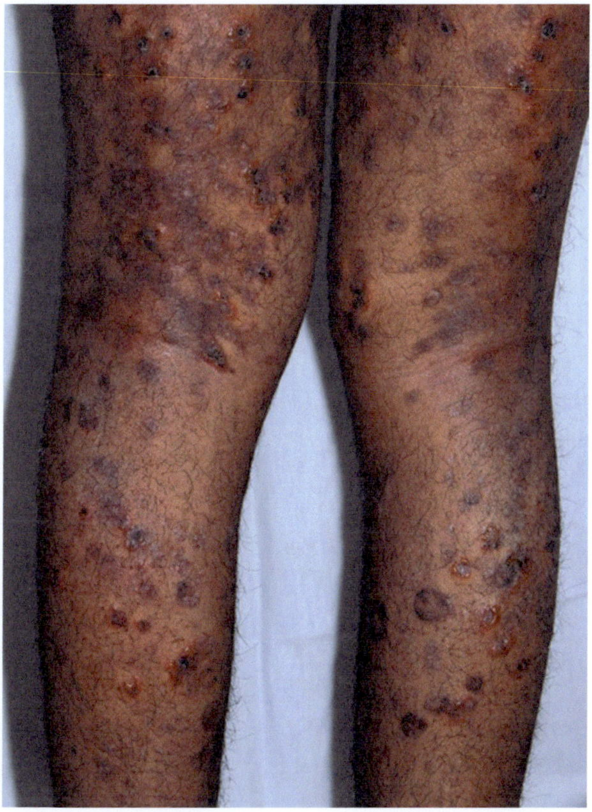

Drug induced pigmentation

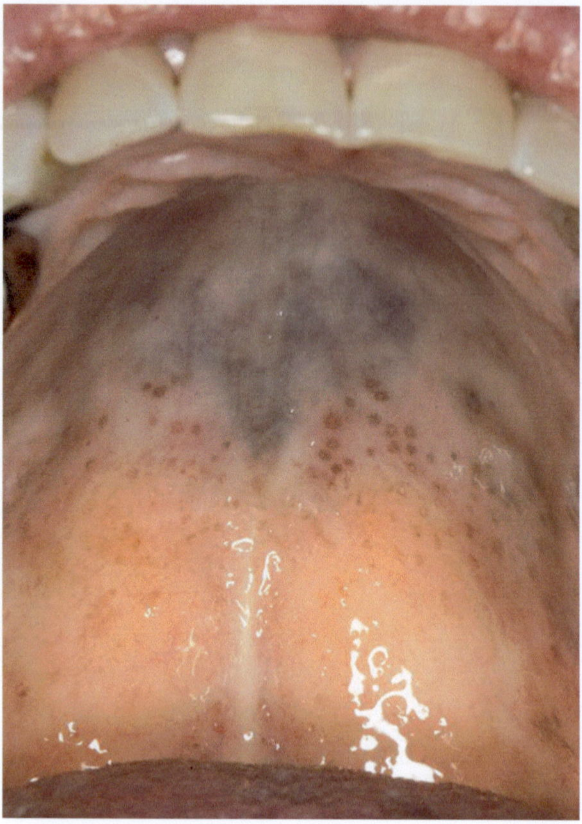

Drug-induced pigmentation

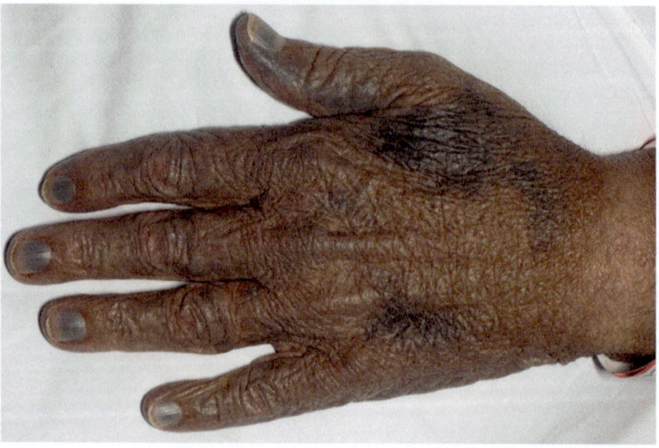

Drug-induced pigmentation

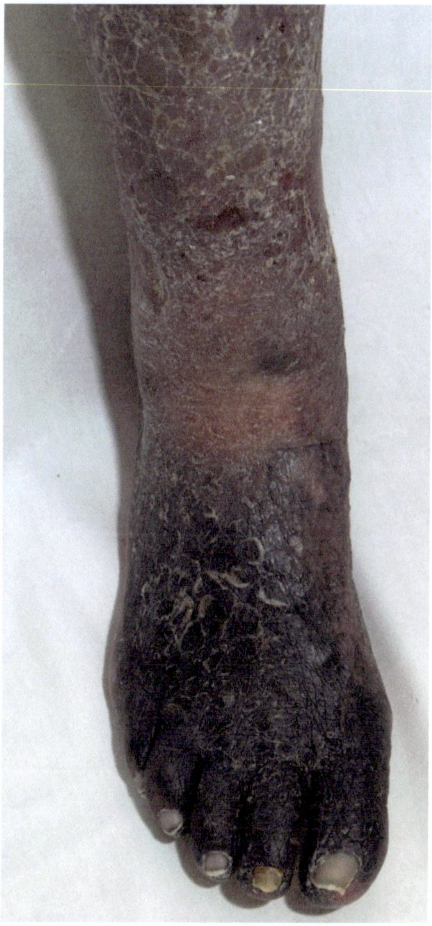

Drug-induced pigmentation

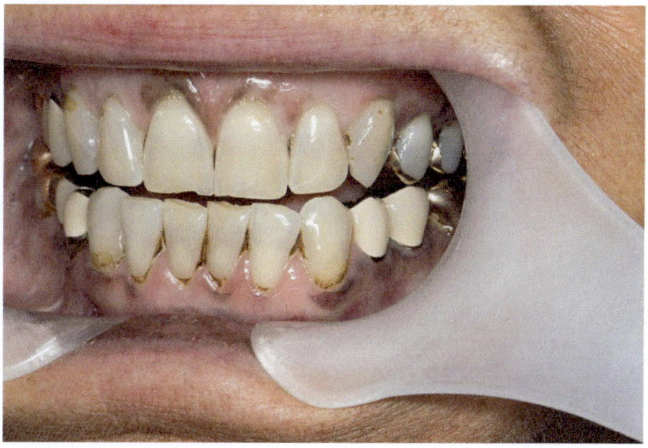

Drug-induced subacute cutaneous lupus erythematosus

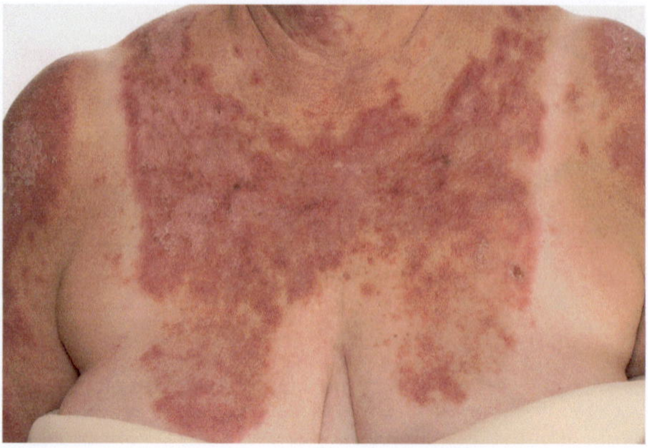

Drug-induced subacute lupus erythematous

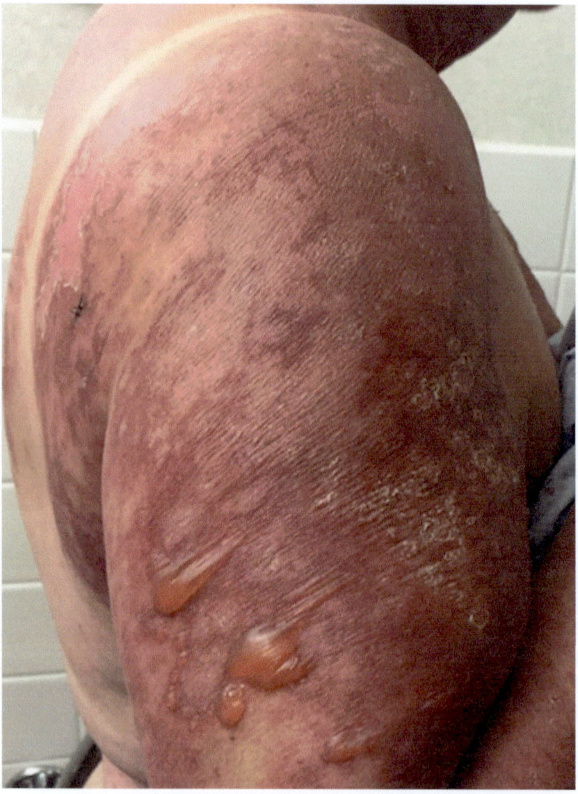

Drug-induced vasculitis

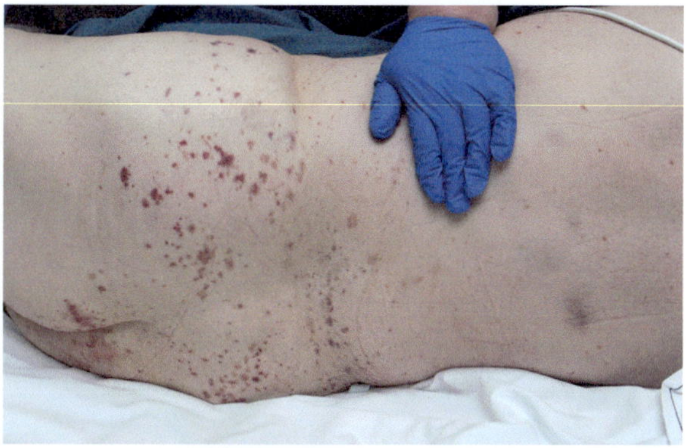

Drug-induced vasculitis

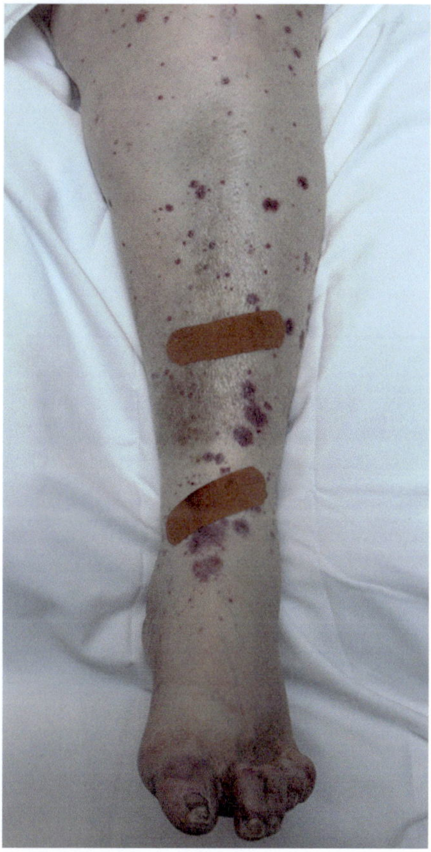

Erythema multiforme

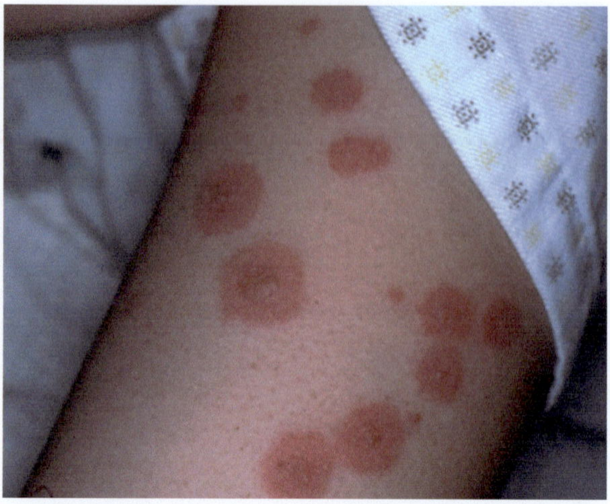

Erythema multiforme

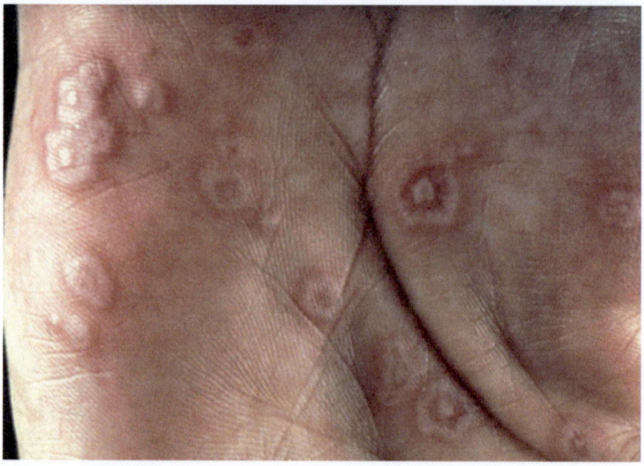

Fixed drug eruption

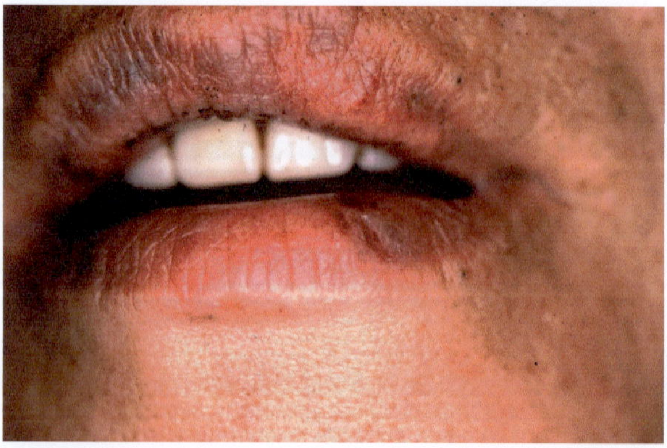

Fixed drug eruption

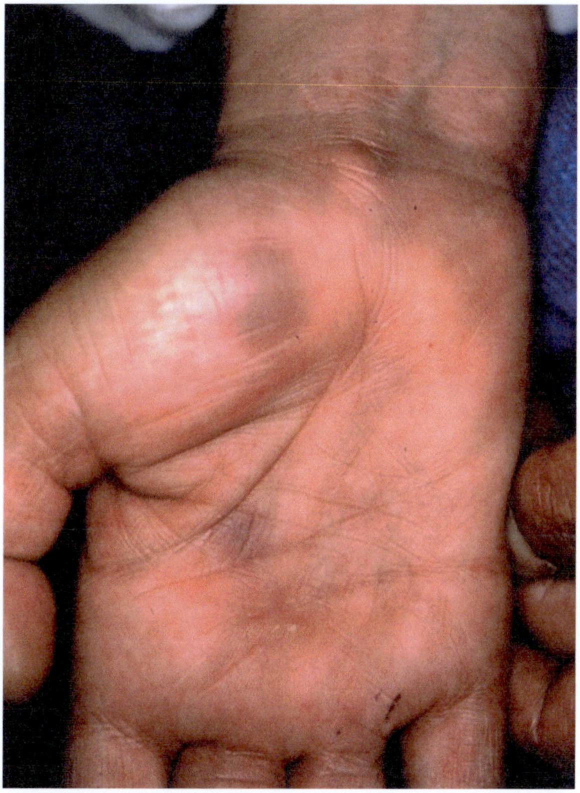

Flagellate blistering eruption

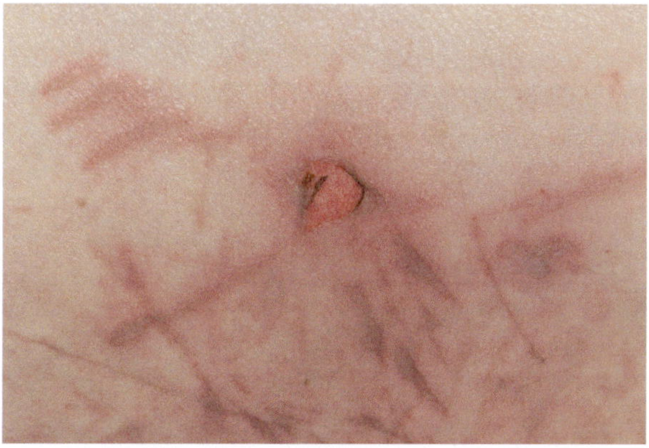

Lichenoid drug reaction

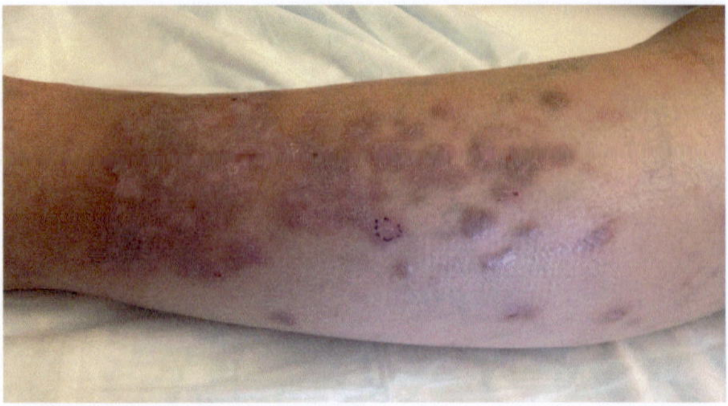

Lichenoid drug reaction

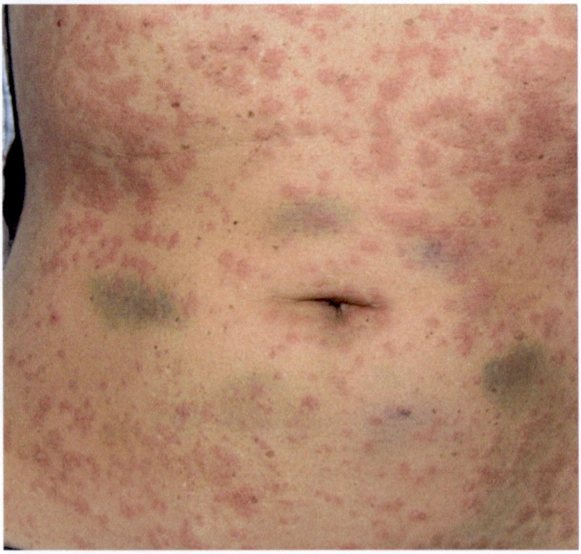

Morbilliform eruption

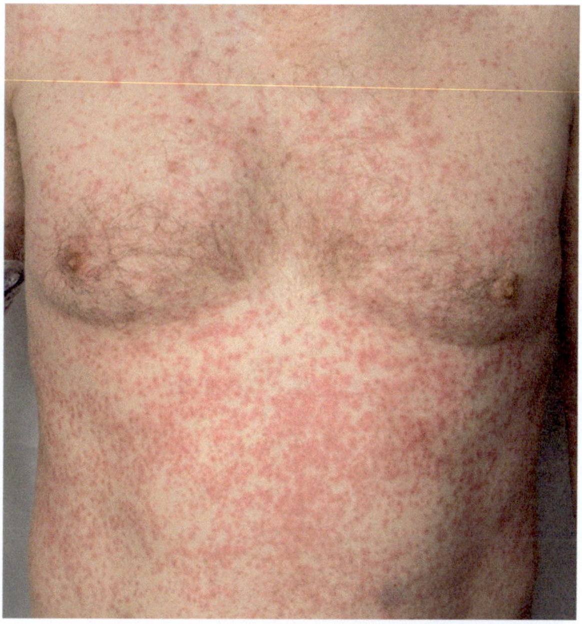

Neutrophilic eccrine hidradenitis

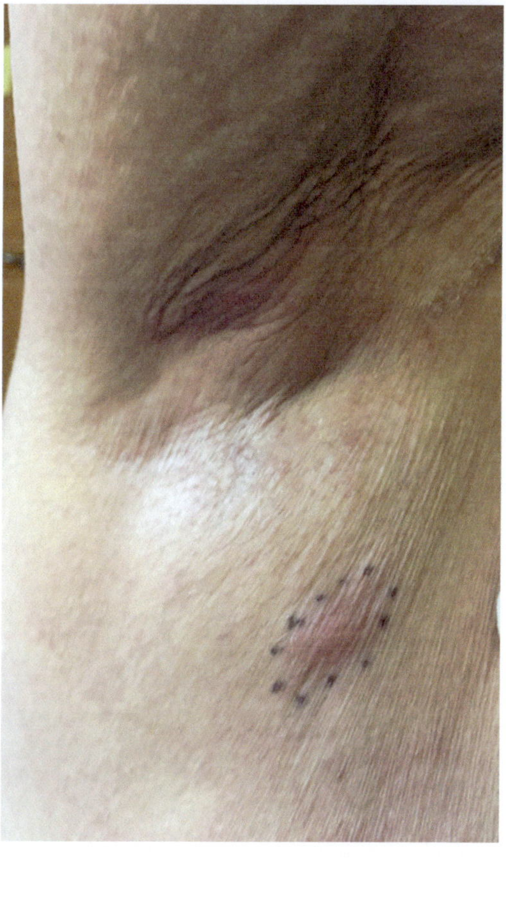

Phototoxic drug reaction

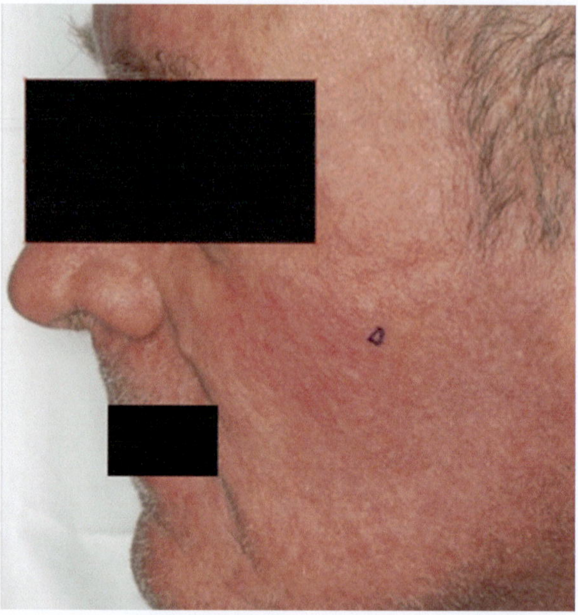

Pseudoporphyria

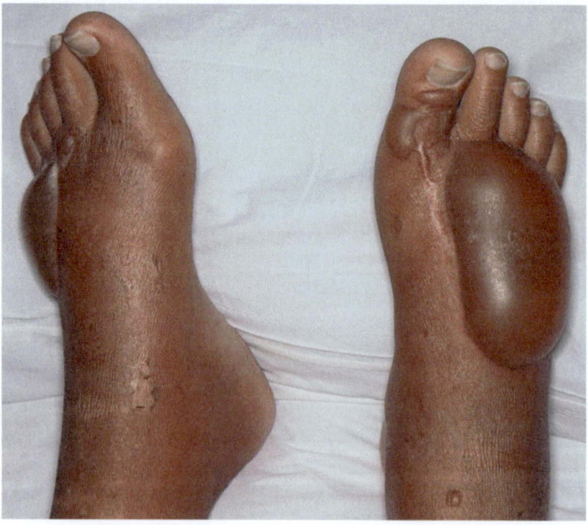

Red man syndrome

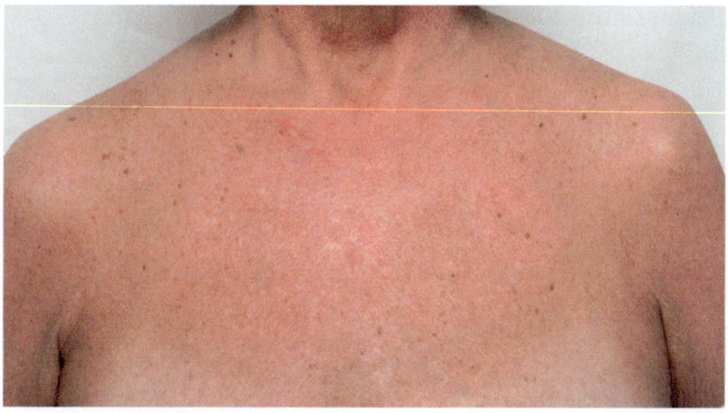

Serum sickness-like reaction

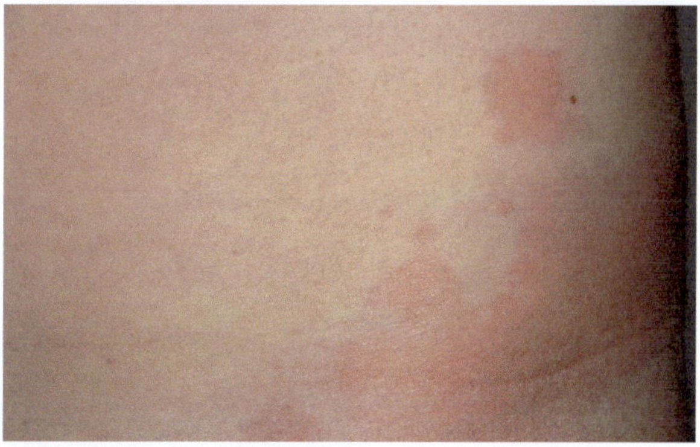

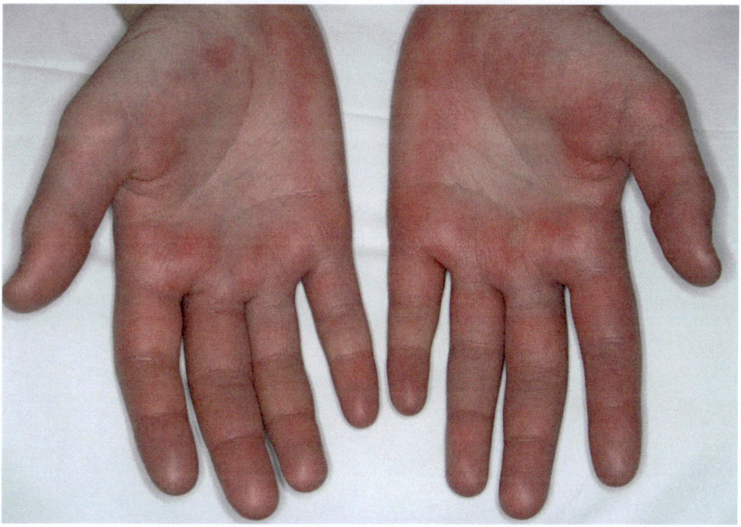

Serum-sickness like reaction

Serum-sickness like reaction

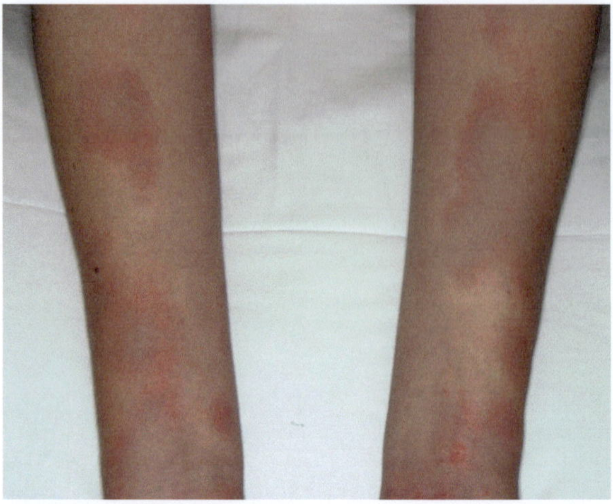

Steroid acne

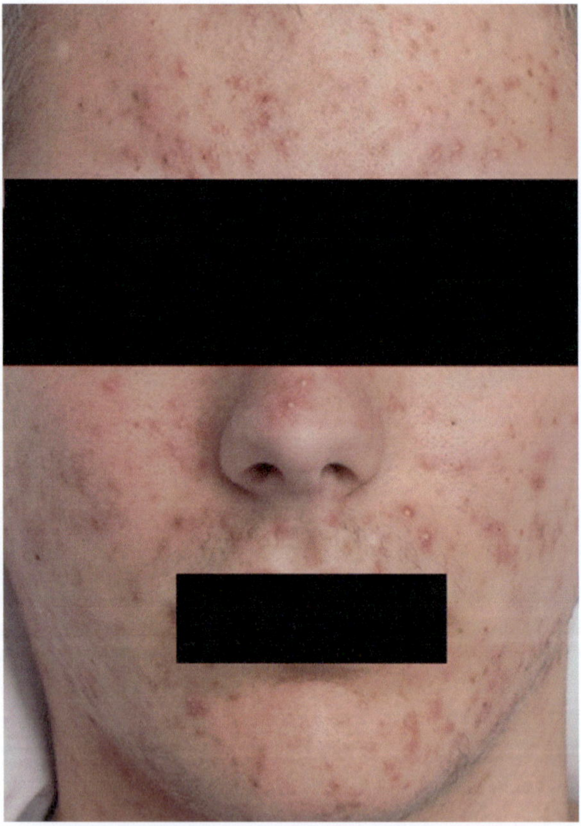

Stevens–Johnson syndrome (SJS)

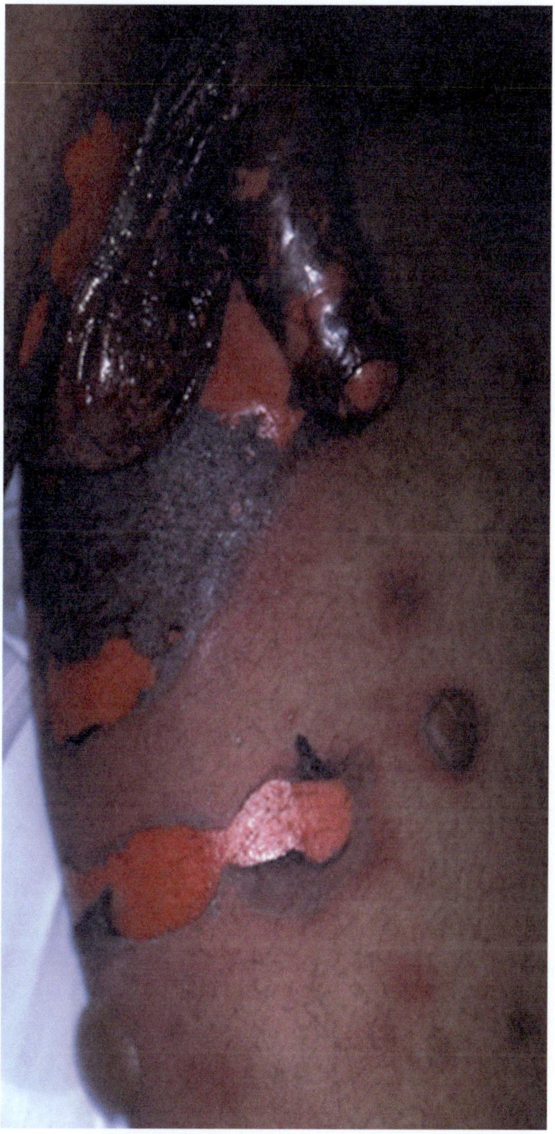

Stevens–Johnson syndrome (SJS)

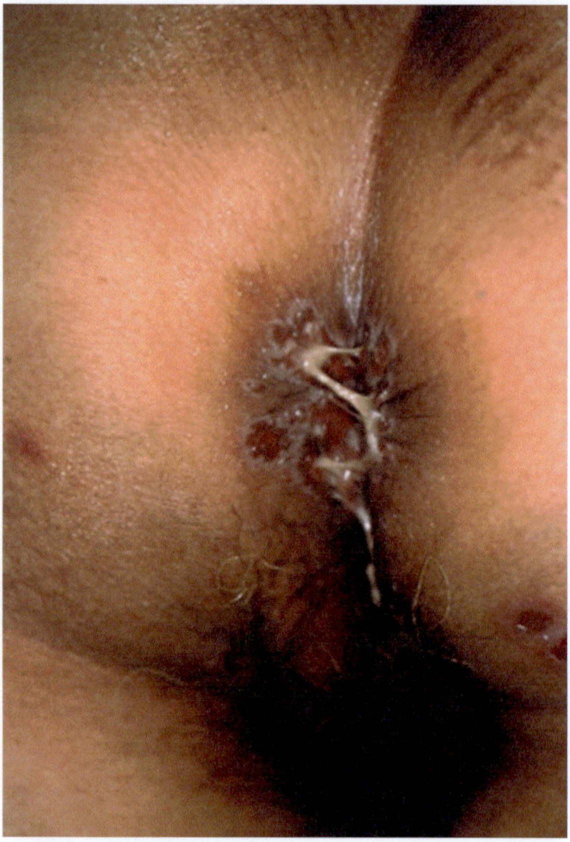

Stevens–Johnson syndrome (SJS)

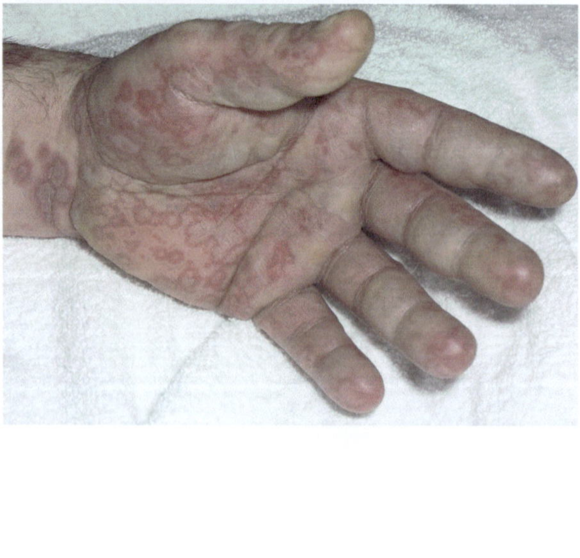

Stevens–Johnson syndrome (SJS)

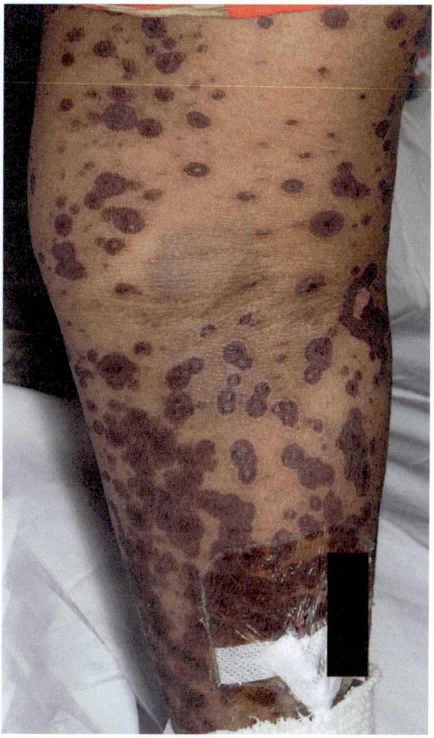

Stevens–Johnson syndrome (SJS)

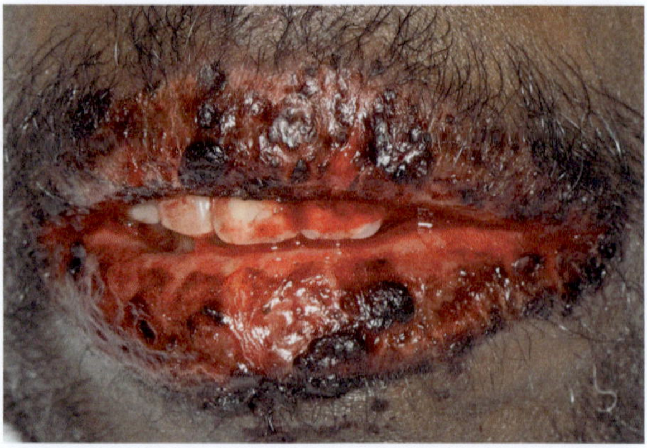

Stevens–Johnson syndrome/Toxic Epidermal Necrolysis

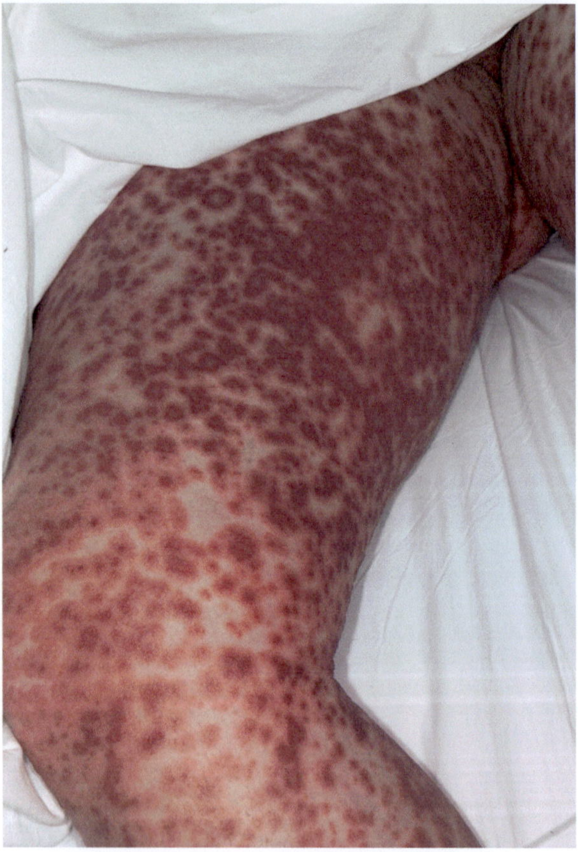

Stevens Johnson syndrome / Toxic Epidermal Necrolysis

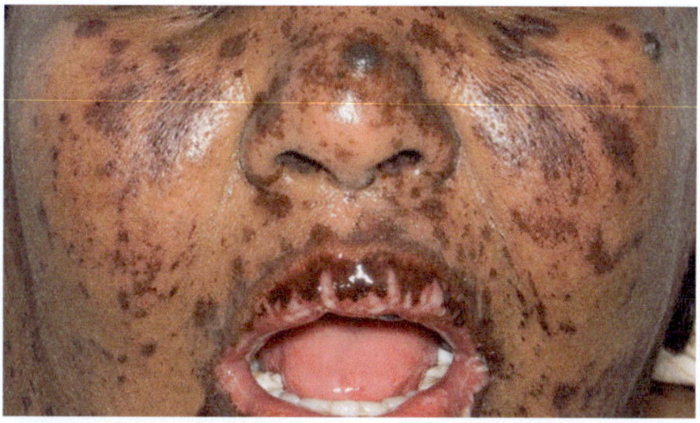

Symmetric Drug-Related Intertriginous and Flexural Exanthema (SDRIFE)

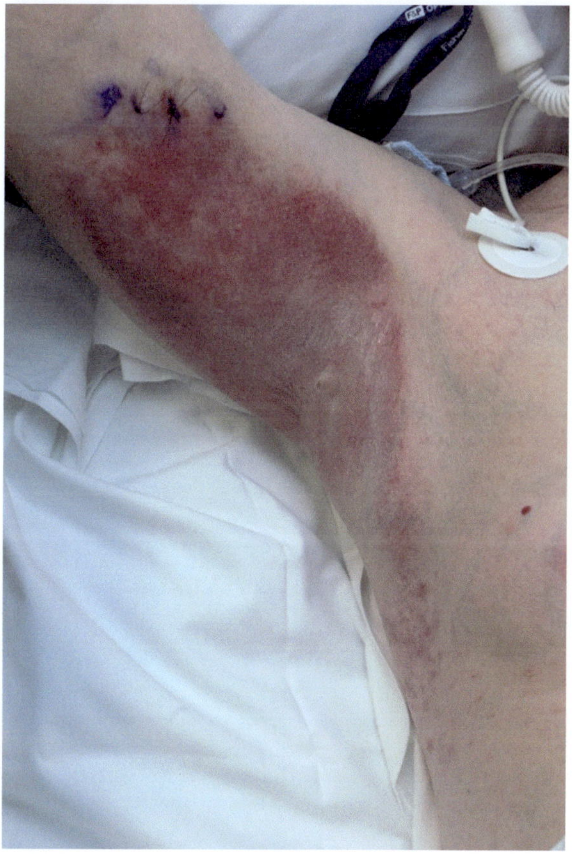

Symmetric Drug-Related Intertriginous and Flexural Exanthema (SDRIFE)

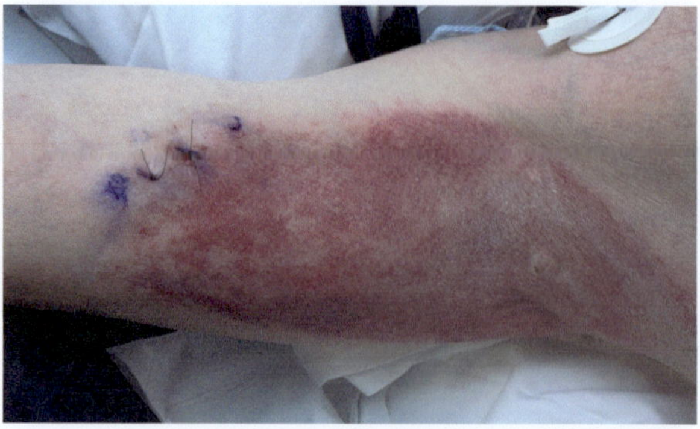

Symmetric Drug-Related Intertriginous and Flexural Exanthema (SDRIFE)

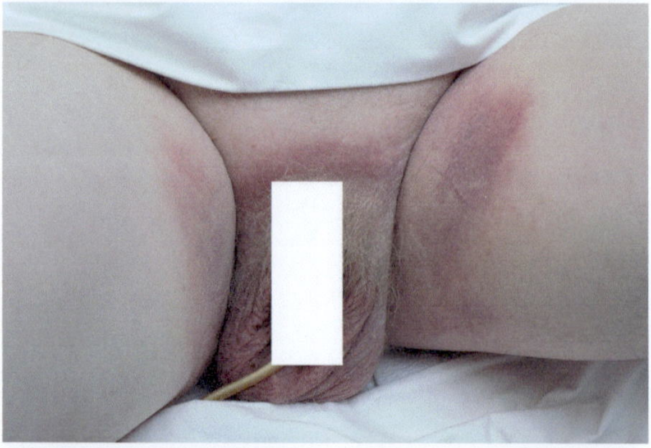

TNFα inhibitor induced lupus-like syndrome (TAILS)

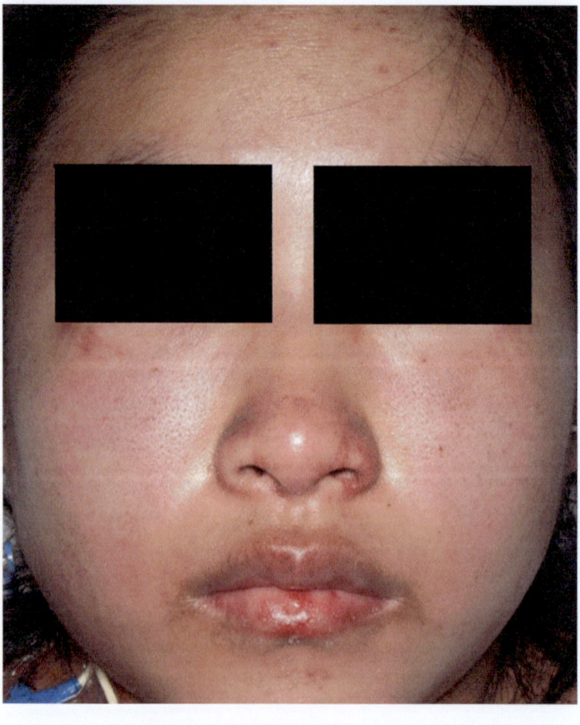

TNFα inhibitor induced lupus-like syndrome (TAILS)

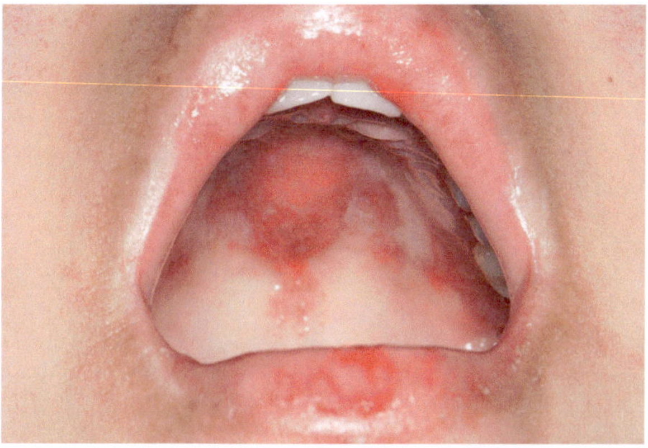

TNFα inhibitor induced lupus-like syndrome (TAILS)

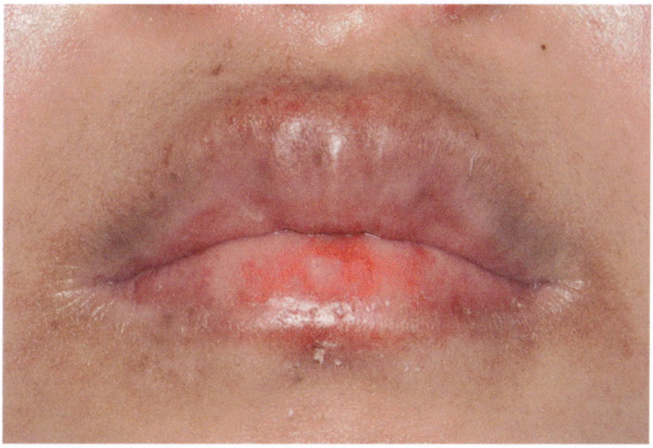

TNFα inhibitor induced lupus-like syndrome (TAILS)

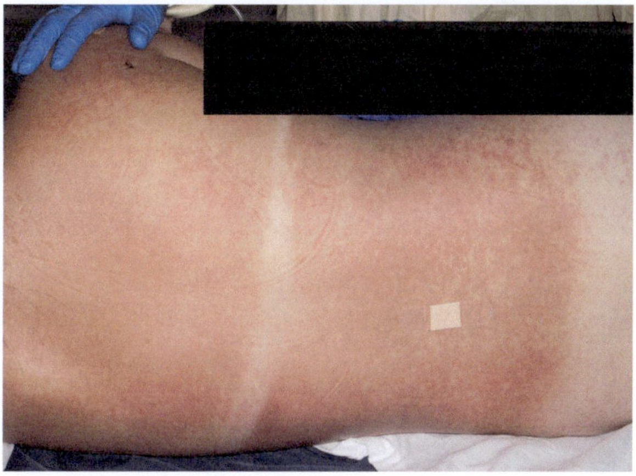

Toxic Epidermal Necrolysis (TEN)

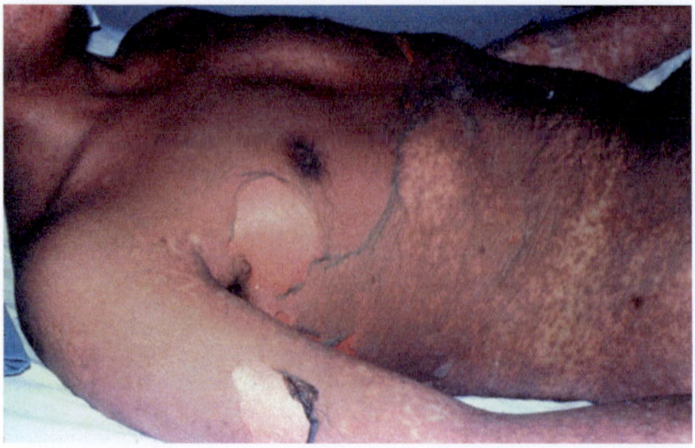

Toxic Epidermal Necrolysis (TEN)

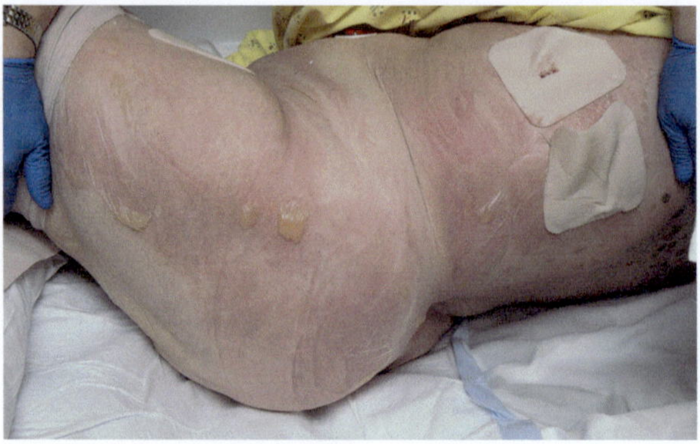

Toxic Epidermal Necrolysis (TEN)

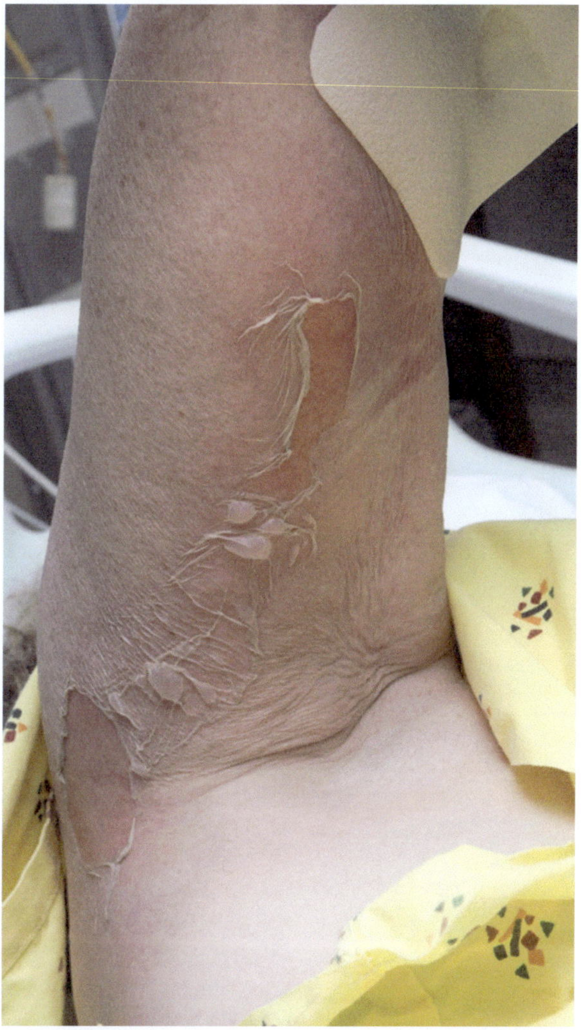

Toxic Epidermal Necrolysis (TEN)

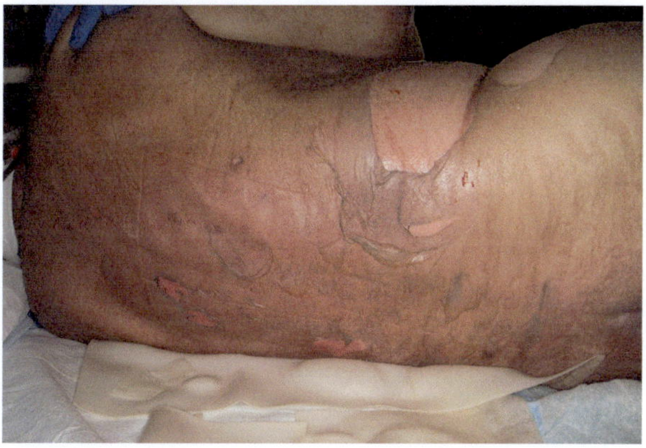

Toxic Erythema of Chemotherapy

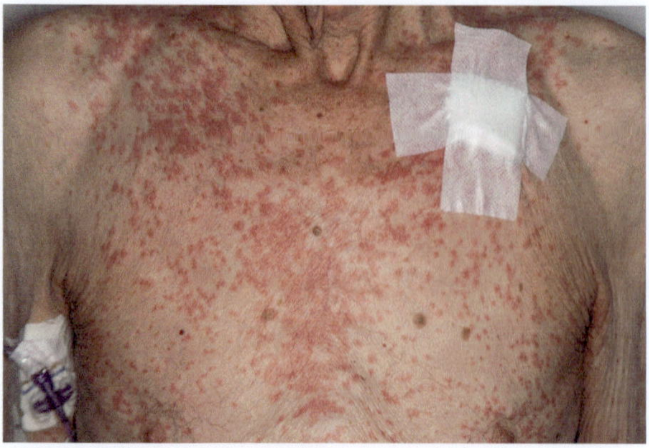

Toxic Erythema of Chemotherapy

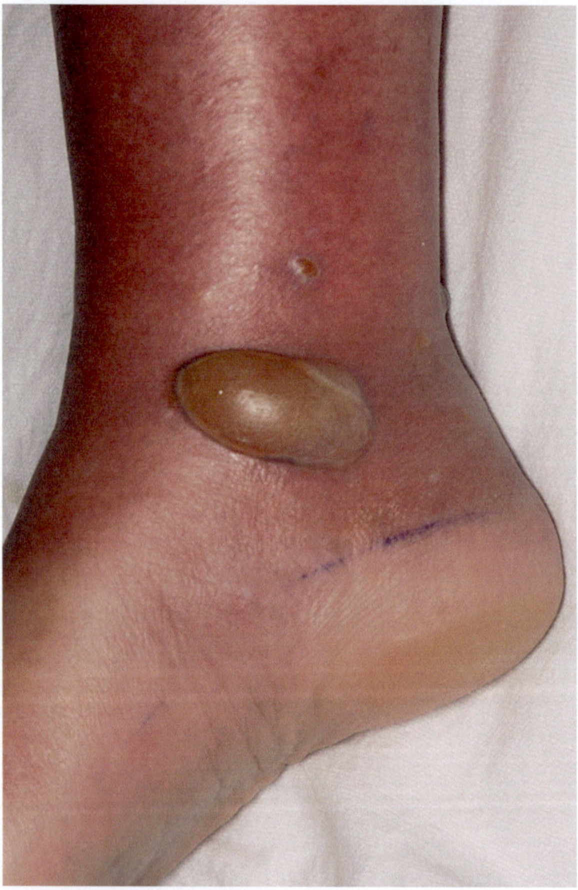

Toxic Erythema of Chemotherapy

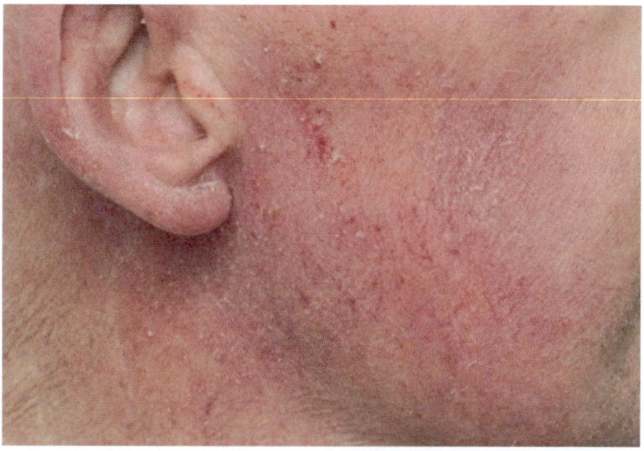

Urticarial drug eruption

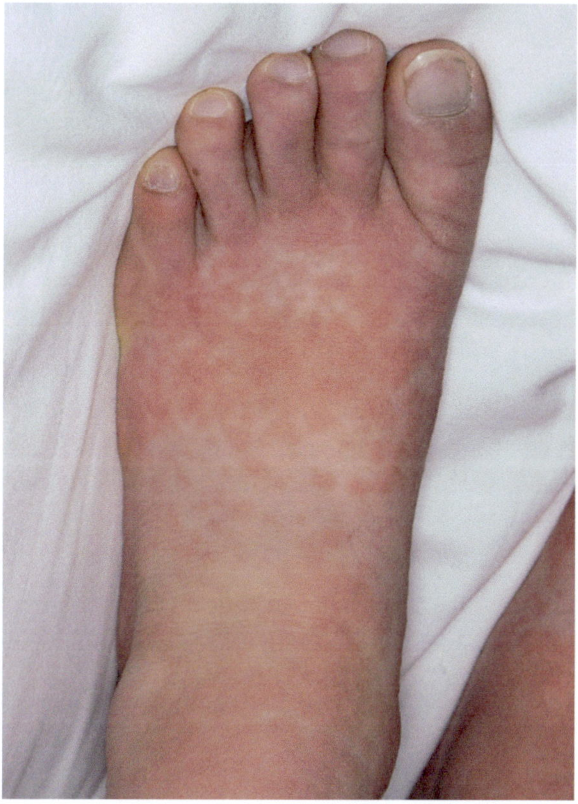

Urticarial drug eruption

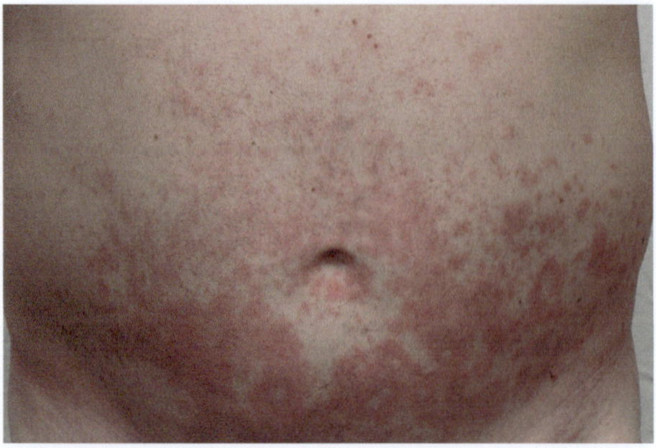

Warfarin necrosis

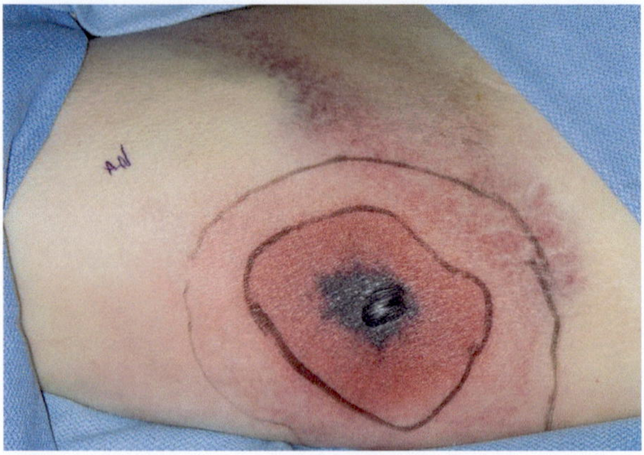

Warfarin necrosis

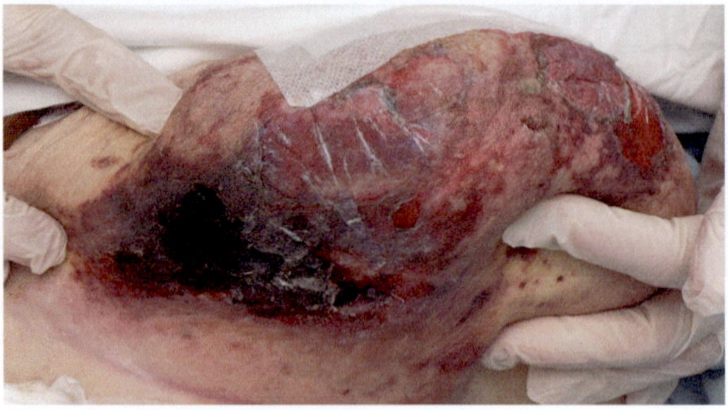